Dr Richard K

"The Age Reduction System"

$17.95a

3
—
5

?

Politics — The wise exercise,
distribution and maintainance
of power.

BEYOND
THE
HELIX

BEYOND
THE
HELIX
—
DNA AND THE
QUEST FOR LONGEVITY

CAROL KAHN

Times
BOOKS

All rights reserved under International and Pan-American Copyright
Conventions. Published in the United States by Times Books,
a division of Random House, Inc., New York, and simultaneously
in Canada by Random House of Canada Limited, Toronto.

Library of Congress Cataloging-in-Publication Data

Kahn, Carol.
Beyond the helix.

Bibliography: p.
Includes index.
1. Longevity—Genetic aspects. 2. Deoxyribonucleic
acid repair. 3. Aging—Genetic aspects. 4. Degeneration
(Pathology)—Genetic aspects. I. Title.
QP85.K34 1985   612'.68   85-40343
ISBN 0-8129-1153-9

Designed by Stephanie Blumenthal
Manufactured in the United States of America
9 8 7 6 5 4 3 2
First Edition

To Ira, Jeremy, and Holen,
with whom I hope to share the next 100 years

Acknowledgments

The close cooperation of many people was required to write this book. I owe a particular debt of gratitude to Ron Hart, Joan Smith-Sonneborn, Phil Lipetz, and Ralph Stephens, who permitted me to observe experiments in their laboratories and were of enormous assistance. For giving unstintingly of their time, I would like especially to thank Dick Cutler, Arthur Schwartz, Jim Trosko, Roy Walford, Jerry Williams, and Bill Regelson. I am grateful to all of them for serving as my teachers in their particular areas of expertise. In certain parts of this book, the dialogue has been reconstructed based on the detailed recollections of the scientists involved.

For interviews I would like to thank Dick Setlow, Leonard Hayflick, Denham Harman, David Harrison, George Martin, Bruce Ames, Donner Denckla, Irwin Fridovich, Ken Munkrees, Caleb Finch, Kathleen Hall, Reubin Andres, Howard Ducoff, Edward Schneider, Don Yarborough, Douglas Brash, Robin Holliday, Vincent Cristofalo, Paul Segall, Lawrence Loeb, David Gershon, Richard Greulich, Stuart Linn, Paul Howard-Flanders, and James Cleaver.

Gathering material for a book of this kind can be very costly, and I greatly appreciate the hospitality that was extended to me by the scientists and their spouses, who prepared memorable meals and in some cases put me up in their homes. In this regard, I would like to thank Jim and Kay Trosko, Phil and Linda Lipetz, Ralph and Irene Stephens, Kathleen and Bill Hall, Joan Smith-Sonneborn, Roy Walford, and, most especially, Dorothea Sacher, who not only opened up her home to me but made available the archives of her late husband, George Sacher. I am grateful to Maggie Channon, whose invitation to stay at her house made it possible for me to attend the 1981 Gerontology Society meeting in Toronto.

Portions of the book as well as the entire manuscript were seen prior to publication by many of the scientists, and I would like to acknowledge their helpful comments and discussions. The book received a line-by-line scientific review by Ron Hart, for which I am most indebted.

For her incredible patience in transcribing hundreds of hours of taped interviews, which often required listening over and over to those sections recorded in conference rooms, hotel lobbies, restaurants, automobiles, and other places with a high level of background noise, I owe a special thanks to Judith Schoenberg.

Having Jonathan Segal as my editor was an exhilarating and rewarding experience. While writers often feel editors literally cramp their style, he encouraged me to expand my vision and to "err on the side of freedom." My thanks also to his associate, Ruth Fecych, for her sensitive editing.

Finally there is my amazing and wonderful family. My son, Jeremy, and my daughter, Holen, who endured my many trips away from home, hours spent at the word processor that would ordinarily have been spent with them, and, especially toward the end, innumerable meals of pizza and takeout chicken—so that I could write "our book," as my son came to call it.

As for my husband, Ira, this book quite simply could not have been written without him. He not only did yeoman duty taking care of the children when I was not available, but he was there for me in every sense of the word whenever I needed him. There were many times when I felt frustrated or discouraged, and he brought me through them with his insights, his compassion, his own considerable literary skills, and, always, his love. Every writer should be as lucky as I to live with a practicing psychotherapist.

"*And so, in discussing the question of life and death, we come at last—as in all provinces of human research—upon problems which appear to us to be, at least for the present, insoluble. In fact, it is the quest after perfected truth, not its possession, that falls to our lot, that gladdens us, fills up the measure of our life, nay! hallows it.*"

—August Weismann, 1881

Contents

BEYOND
THE
HELIX

Introduction

All the pieces were in place, although no one knew it at the time. It was the last meeting of the last session of the 1979 Gerontology Society conference in Washington, D.C., and many of the participants had gone home. Only about thirty people straggled into the small "Military Room" of the Washington Hilton. But they included nearly all the leading players in this particular scientific drama: the search for the mechanism of aging and longevity.

There were Ron Hart, the large, gregarious molecular biologist whose work in DNA repair had started the ball rolling; George Sacher, the genial president of the society, who, along with Hart, had pioneered the longevity-assurance theory; Dick Cutler, guarded and suspicious after all the attacks upon his work, yet still generating excitement with his research; Art Schwartz, slight, earnest, bespectacled, whose revelations at the Gordon Research Conference on Aging earlier in the year had stunned his colleagues; Roy Walford, with his Fu Manchu mustache, shaven head, and leather jacket, as unconventional in thinking as in appearance; Joan Smith-Sonneborn, an exuberant advocate of life extension whose recent experiment provided the first real proof of a longevity mechanism in DNA; Jerry Williams, southern in voice and manner, who would do his real work in the coming years; and last, Phil Lipetz, who wasn't there, but whose tantalizing, albeit preliminary, results heralded a shift in the understanding of the role of DNA in aging.

These were by no means gerontology's elite. Most of them had never held an important post in the Gerontology Society, been chairman of the prestigious Gordon Research Conference on Aging, or sat on the study groups or peer-review committees that decided who got the funding that could make or break a laboratory. Their insights, which helped bring the field to its present state of understanding, had come largely as by-products of their research in cancer, toxicology, and immunology, rather than gerontology. Indeed, most of them had never gotten a penny from the National Institute on Aging (NIA).

The "Symposium on DNA Repair and Aging" began with raucous laughter as the chairman, Ed Schneider of the NIA, jocularly announced, "This is a meeting of the Ron Hart Fan Club." It ended four hours later with the audience chattering excitedly like a flock of birds as they followed the last speaker, Joan Smith-Sonneborn, out of the room. "That meeting was a milestone," remarked a young graduate student in aging research as he rushed to join the others.

How these people had arrived at this point and where they were headed were questions I planned to trace. They are a handful among several hundred scientists doing basic research in the biology of aging, and among the thousands more whose work provides a supporting matrix of experimental results and data. I focused on them and a few others partly because they helped lay the groundwork for one of the most promising avenues of research in gerontology—the idea that aging and life span are controlled by the DNA—and partly because they provide a paradigm of the development and evolution of scientific thought. Only time will tell whether their theories will prevail.

Working independently, in most cases unaware of each other's existence, half a dozen of these scientists were carrying out experiments that overlapped and interlocked in a way that would become apparent only years later. Finally, when they put all their work together, they realized that it provided a basis for concluding that the aging process might not be inexorable, that the mechanisms that kept the genes in proper working order might be subject to manipulation, that the age-old wish to hang on to one's youth for the longest possible period of time might be attainable.

Throughout the time during which I researched and wrote this book, what fascinated me was not the product of the science these people were carrying out, important though that was, but the process. What were the turns and twists in their lives, the people and ideas that influenced them, the sudden flashes of insight, the emotional highs and lows, the successes and failures, the kind of blind faith that allowed them to hold fast when everything seemed to be pointing in the opposite direction? The answers to these questions would have been interesting from any group of scientists embarked on a quest, but these men and women were after nothing less than the basis of human mortality.

" 'We have discovered the secret of life,' [Francis] Crick told everyone within earshot over drinks that noon at the Eagle," reports Horace Freeland Judson in *The Eighth Day of Creation*, when Crick and James Watson had just laid bare the double-helix structure of the DNA—the genetic blueprint for all the cell's functions and the repository of all the traits passed on from generation to generation. When I asked Ron Hart what his reaction was upon realizing that he and Richard Setlow, his former mentor and collaborator, had found a direct correlation between a mechanism for repairing DNA and the life span of seven different species, he said: "Well, we didn't go running out yelling, 'Eureka,' like Francis Crick."

"It wasn't on the same order," I said.

"You never can tell," he replied. "If we found something, a trick, that led to the understanding of the mechanism by which longevity is achieved in mammalian species, it would probably have a greater effect on our lives and our society than the discovery of the double helix. It's true that one could not have proceeded without the other. But then is the discovery of the DNA molecule and its structure of any importance unless that molecule has a major role in some related event?"

The idea I had when I began this book was that the pursuit of a scientific goal, especially one that has such significance in the lives of all of us, including the investigators themselves, contains the elements of a good thriller—the false clues, the blind alleys, the hypotheses that are enthusiastically embraced and discarded, the crescendoing excitement as first one researcher, and then another, picks up the right trail. I would not be writing history but, rather, chronicling events as they unfolded. In the four years I spent crisscrossing the country, going to conferences on aging, visiting researchers in their laboratories, offices, and homes, watching them present their findings at conferences, meeting their students, associates, spouses, and children, I came to know them as scientists and as people. It was a closeup view that I don't think is accorded many people outside the profession. "What's interesting," Art Schwartz told me, "is that you are getting information from people before selective memory has had a chance to work. When people are asked about experiments years after they were carried out, they tend to forget all the botches, the things that went wrong, and remember only the things that worked out."

But there was another aspect of being present for the discoveries. Inevitably, I shared with these scientists their uncertainty about the outcome of their work. Of course, my risk was not theirs. Whatever the results of their experiments, I would have a story—a book. But if the experiments were successful, the potential benefit for all of us would be incalculable.

If these researchers are on the right track—and there are considerable indications that they are—many of us alive today may live to see the elimination or postponement for several decades of age-related diseases such as cancer, diabetes, and arthritis; the extension of health and vigor into old age; an increase in life expectancy; and perhaps even the extension of the maximum human life span itself by another fifty years or more.

To grasp the significance of the last statement, one has to understand what is meant by life extension. Although we seem to be living longer and longer, that is actually not the case. As the Bible notes, the allotted time of man on Earth is three score years and ten. The gains in nutrition and sanitation, and the elimination of most infectious diseases have allowed a far greater percentage of people to reach that benchmark. Whereas most people at birth in Roman times could expect to live about 25 years, now they look forward to about 72 years. It's what gerontologists call "rectangularizing the curve," so that on a chart depicting the life span of a population, instead of a precipitous drop, there is a plateau before the decline. What has not changed throughout the history of man is the maximum life span. This appears to be built in for each species, and for humans it is about 115 years.

Unfortunately, the increase in average life expectancy has not been accompanied by a parallel increase in health. Most of the medical advances have been made in the area of childhood diseases, but the chronic diseases of aging—cancer, arteriosclerosis, arthritis, diabetes, autoimmune diseases, and liver and kidney ailments—have been largely refractory to treatment. The latest review of aging surveys by the National Institute on Aging shows that, contrary to expectations, the rates of sickness and disability among the elderly have not dropped. More people in the United States are living longer, but not better.

Obviously, extending life, if it continues in the same downward progression, is not the answer. As gerontologist Gairdner B. Moment has written, "Few would opt for 800 years of shuffleboard and bingo." What is needed is to change the course of nature itself, to intervene in the genetic plan.

Gerontologists themselves are divided about how far they should or could go. They range from Leonard Hayflick, a pioneer in the field, who studies aging because it is "an interesting scientific puzzle," and sees extending life span as "an undesirable goal," to Paul Segall, a research scientist at Berkeley, who calls himself an "immortalist" and talks of cloning an embryo for each individual, placing it in suspended animation, growing it up to adult size with supernutritious I.V. feedings, and using the golemlike twin as a source for cannibalized parts. But almost all of these scientists are united on one point: The kind of life extension now being practiced in this country—coronary-bypass operations, respirators, pacemakers—is actually prolongation of senescence. What they hope to accomplish is the opposite: prolonging the optimum period of human health and productivity, currently the years between twenty and forty, for as long as possible.

And what of the chronic diseases themselves? Here is where some gerontologists believe they may make the greatest contributions. Since most of these diseases are age-related, slowing the pace at which we grow old may turn out to be the best means of prevention. And since the study of aging involves the study of the fundamental processes of the genes, cells, hormones, and immune functions, the lessons learned from this research may well have payoffs for specific diseases. Indeed, some believe that it is from aging research that the answer to cancer will emerge.

Yet from the outset, many people reject the idea of extending life—even disease-free—for reasons ranging from a religious belief that it goes against God's plan, to an evolutionary view that species improvement depends upon the mortality of the individual, to economic fears that it would disrupt the social security system, to a romantic wish to experience all the seasons of life. But perhaps the real motivation goes much deeper. Chad Everone, director of the Center for Infinite Survival in Berkeley, California, says that a quick diagnostic test of one's psychological orientation to life in general is to ask: " 'How would you like life extension?' If the reaction is, 'Oh, my God, why?' you'll find that basically they don't like life. But if they say something like, 'Wow! Let's get on with it,' they are usually successful, have visions they want to accomplish, and need time."

Perhaps nothing illustrates this point so much as a story told to me by Joan Smith-Sonneborn. She had been on a holiday picnic with a number of friends and was about to leave when a beautiful young woman she had never met before said to her, "I want to commit suicide." Before she could respond, some other people joined them, so she quickly wrote out her address and told the girl to come over. That night they spoke for hours. The girl was having trouble with her boyfriend. Like everyone else in her life, she said, he disappointed her. Gently, Smith-Sonneborn talked her into seeing a psychotherapist. Then, as the girl was leaving, Smith-Sonneborn could contain her curiosity no longer: "Why did you pick me to talk to?"

"Of all the people at the picnic, you looked like someone who loved life. I thought you could tell me what made you love life so much."

"Oh, I just do," Smith-Sonneborn exclaimed. "Because it's so marvelous."

"What do you do?" asked the girl.

Smith-Sonneborn described her research and what she was trying to accomplish. "Oh, my God," said her visitor. "I don't want to live until tomorrow. And here you are trying to extend life."

Chapter One

DNA—The Imperfect Molecule

DNA and the control of aging—it is hard to think of two more compelling subjects in modern science; the first understood only in the past thirty years, the other sought since the dawn of civilization. Is there a vital connection between the two, between the genes that code for all the constituents of the cell and the inevitable, gradual deterioration of these same cells? Could the link be the wear and tear on the DNA that comes from simply living, the daily insults inflicted by everything from sunlight to toxic by-products of oxygen? Might genetic damage be the first step in a multistep process involving all the various levels of biological organization in the body and leading to the slow deterioration of cells, tissues, organs, and organ systems, which we call aging? And, most far-reaching of all, can the built-in mechanisms that protect and repair this damage be harnessed to slow the march of age, stop it in its tracks, perhaps even reverse it?

These questions could not have been asked ten years ago. That DNA could repair itself was only discovered in 1964, while the very structure of DNA had been determined just a decade earlier in 1953. Similarly, the scientific study of the aging process that began a hundred years ago was sidetracked for half a century by a spectacular example of flawed research. Not until 1962 did the idea that aging is fixed in the cells become respectable again, eighty years after August Weismann, a German contemporary of Darwin, first advanced it. All this work, from Weismann's ideas on the evolution of mortality to the current hopes for life extension, first found support in a single experiment by molecular biologists Ronald Hart and Richard Setlow at Oak Ridge National Laboratory that brought together DNA repair, gerontology, and the idea that the control of aging and longevity might reside in our genes.

For all of 1973, on Tuesday mornings when the sky was still filled with stars, Ronald Hart would start the four-hundred-mile trip from Oak Ridge National Laboratory in Tennessee to Ohio State University. Usually he'd arrive in Columbus about nine A.M., just in time to teach his first class. Late Friday afternoon, when everyone was heading home, he'd be back in his car on the return trip, reaching his destination about midnight.

Often during the seventy thousand miles of driving he put in that year, he wondered whether it was worth it. But his doubts stopped at the door of his laboratory at Oak Ridge. In the hushed stillness of this small, almost cell-like room, with its concrete block walls, Formica counters, wooden benches, and a work table that took up most of the space, was the center of his life. As he moved around the lab preparing for the next day's experiment, making notes in his meticulous handwriting, setting up the equipment, he would feel a deep sense of contentment. At the lab bench, life took on a precision that it did not have on the outside. He fantasized that even if all the lights suddenly went out, he could continue working without missing a single beat.

"I seek to know how things work, why they work," he says. "This is my goal in life, the force which drives me. Many scientists in the field of gerontology are seeking immortality, but for me the moment of immortality comes when I understand something new. For that split second I reach the very height of being. That is such an internally satisfying feeling that I am addicted to knowing, addicted to understanding the push, propensity, or tendency of natural systems."

It doesn't even have to be a major finding, he insists, only a new perspective, a different way of thinking, an awakening to possibilities that one never considered before. He remembers first having the feeling as a boy of seven or eight when he came across a shale bed on his grandfather's farm. Bored, he banged one rock against the other, and out popped a fossil. In utter amazement, he stared at the delicate patterns of an ancient trilobite, the traces of a life that had existed millions of years before he was born. That night, while reading about fossils and evolution in his encyclopedia, a crack seemed to open in the world through which he could discern how things came to be.

A man of bearlike dimensions, Hart has a surprisingly boyish face with a forehead fringed with bangs, an upturned nose, and a wide-open grin. "Most people fall into a bimodal distribution regarding Ron," says Jim Trosko, his friend and colleague in DNA repair, meaning they either hate him or love him. His odd combination of bombast, good-ol'-boy country humor, and a nonstop verbal stew of brilliant ideas and insights, digressions, and tangents seems either to alienate him from or endear him to everyone he meets.

Growing up in the 1940s in upstate New York, the only child of a fireman and a beautician, he seemed to have slim chances of being exposed to the world of science. But then on October 4, 1957, when he was fifteen years old, Sputnik, the "fellow traveler" of Earth, was launched along with the race for space. In the ensuing panic that gripped the scientific, technological, and military establishments, millions of dollars were poured into the education of future scientists for the first time in our history.

Among the beneficiaries were the Boy Scouts. Hart became a science explorer scout. His troop was a motley crew of rugged individualists and science enthusiasts, but their leader worked in research and development at the nearby Griffiss Air Force Base, and the group held its meetings in the base's chemical and biological laboratories.

Scouting was never like this. On their one camp-out they refused to tie knots, cook food in aluminum foil, or talk about tanning skins. Instead they concentrated on turning the campsite into their sorely missed comfortable homes. They rigged up a current conductor with salt and water to provide electric light, constructed a pump that saved going down the hill for fresh water, and figured out a heating system to cook the food they had brought from home. It was science for survival, and they all swore, "Never again." Still, according to Hart, the Sputnik-inspired program accomplished its aim, and all the scouts in his troop went into science.

While a freshman in high school, he began experiments in the basement of his house that would prefigure his later research. Having read that ultraviolet light mutated cells, he and his father rigged up a UV light box, and using algae from nearby ponds, he began mutating cells. But his results were strangely inconsistent: Sometimes the rates of mutation were very high and at other times very low. In the classical manner of scientific observation, he went over all the variables and finally hit upon the fact that the low rates of mutation occurred when he did his experiments close to where his mother trained her fluorescent bulbs on her prize-winning African violets. Inadvertently, and quite independently, he had discovered a form of DNA repair, called photoreactivation repair, which was activated by a wavelength of light found in the bulbs.

Ten years later in graduate school, his interest in DNA repair, mutation, and evolution had developed into a passion that found few adherents among his fellow students at the University of Illinois. But in Hart's small group of students in the department of radiation biology, there was a scientific soul mate, Dan Griffith. In their office in the subbasement, he and Griffith would pass journal papers back and forth, speculating on the latest concepts, arguing late into the night. Sometimes they would be joined by their major professor, Howard Ducoff, when he came in to do a late-night experiment.

"He was totally involved in science," says Hart of his mentor. "I don't think it really mattered to him if anyone else in the world cared about his research. He just went on doing it. He was a fabulous teacher, but one of the toughest I've ever had. Once I went into his office and demanded to know why he had taken off double points on every mistake I had made in a test. He said, 'Because you're my student and you're expected to do more than if you were someone else's student. This is going to be your field, not theirs.' "

Hart picked up Ducoff's style of teaching, his meticulous approach to lab work, and a lifelong interest in a very basic question: Where does the control of aging lie?

The central problem for anyone in research on aging is that virtually everything in the body changes over time. Some things go up like the amount of excess sugar in the blood; most things, from vital lung capacity to dreaming, go down; and a few things like the ability to solve complicated problems of logic, remain remarkably stable until about age seventy. But change is the dominant feature. The result is that there has been less agreement among gerontologists about the basic cause of aging—or indeed if there is one basic cause—than among horseplayers on how to pick a winner. In his classic book, *The Biology of Senescence*, Alexander Comfort lists more than fifty authors of theories and their variations. There are deterioration theories, accumulation theories, toxin theories, growth theories, metabolic theories, cosmic-ray theories, sex-gland theories—even the action of gravity has been blamed. As late as 1976, Leonard Hayflick was moved to write, in an article for *Natural History* magazine, "There is probably no other area of scientific inquiry that abounds with as many untested or untestable theories as the biology of aging."

But in Hart's graduate-school days in the late 1960s, several hypotheses loosely gathered under the rubric of "somatic mutation" stood out from the crowd. They were elegant, timely, and, most desirable of all, could be tested in the laboratory. The idea behind them, that changes in the somatic cells of the body were responsible for aging, was a very old one dating back to August Weismann in 1881. But in the annals of science, where progress is often illusory and the path to knowledge tortuous under the best of circumstances, the checkered history of the role of cells in aging was almost without parallel.

August Weismann, who might be called the "Father of Somatic Mutation Theory," was a towering figure of nineteenth-century thought. A scientist, writer, and philosopher at home with the ultimate questions of life and death, he lived in the shadow of his great contemporary, Charles Darwin, whose cause he championed. Ironically, while most anyone who has taken a high-school biology course remembers Lamarck as the man who failed the question of which came first, the chicken or the egg, few recall Weismann, the German evolutionist who proved Lamarck wrong.

Weismann's ideas on aging, which today are enjoying a revival, arose from his own important contribution to evolutionary theory—the division of the body into germ and soma; that is, those cells involved directly in the reproduction of new individuals, and the rest of the cells in the body. As he saw it, the germ cells were perfect and immortal, stretching back in time in an unbroken chain to the first living cell. Everything that happened in life affected only the soma, which surrounded and protected the germ. When the body died, all of its habits, changes, adaptations, efforts died with it. Only the germ cell was passed on during reproduction. Heredity was a one-way street—from the germ out. "From the moment when the phenomena which precede segmentation commence in the egg, the exact kind of organism which will be developed is already determined—whether it will be larger or smaller, more like its father or its mother, which of its parts will resemble the one and which the other even to the minutest detail," he wrote.

In this way Weismann knocked down the idea, first advanced by Lamarck (even conceded by Darwin when he beat a confused retreat from his earlier writings), that environmental influences on an individual during its lifetime could be inherited. To prove his point, Weismann, like the farmer's wife, cut off the tails of twenty generations of mice, and not one of the offspring was born tailless. He had resolved the chicken-and-egg conundrum, proving that if any change took place, it had to occur first in the egg in order to be passed on.

The question that Weismann posed was this: If the germ cell, the seed for the entire individual, was perfect and immortal, how did it give rise to the mortal soma? His answer, like his answer to all of life, was contained in the evolutionary process. Aging and death were not, as poets, philosophers, and scientists throughout the ages had always assumed, a fundamental part of the scheme of things. Rather, these unwanted gifts had evolved as a by-product of natural selection.

At its heart Weismann's theory of aging was a secular retelling of Genesis: In the beginning, life was immortal, the capacity for reproduction infinite. One-celled animals, such as paramecia, he believed, still enjoyed this state. But as multicellular organisms evolved, a division of labor took place, with some cells reserved for reproduction and the rest doing the specialized work of the body. The price of the differentiation of the somatic cells was the loss of the infinite capacity for division and renewal. Aging and death had entered paradise. All that remains of that primeval perfection in higher organisms is the germ cell, the tiny piece of immortality passed on from generation to generation.

"Death takes place," Weismann told the Association of German Naturalists in Salzburg in 1881, "because a worn-out tissue cannot forever renew itself and because a capacity for increase by means of cell division is not everlasting, but finite." Weismann had his audience imagine a situation in which some members of a higher-order species were immortal. Although impervious to disease, they could not avoid injury to one or another part of the body. Eventually these individuals would become decrepit, but would continue to compete with the rest of the population for the food supply.

"From this follows," he said, "on the one hand, the necessity of reproduction, and, on the other hand, the utility of death. Worn-out individuals are not only valueless to the species, but they are even harmful, for they take the place of those which are sound. Hence, by the operation of natural selection, the life of our hypothetically immortal individual would be shortened by the amount which was useless to the species. It would be reduced to a length which would afford the most favorable conditions for the existence of as large a number as possible of vigorous individuals at the same time."

Going against the traditional view of death as integral to "organic nature," he averred: "I consider that death is not a primary necessity but that it has been secondarily acquired as an adaptation. I believe that life is endowed with a fixed duration, not because it is contrary to its nature to be unlimited, but because the unlimited existence of individuals would be a luxury without a corresponding advantage."

Considering that he lacked the means to test his ideas, Weismann was amazingly prescient about the cornerstone of his theory—the mortality of somatic cells. It would take exactly eighty years to prove him right. The study of aging, which had such a bright beginning but fell rapidly into a kind of dark age, involved one of the most publicized experiments of the twentieth century.

In 1912, Alexis Carrel, a French surgeon working at the Rockefeller Institute in New York, announced that he had succeeded in culturing tissue from a chick embryo heart. Although the culture was only eighty-five days old, with characteristic presumption he entitled his paper, which appeared in the prestigious *Journal of Experimental Medicine*, "On the Permanent Life of Tissues Outside the Organism." Throwing down the gauntlet for would-be challengers, he wrote, "It is even conceivable that the length of the life of a tissue outside of the organism could exceed greatly its normal duration in the body because elemental death might be postponed indefinitely by proper artificial nutrition."

Until Carrel's experiment, the life of a tissue culture had been categorically brief, usually lasting from three to fifteen days, before the cells started to die off. Now the proud, intense scientist who had earlier carried out revolutionary experiments in organ transplants on animals claimed that he had realized the dream of biologists to grow outside the body cells that fed on the culture medium and multiplied indefinitely.

Thanks to Carrel's flair for publicity and his winning of a Nobel Prize for entirely unrelated work in blood-vessel repair, the cells captured the imagination of the world. For thirty-four years their existence was chronicled in newspaper and magazine accounts until they were voluntarily "retired." Legends grew up surrounding them, but nothing was as bizarre as the truth itself.

Visitors were barred from the laboratory, and even reporters had to be content with peeks through glass "portholes" into the sanctum sanctorum. Inside this sterile operating theater whose walls and ceilings were painted black (to reduce the probability of microbial contamination), technicians capped and gowned in black, like the votaries of some medieval religious sect, tended their "immortal" cells.

If his methods were effective in preventing access to his data, they were equally effective in inhibiting independent research. Scientists were awed by the mystique surrounding his work, impressed by the difficulty of tissue-culture technique, and few of them wished to practice what seemed literally a "black art." Carrel's influence prevailed, and progress in the fields of both tissue culture and gerontology languished for half a century. Although no laboratory succeeded in confirming his results, his contention that his chick heart cells were immortal went virtually without challenge. It became the dogma of the day. In aging research, his work did double damage. First, it implied that although individuals were mortal, their cells, freed from the constraints of the body, were not. Second, it led investigators interested in the basic cause of senescence to look anywhere but at the cells.

Extracellular theories abounded along with matching "remedies." Elie Metchnikoff, an associate of Louis Pasteur, believed that aging was a kind of fermentation process set in motion by intestinal bacteria, and he launched a yogurt-eating craze. Alexander Bogomolets, a Russian scientist, claimed to have discovered a "serum" that regenerated worn-out connective tissue. Serge Voronoff of the College of France advocated transplanting monkey sex glands to restore old men to their youthful vigor.

In the late 1950s, about a decade and a half after Carrel's death, Leonard Hayflick, a young microbiologist at the Wistar Institute in Philadelphia, was looking for the viral cause of cancer. He wanted to transfer fluid from cancer-cell cultures to the media of normal human cells. If the cancer cells contained a virus, he reasoned they might convert the normal cell to a malignant one.

But he and his collaborator, Paul Moorhead, soon discovered a snag. No one had succeeded in growing human cells that maintained their normal state for an extended period of time. They would either stop multiplying in culture after several months, eventually dying out, or become "transformed." Different scientists have different criteria for the abnormal state known as transformation. For Hayflick, it is a cell whose chromosomes have an atypical number or shape, which frequently produces tumors when introduced into test animals, and which grows indefinitely. By this time, immortal cell populations from at least 225 mammalian tissues had been cultivated and all of them were transformed. (It has never been established whether Carrel's chicken cells, which appeared normal, were actually transformed.) Using ten different criteria devised by Hayflick and Moorhead, every "immortal" culture the Philadelphia scientists examined was found to grow and behave in ways associated with cancer cells.

Since Hayflick's goal was to look for human cancer viruses, he decided to start with the "cleanest" possible tissue—that taken from an embryo. He obtained the bulk of the tissue from Sweden, one of the few countries in which abortion had been legalized. As soon as a package arrived, they put the cells into culture, but sometimes weeks passed before fresh tissue was available. It was this odd happenstance of timing, both political and biological, that provided Hayflick with his first clue. One day, about six months into their experiments, they found that some of their cultures were dying off. At first this did not surprise them. The difficulties of maintaining life *in vitro* were well known. For instance, Theodore T. Puck, a pioneer in the field who had also been cultivating human cells, had stressed in his papers the need to screen each batch of fetal bovine serum—a major component of the medium—for the presence of toxic substances. But despite his precautions, Puck's human cell cultures with the proper number of chromosomes stopped dividing within a year. And not only had Hayflick and Moorhead not bothered to test the serum, they used commercial serum right off the shelf.

"I was raised with the dogma that said if cells are grown in culture several weeks and if you lose them after that time, it is because you did something wrong," says Hayflick. "You either didn't prepare the culture media properly, or the glassware wasn't clean enough, or the phases of the moon were wrong, or the technician was drunk the night before. All kinds of excuses had been invoked for fifty years to explain the loss of cultures." But he was not quite prepared to join the ranks of the faithful, because, as he puts it, "one of the observations I made didn't fit the dogma. What we saw was that the oldest strains, the ones that had been in culture the longest, were the ones that were dying. The ones that we had just received were fine, despite the fact that the same technician using the same medium with the same glassware was working with them. That was the tipoff."

From there it was just a matter of proving to himself that he was right. After determining that the cells went through fifty population doublings before they stopped dividing altogether, he began freezing some of the cells after a few weeks of growth. When these cells were thawed and put back into culture, they actually "remembered" the doubling number at which they had been arrested and continued from there until reaching a total of about fifty doublings. The conclusion was inescapable: According to Hayflick, *cells died because they were as mortal as the body they came from.* The only immortal cell cultures were those that were transformed; that is, they had all the characteristics of cancer cells.

Hayflick and Moorhead had upended fifty years of wrong thinking. "It is amazing how people get brainwashed," says Hayflick. "Your mind is not prepared when it has been subjugated by dogma. The loss of cells after several months in culture was known before I was born. So I didn't discover anything new in the sense of a new phenomenon. What I discovered was a different way of thinking about a phenomenon that had been seen but never appreciated because it had always been attributed to human failure."

He had solved the mystery of why cells died in culture but had to sell it to his colleagues. As he saw it, it was a case of a "kid fresh out of school confronting the gray eminences." In his role of heretic, Hayflick was aided by a streak of stubbornness, a combative nature, and the unshakable conviction that he was right. His first presentations at scientific meetings in 1960 were met with ridicule, skepticism, and disbelief.

So great was the resistance to his findings that Hayflick decided to do one further experiment before putting them into print. He sent his cultures when they were three months old to some leading cell biologists. Knowing the cells had a nine-month limit, he informed them that on a certain day six months hence, some of the cultures were going to die. "Of course they all thought I was crazy," he says. "But when the phone started ringing on the very week I had predicted, I decided to publish."

He sent the paper off to the *Journal of Experimental Medicine*, the publication in which Carrel's work had appeared. The letter of rejection, signed by its editor, Francis Peyton Rous, a giant in virology and tissue culture, now hangs framed on Hayflick's wall. There are two passages he loves to quote: "The largest fact to have come out from tissue culture in the last fifty years is that cells inherently capable of multiplying will do so indefinitely if supplied with the right milieu *in vitro*"; and, "To suggest that this phenomenon has anything to do with aging is notably rash." Hayflick next submitted the manuscript to *Experimental Cell Research*, which published it in 1961. The article, in which he redefined a number of terms that are now common usage, became a classic in biology, and in a gesture of sweet triumph, Hayflick sent a copy of his one thousandth reprint request to Rous.

It took another decade and the confirmation of his results in hundreds of labs worldwide before Hayflick's work was fully accepted. Later experiments by George Martin at the University of Washington in Seattle, and by Ed Schneider, now deputy director of the National Institute on Aging, confirmed and extended Hayflick's work showing a rough correlation between the number of cell divisions in culture and the age of the person from whom the cells were obtained. Cells from younger individuals divided more vigorously and went through more population doublings than cells from older people. But even now some critics argue that it is the hardships endured by the cells, being wrenched from the body and placed into the unnatural condition of culture, that limits growth, not any inherent mortality. Others continue to insist, as Carrel did, that given the "proper artificial nutrition" they would flourish forever. "It is the fountain-of-youth idea," snorts Hayflick contemptuously. "If you believe that there is a fountain of youth, I will believe that there is such a medium.

"It really is a psychological rather than a scientific problem," he contends. "Everyone knows intuitively that intact whole animals like you and me are going to die someday, but when you see the cells taken from you and me in a bottle dying, there is some psychological reason for resisting that obvious fact. I believe it is based on the fact—and I do not understand this—that here these cells are growing beautifully, dividing every other day, and they look absolutely spectacular in the bottle. They grow for weeks and months and all of a sudden they quit. I don't understand it because you and I are doing the same thing. We are growing beautifully and we are living marvelously week in and week out, year in and year out, and all of a sudden you and I are going to get old and die. Now why in the hell do we accept that, and not when we see it happening in the bottle? That is my dilemma and that is my argument."

But just how did Carrel keep his cell cultures going so long? While he lacks solid proof, Hayflick has a possible explanation. One day, after a lecture at the University of Puerto Rico, he was approached by a woman of about sixty who was working at the school. "I was Alexis Carrel's chief technician, and I agree with you completely that his work is probably not true," she said. The woman revealed how the cell-culture medium was prepared. The technicians took live chick embryos, macerated them, then put them into a centrifuge to separate the cellular material from the embryo juice. But the speed of the centrifuge in those days was very low, and when they extracted the clear fluid floating on the top of the test tube, they also picked up viable embryo cells that were supposed to have clumped on the bottom. Each time they fed the culture, they were actually adding new live chick cells. And, if this were true, the immortal culture contained cells as young as that day's feeding.

Whether or not Carrel knew what was happening is another story. Most of his technicians were, at one and the same time, fanatically dedicated to and afraid of him. "There is reason to believe," says Hayflick, "that they would be absolutely fearful to tell him about the cells after he made his worldwide reputation substantially on the basis on the so-called immortal cell population. So I've suggested that the technicians knew and, to give him the benefit of the doubt since he isn't here to defend himself, that he, himself, did not know."

The discovery by Hayflick and Moorhead that normal cells in culture die out was a watershed in gerontology. Indeed, a number of scientists believe that modern aging research began with that revelation. Regardless of the interpretation of what has come to be known as the "Hayflick limit"—and there are several conflicting ones—the proof of its existence did several things: It showed that cells in culture were as mortal as the body they came from; it provided a means for studying "aging under glass"; it established the idea of an aging "clock" that starts ticking away in our cells from the time of birth; and most important of all, it refocused aging study on the cellular level, where Weismann had left it eighty years earlier.

Although no theory claims to be all-inclusive or to answer every question, by the late 1960s, gerontologists were loosely divided into two camps: those who hold that the cause of aging is fundamentally *intrinsic*, that is, inside the cell; and those who look to outside, or *extrinsic*, factors, such as hormones, which in turn bring about age changes in the cell. An example of the latter is the hypothesis advanced by Vladimir Dilman in the Soviet Union, A. V. Everitt of Australia, and Caleb Finch of the University of Southern California: that the brain, the conductor of the orchestral body, also sets the tempo for senescence. Finch's candidate for the aging clock is the hypothalamus, a Jack-of-all-trades structure, which among other things helps regulate body temperature, appetite, thirst, sleep and wakefulness, blood-sugar level, and salt and water content, as well as the emotions.

If aging is located primarily in the cell, there are two further possibilities: Either it is a "programmed" event, a kind of genetic determinism in which the decrements of age, from skin wrinkles to senility, are timed in the cell in the same way as the development of the heart, spinal cord, and limbs are timed in the fetus; or it is random, untimed, the result of wear and tear on the cell, like friction on a tire.

"Molecular" theories became popular at that time for two major reasons. First, knowledge was emerging about DNA as the command center of the cell; and second, experiments in national atomic laboratories showed that ionizing radiation shortened life span, induced mutations, and caused cancer, an age-related disease. While other agents are known to do this, the striking thing about X-rays was that their effect was dose-related—the greater the dose, the more aging was accelerated. The evidence was circumstantial—ionizing radiation caused mutations and shortened life span—but it put the suspect, somatic mutation (the accumulation of errors in the body's cells over an individual's lifetime) at the scene of the crime.

One of the first people to advance a somatic mutation theory of aging was Leo Szilard, who helped design the first nuclear reactor and had a reputation for original thinking even among the select group of atomic physicists. Turning his fertile mind from atomic decay to biological decay, he proposed in 1959 that aging was the result of chance mutations, perhaps from background radiation, which inactivated chromosomes or chromosomal segments. While the effect of one "aging hit" on a cell was negligible, the accumulation eventually took its toll in the general breakdown of the body.

Four years later Leslie Orgel, a leading molecular biologist, proposed an ingenious refinement of Szilard's idea: Aging was a kind of accelerating feedback mechanism in which one mishap led to another. In this case the errors were in the protein-making machinery of the cell. Since some of the proteins are involved in making new DNA, which in turn codes for the production of new proteins, any errors that crept in would be self-perpetuating, eventually ending in an "error catastrophe." As F. Macfarlane Burnet, another somatic mutation theorist, wrote in his book *Intrinsic Mutagenesis*, "Error in a proportion of end products of some complex and coordinated process, whether molecules, cells, or industrial products, is always tolerable, but error in the 'design stages' can be fatal, since it is reflected in *all* the products."

By 1967, when Ronald Hart came to the University of Illinois, another factor had to be considered. While it was true that DNA could be damaged by many different physical and chemical agents including X-rays, ultraviolet light, industrial pollutants, body heat, and the chemical breakdown of oxygen in the cells, it could also fight back. Four years earlier, two groups of scientists had found that the cell contained enzymes that recognized and repaired damage to the DNA. Although they had shown this only in bacteria, Hart and others felt quite certain that it occurred in the cells of all living organisms.

At their nightly sessions Hart and Griffith would toss around their ideas on how DNA damage might contribute to the aging process and to the development of cancer. There was the work of Ducoff and others showing that X-rays, which induced mutations, also caused cancer and shortened life span. There were the studies of Arthur Upton at Oak Ridge revealing that radiation and cancer-causing chemicals, which acted in the body like radiation, played a role in many age-related conditions such as cataracts, degenerative diseases of certain tissues, and atrophy of the gonads. And there were all the clinical studies indicating that aging was to some extent inherited.

Every species looked at appears to have a built-in maximum life span. Moreover, longevity appears to run in families. In one famous study in 1934, about 87 percent of people over ninety years old had at least one similarly long-lived parent, and more than half had two such parents.

Thirty years later when better medical care and the elimination of childhood diseases had an equalizing effect upon the population, the grandchildren of the original group still enjoyed a six-year advantage in survival over the control group. Even more compelling, a study of one thousand pairs of twins, both identical and fraternal, found that the age of death for twins who shared the same genes was far closer than for twins who shared only the same womb.

But where did DNA repair fit into the picture? they wondered. Could it be that the rate of repair controlled the rate at which DNA damage accumulated in the cell? And did this rate of damage accumulation, in turn, modulate the rate of aging? Were there other aging modulators, which acted to protect the DNA before it was damaged? Would differences in the efficiency of these aging modulators account for the difference in life span among various species?

Scientists as a rule fall into two categories—analyzers and synthesizers: those who focus narrowly on one particular area, painstakingly acquiring bits of data, contenting themselves with exploring one small facet of a much larger issue; and those who expand their search for information in many directions, picking out this fact and that experiment and putting it into a larger framework. The difference is a matter of temperament, and neither one kind nor the other is intrinsically better, any more than, say, a finely wrought piece of needlepoint is preferable to a bold tapestry. But the fact remains that there are these two groups—and they are almost always at odds. Says Hart: "I remember one time when I stated in a seminar that DNA damage and repair could have a causal role in cancer and aging—this was at the time when everyone was on the path of the great cancer virus—and a couple of professors who will go unnamed said, 'Yeah, yeah, it's easy to come up with theories' and started laughing about the whole thing. And everybody thought it was a joke, because everybody knew that cancer came from a virus. I think that if I did not have a certain intrinsic belief in myself, I would have been totally squelched by the reception to my ideas."

Sometimes Hart's exuberant and vociferous defense of his ideas threatened to get him into trouble, Ducoff recalls. "Hart was very harsh on his fellow students. He could not understand anyone going into science who wasn't willing to work seven days a week."

While Hart was in graduate school, two things happened to him that had a profound effect on his life. The first was when Ducoff took his students to the biomedical division of the nearby Argonne National Laboratory. One of those who addressed the students was George Sacher, a tall, gentle, soft-spoken scientist who immediately impressed Hart with the depth of his thought and the breadth of his data on aging theory. While most of his class wandered off to talk with other people, he stayed behind to meet Sacher.

The second incident occurred in his last year at Illinois. In 1970, as chairman of the seminar committee in the Department of Physiology and Biophysics, he had invited Jane Setlow, a biophysicist who had done some of the early work on DNA repair, to give a talk. He spoke to her of his interest in DNA repair and asked about doing postdoctoral research with her. Her husband was now working with mammalian cells, she said, adding, "Really, he is the person you should speak to."

Only six years earlier, Richard Setlow had stunned the scientific world when he and his coworker, William Carrier, at Oak Ridge National Laboratory in Tennessee, and another team, from Yale University, Paul Howard-Flanders and Richard Boyce, simultaneously reported the discovery of a DNA repair mechanism. Until then the idea that the DNA contained enzymes that recognized damage to itself and went about repairing it, the way a handyman might replace a broken shingle, was not even suspected.

Short and lithe, with a whitish-gray mustache, Setlow is a dapper man with a charming, cultivated manner. In his early sixties, he is still a bench scientist, preferring to collaborate with one or two peers rather than administer a stable of postdocs, graduate students, and technicians. His interest is in "pure" science, asking interesting questions—the equivalent of climbing a mountain because it is there.

Pure science is what led him serendipitously to the discovery of DNA repair. Like most breakthroughs, it occurred in a jumble of happenstance, mishaps, and misconceptions. It is the story of people literally working in the dark, with little idea of what they were after, how to go about it, or the possible significance their work would have in the further understanding of disease, aging, and perhaps evolution itself.

Setlow began his doctoral work in physics at Yale just before World War II, taught physics to Navy personnel during the war, and, by the time the war was over, had decided to change fields. "Physics had shot its bolt," he says. "It had reached one of those plateaus where a lot of things had been found out and people were cleaning up odds and ends. Biology looked much more exciting. Not very much was known, and a number of people with physics backgrounds were going into it."

Like Leo Szilard, Francis Crick, George Gamow, and others, Setlow crossed the line from the inanimate to the animate, bringing with him a "quantitative way of thinking about problems" to the dizzying complexity of living systems. Together with his fellow travelers at Yale University, he helped found the hybrid that is known as biophysics. Although today biophysics is practically synonymous with molecular biology, at that time, says Setlow, "it was whatever physicists were interested in."

Setlow's interest was in an area where physics and biology came together. How did a physical force—in this case, ultraviolet light—kill living cells? Since 1877 it had been known that ultraviolet light, the invisible, extremely short wavelengths of light beyond the violet end of the rainbow, could kill bacteria, and germicidal UV lamps are still used for that purpose. Later studies showed that the rays could also mutate the cells.

In 1928, Alexander Hollaender found that the most mutagenic wavelength of ultraviolet light corresponded to the wavelength most readily absorbed by the nucleic acids (DNA and RNA) in the nucleus of the cell. But for the most part, the scientific community was as blind to the significance of this fact as the human eye is to ultraviolet light. Even Hollaender did not fully appreciate the significance of his own finding. "It is probably somewhat dangerous to overemphasize the importance of nucleic acid in the study of radiation effects on living cells," he and his coworker C.W. Emmons wrote in 1941. "It is very well possible that in radiation produced mutations the nucleic acid is only the 'absorbent' agent, then transfers the absorbed energy to the protein closely associated with it." Protein, not DNA, was considered the important part of the chromosome. And that is where Setlow trained his ultraviolet light when he first began his studies in the late 1940s.

Such a blind spot is extremely common in science. In fact, according to Thomas Kuhn in his influential book, *The Structure of Scientific Revolutions*, it is the rule rather than the exception. In Kuhn's view, science proceeds not in a gradual fashion with a slow accretion of facts, logically building one upon the other, but in sudden jumps, from revolution to revolution, upheaval to upheaval. If new conceptions are to replace old ones, there must be a shift in the paradigm—a scientific model that has the ability to link together discrete findings into a unifying framework. Before such a shift takes place, there are many anomalous findings, which herald the coming change. But because they do not make sense in terms of the prevailing paradigm, they are almost invisible. Like the scene in Steven Spielberg's film in which E.T. hides in the closet, "camouflaged" behind a jungle of stuffed animals, they are not seen for what they are.

The problem in this case was that no one knew DNA was the genetic material, the necklace on which the genes were strung. In the 1940s most scientists assigned that role to the proteins in the chromosome. Protein, which takes its name from the Greek *protus* for "first," was considered of prime importance to the cell. It comes in a dazzling variety of molecular sizes and shapes, while DNA is made up of four component parts called bases, which, it was believed, occurred in monotonous repeated sequences like a wallpaper pattern. But as with the data from ultraviolet light, there were anomalous findings dating back two decades that appeared to put DNA, rather than protein, in the driver's seat.

In 1944 an experiment was performed that should have settled the matter once and for all. Three Rockefeller Institute scientists, Oswald Avery, Colin MacLeod, and Maclyn McCarty, showed that an extract from a virulent pneumococcus bacteria could transform a harmless strain into a killer one. Since the extract contained only DNA, it, and it alone, was the "transforming principal." There it was, indisputable evidence that DNA, not protein, was the carrier of heredity. And yet scientists, for the most part, responded with outright skepticism. The protein-holdouts insisted that Avery's extract was contaminated, that a trace of protein had caused the transformation, and that DNA could not possibly comprise the genetic library.

But for Jim Watson, a twenty-three-year-old American biologist working at Cambridge University, the Rockefeller experiment was a beacon by which to set the course of his research. In 1953, he and Francis Crick, an English physicist, proposed a model of the double helix that not only showed how the bases were stacked, but offered "the explanation of the real nature of heredity" that Weismann had sought. In their historic two-page report in the April 25, 1953, issue of *Nature*, they included a sentence widely considered the last word in scientific coyness: "It has not escaped our notice that the specific pairing we have postulated immediately suggests a possible copying mechanism for the genetic material."

They had split the molecule as surely as the physicists before them had split the atom, with similar possibilities for enormous good or enormous evil. They were rewriting the Book of Genesis. In the beginning was adenine, thymine, guanine, and cytosine—and there was life.

What they found had the internal logic and consistency of the Periodic Table of Elements. The double helix of DNA in their model looks something like two spiral staircases that coil around each other. Crick has compared the two strands to entwined lovers. Other scientists are fond of ing one DNA strand Crick and the other Watson.

The backbones of the DNA strands are composed of a combination of sugar and phosphate molecules. Jutting out from each backbone is a series of four chemical groups called nucleic acid bases: the purines—adenine (A) and guanine (G); and the pyrimidines—cytosine (C) and thymine (T). If the strands are lovers, then the bases are going steady. Adenine can link up only with thymine on the opposite strand, guanine with cytosine. This specificity, as Watson and Crick noted, makes possible the replication of DNA. When the strands separate, like two ropes uncoiling, each DNA chain serves as a template for the synthesis of a new chain. The process has such striking simplicity: A goes with T, G goes with C.

But just as three primary colors can be combined to make a Monet painting; or twelve different notes of the chromatic scale to make a Beethoven symphony; or twenty-six letters of the alphabet, a Shakespearean play, the four nucleic acid bases comprise the code for the constituents of every living cell from plant to man. DNA is the four-letter alphabet of the body's proteins. Three nucleic acid bases make a "word"—in this case, an amino acid. The amino acids, in turn, are strung together to form a "sentence"—the protein. There are, in all, sixty-four combinations of nucleic acid triplets that code for twenty amino acids as well as a "stop" signal. This is the "genetic code," a molecular Rosetta Stone with the nucleic acid language on one side and the amino acid language on the other.

With the further contribution of a number of other scientists, many of whom won Nobel Prizes for their work, the mystery of how the gene worked was soon unraveled. By the simplest explanation, the gene is a segment of DNA, which codes for a protein—one gene, one protein. The message of the gene is copied by "messenger" RNA using the same base-pairing mechanism as DNA, only in this case uracil is substituted for thymine. This stage, appropriately enough, is called "transcription." "Messenger" RNA then shuttles the information across the nucleus into the cytoplasm of the cell, where "transfer" RNA matches it up with the correct amino acid—a step called "translation." The final act is "synthesis," when the amino acids join together to form the protein. "Transcription, translation, protein synthesis—this is the modern Holy Trinity," one gerontologist, crossing himself, told me half-seriously.

Now the true meaning of a mutation became clear. An "error" in just one base would change the meaning of the amino acid word, which in turn would alter the protein sentence, with consequences for the cell ranging from beneficial to lethal. Moreover, since the mistake would be repeated every time the DNA was replicated to make a new cell, the error would be permanent. In fact, a mutation has come to mean any change in base sequence that is passed on when the cell divides.

By 1960, Setlow, who had moved to Oak Ridge National Laboratory, was an expert on the effect of ultraviolet light on DNA. He knew which wavelengths mutated cells and which killed them. But neither he nor anyone else knew why UV at these wavelengths was so detrimental. Even more provocative were suggestions, sprinkled throughout the scientific literature, of a mysterious "recovery system" that allowed cells sometimes to survive toxic doses of radiation. There were reports of lethally irradiated fungus spores that recovered after being incubated in various chemical solutions; of viruses inactivated by UV light and brought back to life after being grown on bacteria; and of chromosomes rejoining after they had been broken by X-rays. There was even one poorly understood recovery process called "photoreactivation repair," which had been discovered decades earlier. In this process, UV-irradiated cells could be revived if they were *exposed* to light—in this case, the spectrum of light visible to the naked eye.

Retrospectively, Setlow points out, no one really thought in terms of damage and repair of DNA. "The reason was, no one knew what to look at," he says. "You must have a product. It's all well and good to say that the DNA is being damaged and repaired, but you have to know what to look at in the DNA to find out if it is being repaired."

Scarcely had Setlow set up his lab at Oak Ridge when his big break came. Two Dutch scientists announced their finding of an "irradiation product." According to Setlow, the Dutchmen, R. Beukers and W. Berends, had been irradiating different substances in various water conditions because they believed water to be the key to life. This led them to extract thymine bases from DNA, freeze them, and then bombard the frozen thymine with ultraviolet light. The result was the creation of a very strange compound— pairs of thymines stuck together like Siamese twins. Unwittingly they had created thymine dimers, the first physical evidence, like a wound on the DNA, of ultraviolet-light damage.

Now Setlow could begin studying UV-light damage in a systematic fashion. He not only learned the wavelengths that were most effective in creating thymine dimers, he also found that other wavelengths had the opposite effect, splitting the dimers back into individual thymines. After a year of work, in which he learned to make or break dimers with just a twist of his

UV light box, he was ready to ask the real question: Did the dimer have any biological significance?

At that time he shared the laboratory with John Jagger, a well-known photobiologist, who was working with purified bacterial DNA. This was known as "transforming DNA" because it could transfer the genetic properties—in this case, resistance to a particular antibiotic—from one strain of bacteria to another. Setlow realized if he showed that thymine dimers could knock out the activity of transforming DNA, it would make his case. Collaborating with his wife, Jane, an expert in assaying for DNA transformation activity, he did the experiment. Two days later, Jane came flying down the corridor yelling, "It worked."

Exactly as Setlow had predicted, UV at a wavelength of 2,800 angstroms knocked out the transforming activity of the DNA, while UV at 2,300 angstroms restored it. The former wavelength caused dimers to form while the latter wavelength split dimers apart. They had shown for the first time that a physical product of DNA damage could stop biological activity cold.

There are very few times in most scientists' lives when for one glorious moment it all comes together. It is the ultimate high. "It was what you call a sexy experiment," Setlow says. "You have a prediction, you get your results in one or two days, and it works. It happens suddenly. I think the real thrill comes from the rate at which things occur, not just finding them."

The rest was not to come so easily. It would take two years of effort with setbacks, like the time a leading researcher declared unequivocally that dimers were not the important damage product of ultraviolet light; but Setlow was ready to ride this one out, certain that it had to be due to "the principle of the big booboo," as he calls it. "It always happens," he says. "Science is full of examples"—in this case a mislabeled vial of artificially synthesized DNA that gave the wrong answer.

One of the reasons Setlow felt confident that dimers were the culprit was that he and his associate Fred Bollum had figured out how UV light killed cells. Dimers slow the synthesis of new DNA in a cell and might even stop it altogether. The unnatural pairing of two thymine bases creates a bulge that distorts the DNA strand. During cell division, enzymes move up and down the strands of DNA, using them as templates to make new genetic material. If a strand contains one of these bumps, the enzyme has no more chance of moving over it than a train would over a track with two bulging ties stuck together. Or as Setlow's student Jim Trosko would describe it many years later, a dimer in the DNA is like having the fly of one's pants caught in the zipper.

During this time, another set of experiments was going on that provided one of those lucky breaks on which so much scientific discovery depends. Ruth Hill, a bacterial geneticist at Columbia University, had been looking for bacteria that were more than usually resistant to UV, but instead found bacteria that were highly *sensitive*. Very small doses of UV light, which had no effect on normal bacteria, would kill them. Her work provided the first indication that normal bacteria might have an enzyme, which the sensitives lacked, that allowed them to overcome UV damage.

Setlow was not the only one to recognize the significance of Hill's observation. Paul Howard-Flanders, a British biophysicist who had come to Yale from England in 1959, the year before Setlow left, met Hill at a "Symposium on Biology" at Brookhaven National Laboratory in Upton, New York, in 1961. When she told him about her sensitive mutants that could not recover from the damaging effects of ultraviolet light, he was amazed. "Here was a very clear indication," he says, "that what had been so casually suspected—the existence of repair enzymes—might indeed be the case." He returned to Yale determined to repeat Hill's results and look for mutants in another bacterial strain that was easier to analyze genetically.

Meanwhile, Setlow obtained samples of both the normal and the sensitive bacteria from his friend Hill and began to zero in on the differences between the normal and the sensitive. He soon learned that the ultraviolet light knocked out DNA synthesis in both types of bacteria, but whereas normal bacteria recovered in about half an hour, the sensitives never revived. Something inside the cell of normal bacteria was removing the dimers. It could not be the recovery process known as photoreactivation repair since that worked only in the presence of visible light, and all his cells were kept in the dark. Furthermore, while photoreactivation split the dimers back into individual thymines, his experiments revealed that in some unknown way the dimers were not being cleaved but were actually leaving the DNA. Now all he had to do was find some way to reach into the cell and show what was happening.

What should have been clear sailing for Setlow turned into a most bumpy trip. For four years he had been firing away at DNA particles and cells with his UV rays, filling in the missing numbers on the wavelengths that turned biological activity on and off, dreaming up experimental proofs that were irrefutable; and now, although he believed he knew the answer to the recovery problem, he had no idea of how to demonstrate it experimentally. He tried one technique after another, filling up lab notebooks with "It didn't work"; and then one day, for no reason at all that he can remember, the idea came to him in a snap—just separate the cell into two parts. "That's the way it is with all great ideas," he says. "In retrospect they're trivial."

From Fred Bollum he had learned that the easiest way to separate various components of DNA was with trichloroacetic acid. Big pieces of DNA were insoluble in the acid and would sink to the bottom of the test tube. Small pieces of DNA, which were acid-soluble, would float to the top of the solution. The sum of the two contents in the fractions is, of course, always the same. Therefore, anything lost from the insoluble fraction would show up floating in the soluble fraction. The thymine dimers themselves were easy to detect because one can "tag" them with a compound called tritiated thymidine, which causes the dimers to be radioactive.

This was no moment-of-truth experiment. It was just a matter of refining the techniques, running the tests over and over, accumulating the evidence until it was irrefutable. "A lot has to do with knowing how to do an experiment and, in part, knowing what results you want to look for," says Setlow. "You have to design an experiment so you can see what you want to see. In a way it is cheating, but unless you do, there's too much noise. It is like listening for a certain voice on a tape through all the background clatter. It's like hearing the music in that voice."

He and his coworker Carrier found that in the time it took DNA synthesis to resume in normal bacteria, dimers were slowly disappearing from the big DNA insoluble fraction and appearing in the soluble fraction. The scenario was clear: Dimers were not being split or changed in any way, they were being excised from the DNA chain. And not just the dimers were leaving, but several bases on either side as well. A little patch of DNA was being cut out with each dimer. The final proof that the removal of dimers from the DNA was responsible for recovery from UV damage was that this migration took place only in the DNA from UV-resistant bacteria.

They were witnessing "excision repair," as it later came to be known. Setlow immediately recognized that this process might be the mysterious "recovery system" that had been sighted by scientists for decades. The idea that DNA not only controlled the embryonic development, coded for proteins, and duplicated itself, but also recognized and repaired its own damage, was still so new that he realized it had to be sold to the scientific community: "You have to do a PR job. I can't write like Watson and Crick, so I put in a catchy title: 'The Disappearance of Thymine Dimers from DNA: An Error-Correcting Mechanism.' This said that mistakes in

DNA are not permanent, that they can be corrected. Therefore, if this works on UV damage, there ought to be other mechanisms that can correct other kinds of damage."

At about the time Setlow submitted his paper, which was coauthored with Carrier, to the *Proceedings of the National Academy of Sciences (PNAS)*, Richard Boyce and Paul Howard-Flanders of Yale submitted one entitled "Release of Ultraviolet Light-Induced Thymine Dimers from DNA in E. Coli-K12." Same experiment, different bacterial strains. Both papers ran in the same issue of *PNAS*, and all the authors have gone down in scientific history as codiscoverers of excision repair.

Setlow is unhappy at sharing the glory. He feels the others don't deserve it. According to him, Boyce, a former student of his, had called Jane for help some months earlier. Revealing for the first time that he and Howard-Flanders, the head of the laboratory, were working on the same problem as the Oak Ridge team, Boyce admitted that they were stuck at the same point as Setlow had been—how to show what was happening to the dimers.

"Unless you had a way to show that," says Setlow, "someone could always say that they were being cleaved. Jane asked me, 'Can I tell them the way to do it?' And I said, 'Sure,' so she told them and they did it. They acknowledged Jane and me for helpful discussions in their paper, but they just couldn't have done it without us."

Paul Howard-Flanders had begun his own search for what was happening to dimers after hearing Ruth Hill speak about her sensitive mutants in 1961. Using a strain of bacteria that was better suited to genetic analysis than Hill's, he and his group at Yale identified three genes that were necessary for recovery from UV-light damage. His first idea, that the dimers were being split during the recovery process, was shot down by hearing Setlow speak at a meeting of the Radiation Research Society, where he described his inability to find evidence of dimer-splitting in UV-irradiated bacteria that were kept in the dark. Boyce and Howard-Flanders immediately realized that if the dimers were not being cleaved, they must be released intact by the DNA repair enzymes. Using their newly isolated mutants, they focused on trying to follow the dimers as they left the bacterial DNA.

According to Howard-Flanders, he and Boyce prepared a manuscript on their work and sent it to Setlow for comments with the suggestion that his paper be published so that it appeared before the Yale paper in the same *PNAS* issue. However, Setlow did not like the idea of submitting the papers together and they were submitted independently to the journal.

"They were not done together and I really didn't want anything to do with it," says Setlow. It wasn't the amount of time or work spent on solving the problem of "dark repair" that had and still has Setlow exercised, but rather his feeling that the Yale scientists jumped on his idea to finish in a dead heat with the Oak Ridge team. "Most of science is made of small things," he says, "like the use of trichloroacetic acid to separate the DNA. They're all simple ideas. That's why we're proprietary about them. Once they're published, they're everyone's ideas."

But Howard-Flanders sees it differently. The problem for the Yale group, he says, was to get the skills needed for biochemical analysis and to overcome difficulties due to poor equipment for counting the radioactive tritiated thymidine label, which they used to measure the dimers. "We felt indebted to the Setlows for their help in methodology," he says, "but we knew our ideas to be our own. The essential ideas were evident to me once Ruth Hill told me of her work and Dick Setlow spoke of his failure to detect dimer-splitting. Setlow is not correct in saying that we could not have done it without them. We would have been slower and hence felt that Setlow's publication should be ahead of ours, which indeed it was [that is, in the same issue]."

He also points out that the work done by the Yale team, identifying the three genes involved in UV excision repair, was crucial to several key pieces of future research. It enabled him to go on and discover a second repair system, called postreplication repair, which comes into play when excision repair fails to catch the error the first time around. And it paid off fifteen years later, when Azi Sancur and W. Dean Rupp, also at Yale, identified and purified the products made by the three genes and showed the role each played in excising dimers.

"I think that Dick Setlow would have liked to have been the sole discoverer of excision repair," says Howard-Flanders. "I remember that he spoke at the Radiation Research Society meeting about trying to look for the monomerization [splitting] of the dimers *in situ* and they couldn't be found there. And that was kind of a helpful piece of information to us.

"I think it is true that I wouldn't have been interested in UV light if it hadn't been for his wife working as a postdoc in my lab in the previous year. It is certainly true that through Dick Setlow I was aware of Beukers's and Berends's experiments [showing the thymine dimers], because he was going around everywhere talking about them. So that debt is owed to him."

It was Setlow's feeling that once the Yale team had gotten their results, they had pushed for early publication, but according to a published piece of writing by Richard Boyce, the person who did the pushing was the late Max Delbruck, one of the founders of molecular biology. In 1980, when the original paper Boyce and Howard-Flanders wrote on excision repair was singled out as a "Citation Classic" (it had been cited in the scientific literature 730 times) by the publication *Current Contents*, Boyce was asked to describe the events surrounding the discovery. At the end of his short essay, he wrote a paragraph that comes about as close as scientists get to acknowledging a priority dispute: "The paper by Setlow and Carrier describing essentially the same results with Hill's strains of *E Coli* B deserves at least equal recognition. This work, published in the same issue of the *Proceedings [PNAS]* predated our own by at least a month. Max Delbruck [a member of the National Academy of Sciences] expeditiously communicated our paper in order that both would appear simultaneously."

After Ron Hart brought Jane Setlow to the University of Illinois to speak and discussed with her his interest in DNA repair and her husband's work in the field, he drove through the night to New Orleans, where the annual meeting of the Biophysics Society was being held. There, as Jane had suggested, he would talk to Dick Setlow about being taken on as a postdoctoral student. They met and talked, but Hart left without a commitment from Setlow. Like an actor waiting for a callback, Hart sweated it out until the next night, when Setlow asked him to dinner. Once more, he "auditioned," presenting his ideas on DNA repair and aging to the other scientists at the table. Finally, a few days later, Setlow asked him what he would do for an experiment, and then offered to help write it up for a National Science Foundation (NSF) postdoctoral fellowship.

Although the usual route for a research scientist is to spend a year or two between getting a doctorate and taking an actual job doing postdoctoral work—a rough equivalent to a medical residency—Hart was worried abut the prospect. He had run out of money after living on a graduate's stipend of $3,000, and the NSF fellowship—only $6,000—had yet to come through. In addition, the job market, following a period during which a talented grad student could practically throw a dart at a map of the country and say, "I think I'll work there," was starting to shrink. Sputnik had done its work only too well. The universities were pouring out Ph.D.s in science, and good positions were becoming scarce. Moreover, in choosing to work in DNA repair, he was going into a new field with few practitioners, a difficult position to be in when one is just starting out. Despite all his fears, he was accepted on the faculties of several universities. One was Ohio State (OSU) in Columbus, not particularly known for basic research; but it offered a decent position in clinical radiation biology, some teaching duties, and a lot of time for research. There was a laboratory, equipment, a technician, and a salary that sounded astronomical—$16,000.

The temptation to take the job was great, but he still wanted to postdoc with Setlow. Resolving the conflict in a typical manner, he decided to do both. Setlow worked out a deal with the chairman of the radiology department at Ohio State, in which Hart would take the position at Columbus while also doing research at Oak Ridge, Tennessee, four hundred miles away.

The arrangement turned out to be a godsend, because when he arrived at Ohio State in October 1971, his laboratory was no longer there. Like the famous scene in Hitchcock's *The Lady Vanishes*, everything was gone—the laboratory, equipment, and technician. It was for Hart a rapid introduction to the cutthroat world of scientific academia, where grants speak louder than words, and where lab space is a turf that must constantly be defended against encroachment.

Hart explains that one of the researchers at OSU had just gotten a large grant himself and had taken all the equipment and the technician with him to another lab. Worst of all, lab space was awarded on the basis of the number of animals used for experiments. As a molecular biologist, Hart was at a distinct disadvantage. As he says, "I had to compete with someone using, say, a hundred dogs a year, while for me, one mouse provides all the cells I need."

Universities pay their faculty members money to live on, but nothing else. For research funds, they must look elsewhere. So Hart began life at OSU, as researchers always do, by writing a grant proposal, which finally came through in 1973. He lured a young technician, Terry Hoskins, and with her help and that of another tech, Hart began clearing out a storage room to which he had laid claim. They removed the dilapidated cabinets, scrubbed, puttied, and painted, scoured rooms and corridors for old tables and desks, and made do with other people's cast-off equipment. It wasn't much, but it was home, and he began applying for more grants. All this time, he was making the exhausting weekly trip to and from Oak Ridge, where he was carrying on three major experiments simultaneously: examining cell transformation—the mysterious switch of a normal cell into a cancerous one; trying to show in fish that DNA damage induces tumors; and investigating whether the amount of repair in human cells was the same across the DNA chain or whether it occurred more in one place than another.

He would spend a morning on the cell-transformation study with Setlow, putting into culture the cells he had extracted from mice and from humans. After lunch he would either start working on the fish experiment, injecting tiny white Amazon mollies with cells from other members of the same species that had been irradiated with UV, or would drop into another lab for the third experiment, where he would strip the protein that normally covers parts of the DNA, to see whether repair was any different there than it was on the DNA not normally covered by protein. At night he often spent hours in the library reading up on the literature.

By 1973, even Hart had had it with being in two places at once. He took a six-month sabbatical from OSU, and moved to Oak Ridge, where his research in cell transformation was becoming very interesting. Normally when cells are grown in culture, they will divide until they reach the edge of the laboratory dish, a point known as confluence. In order to start the cells cycling again, it is necessary to move, or "pass," a few of them to another dish. Occasionally, for reasons that are still to be fully explained, a normal cell line becomes transformed, and the cells ignore the stoplight when they reach confluence and continue to pile up helter-skelter in layers until they suffocate the cells at the bottom. Transformed, or malignant, cells do not obey the Hayflick limit, where cells stop dividing after a certain number of passages from dish to dish, but seemingly go on forever in culture. At that time several researchers had observed that the rates of spontaneous transformation were different for different species. For instance, in mouse cell cultures, after about ten or fifteen "passages," cells would enter this uncontrolled state, while in human cell cultures this almost never happened. Hart was intrigued by this finding as well as by Alexander Comfort's observation that various species, such as dogs, mice, cats, and man, all had about the same number of tumors over their life spans and that these tumors occurred at approximately the same point in their lives; that is, after the same percentage of their life span had been expended.

Here, thought Hart, you have a situation in which man lives fifty times longer than a mouse and has ten thousand times more cells, any one of which could become transformed, and yet he has no more tumors over his lifetime than the rodent in its lifetime. Could the difference be due to man's having a better repair system than a mouse? And does superior repair in humans account for the low transformation rate of cells in culture and the relatively small number of tumors over the life span when compared with mice? One way to answer these questions, he decided, would be to measure the rate of excision repair of various species with different life spans to see if they matched the differences he saw in transformation of their cells in culture.

Since the original work on excision repair, Setlow and other scientists had been filling in the missing steps. It was a remarkably coordinated process, in which enzymes, like the shoemaker's elves, whisked in and out of the DNA, doing their specialized jobs: clipping, excising, synthesizing, and sewing. In the first step, enzymes known as endonucleases recognize the bulging dimer and snip the strand of DNA at that point. Other enzymes called exonucleases cut out the dimer and some of the surrounding bases, leaving a hole. The DNA polymerases then make a new patch of DNA using the bases on the opposite strand as their pattern. Finally, the ligase enzymes sew the ends of the new bases back into the strand.

While Hart was preparing cultures from several animal species that were available at Oak Ridge, another set of experiments had just been completed in Setlow's division that appeared to bolster Hart's ideas. Earlier Fred Bollum had developed a very sensitive method for measuring the breaks in the DNA strand made by enzymes in the first step of excision repair. Taking advantage of this new technique, Takadi Makinodan, a pioneer in gerontological research, and his graduate student at the time, Gerald Price, decided to measure the number of strand breaks in young and old mice. If DNA damage did play a role in aging, as suggested by somatic mutation and error theories, then the amount of damage, as shown by strand breaks, should accumulate with age. And this is what they found when they compared tissue from young and old animals.

"Ron Hart always likes to jump into the fire much faster than I do," says Setlow. "So when he heard the results of Price and Makinodan's experiment, he said, 'Ah, the older animals have more damage because their repair system decays as they age, and since damage is always occurring, the older cells ultimately accumulate more damage. It isn't that they receive more damage, it's that they don't repair as well.' So that started Ron looking at tissues from animals of different life span."

But Hart disagrees. In his recollection, it was Setlow who suggested that DNA repair might decline with age. All he wanted to do was to see if there were differences between species and if these could account for differences in transformation of the cells in culture. "The way Dick recalls it, it is as if what I was doing was purposeful, as if I were going after it. But at that point I wasn't that interested in aging. I was interested in cancer."

In Setlow's comment about Hart, one can hear the age-old complaint of father about son: Setlow, the careful, conservative scientist, never leaping beyond the data, taking one step at a time, slowly building his case, versus Hart, jumping into the fire. And yet it was Setlow who talked about the advantage young scientists had over their older peers. "They haven't been thinking about the same thing for so long," he said. "An older scientist may have more technique and knowledge, but he doesn't have that ability to flip things around, to say, 'Oh, we got it backwards.' " (Ten years later, when Hart had his own students, he would chide them for jumping too easily to conclusions. Then he would put on the hat of a conservative scientist, eschewing theories in favor of a meticulous step-by-step, slow accumulation of data.)

The way of science, which has for so long been dominated by men, often tends to be a kind of Oedipal drama, in which father and son, locked into a love-hate relationship, battle with each other for supremacy. The older man, the mentor, the advisor, the imparter of knowledge, struggles to maintain the position that has taken him so long to secure. Yet at the same time, he yearns for a student/son who will carry on his work after him, conferring upon the older man a kind of immortality. The student, a willing apprentice, eager to learn, dependent on his advisor for emotional, mental, and professional sustenance, both loves and resents this most powerful figure. His conflict is to win this person's love and respect and, at the same time, overthrow him by surpassing him in accomplishment. It may take years—during which time the younger man has climbed the academic ladder, published in the right journals, made his own reputation, and most important of all, had his own students—for these feelings to sort themselves out and both men to achieve a kind of equilibrium based upon mutual respect.

Setlow and Ducoff tended to be strong taskmasters for Hart, demanding a kind of perfection from their students that they didn't from others who mattered less to them. And if anything, life at Oak Ridge was more intense than at the University of Illinois. Given two compulsive, strong-minded people working closely together, clashes were inevitable. "We used to argue about everything," says Hart: "What the correct procedure was for labeling cells, whether a pipette should be washed out two times or three. We'd read an article, and I'd say, 'That was a good piece of work,' and Dick would say, 'That piece of crap!' Or you'd tell him something, and he'd say, 'How do you know that's the case? Show me your reference.' And you'd bring it to him, and he'd say, 'That's not a good reference, bring me four more.' Any statement you made, any piece of data you showed him, anything that you wrote, Dick cross-examined five hundred ways. And that was very good, because it made your work have better and better quality. But at the same time, it constantly made you feel, Doesn't he think I know *anything?*"

It was at Setlow's lab that Hart developed a style that he passed on to his own students: perfectionistic, demanding, intolerant of mistakes, failure, or sloppiness in either thinking or execution, generous with criticism, and parsimonious with compliments. "Dick did very little positive reinforcement, very little stroking," says Hart. "There were times when I hated that man passionately, and there were times that I was so much in love with him. I mean he was more important to me than any person in the world. But I could not appreciate totally his psyche until I had matured myself."

Hart began his experiments with cells from five species that were readily available at Oak Ridge. To test for excision repair, he added hydroxyurea to the media, a compound that inhibits normal DNA replication but does not stop unscheduled DNA synthesis (UDS), the new DNA formed during the process of repair. He then irradiated the cells with ultraviolet light from a germicidal lamp. To detect the presence of repair, he incubated the cells in the radioactive isotope, tritiated thymidine. If repair took place, the tritiated thymidine was incorporated into the new DNA synthesized during the repair process. If no repair occurred, then the radioactive thymidine was not picked up. Over the cells, he layered a fine photographic emulsion. As particles from the radioactive decay of tritiated thymidine traveled through the emulsion, it produced a dark silver grain, which could be seen in a microscope. By counting the number of grains per cell nucleus, which at that time was done painstakingly by hand, he could determine the amount of unscheduled DNA synthesis as a measure of the amount of DNA repair in the cells.

When he got the results, he could not help feeling somewhat disappointed. The animals with high rates of repair did have lower rates of spontaneous transformation, but there didn't appear to be any correlation between DNA repair and life span. Although he claims that his interest at the time was in cancer and the phenomenon of spontaneous transformation, rather than aging, he admits that "somewhere it was in the back of my mind." But the data squelched such speculations.

A short time later, while talking to George Sacher on the phone about some business involving the Argonne University Associates Biology Committee, on which they both sat, he mentioned the experiments on DNA repair. According to Hart, the conversation went something like this:

"George," said Hart, "you have the best records available on maximum achievable life span; do you have anything on spontaneous transformation?"

"No, I don't," said George. "Why?"

"Well, I did this study on different animals, but there certainly doesn't appear to be much of a correlation with life span."

"What'd you find out?"

"It can't be right. The rodents are low and man is high, but we also get a high repair capacity for the cow."

"So?"

"Well, a cow only lives four or five years."

"Where in the world did you get that information?" asked Sacher incredulously.

"Well, on my grandfather's farm we always butchered them when they were about five years old."

"Hell, a cow lives thirty years!"

Hart roared with laughter. "So who would eat a cow that old?"

While Sacher read him the life-span data, he began plotting the extent of unscheduled DNA synthesis versus how long each of the animals lived. When he was finished, he just stared at the paper. There was an almost perfect correlation between the repair capacity of an animal and its maximum achievable life span. Since Weismann's time, people had been looking for correlations between life span of a species and one physiological factor or another. But, in fact, there were very few: An inverse association with metabolic rate; a correlation Sacher had developed using metabolism as well as the ratio of brain size to body size; and now it appeared that DNA repair, at least as it related to UV-induced damage, might be a third.

It was for Hart a most exquisite moment: "The feeling is like . . . there is something that no person has ever seen before. And you wonder, can it be real? Is it really right? See, at first there's amazement and then there's the questioning: 'Did we do all the controls properly? We better repeat certain points. Maybe we should test it another way.' But for that one moment before all the questioning begins, it is a matter of wonder that nature is discernible, that we don't live in a disorganized universe, that you can understand things. It's that touching of infinity, that being one with the cosmos. You see, that's the heart of science. There's that part of science that is the hours and days and weeks and months in the lab collecting data, just collecting and collecting, and then you put it all together."

That night Hart told Setlow about his conversation with Sacher and the fascinating outcome. And that is when, according to Hart, Setlow shared with him the findings of Price and Makinodan. "Did they look at different species?" Hart wanted to know.

"No," said Setlow.

"Well, wouldn't it be interesting if the rate of accumulation of damage varied between different species and correlated with life span?"

It would, Setlow agreed. But they would need more species to prove their point. It took the full six months of Hart's sabbatical from OSU to work on that one experiment to get it done. As usual, Setlow stood over his shoulder asking the exasperating, but necessary, questions. Was he certain that all the animals in the sample had expended the same amount of their maximum achievable life span? Were the biopsies all taken from the same area? Adhering to these exacting criteria, they ended up with seven species in all, ranging from the tiny shrew, which lives about a year and a half, to man, who lives about ninety-five years. And the amount of DNA repair of every species tested was directly proportional to its maximum achievable life span.

What they found was a correlation, nothing more and nothing less—a kind of tantalizing glimpse of the underlying order that Hart seeks. But correlations are not causality. The cock crows at dawn, but he doesn't make the sun come up. On the other hand, there is a high correlation between cigarette smoking and lung cancer, and the scientific evidence collected since that association was first shown supports the contention that the former causes the latter.

But the experiment was important for other reasons: It brought together for the first time the fields of gerontology and DNA repair. It continued the rehabilitation of a cellular and genetic theory of aging begun by Hayflick after the Carrel debacle. It elevated the status of molecular biology in aging research, and as all good experiments should do, it stimulated the thinking of other scientists.

If Hart was correct, if DNA repair played a role in the longer life spans seen as one climbed up the evolutionary ladder, at least in terms of warm-blooded mammals from mice to man, then this fact had implications not only for aging and life span but for the very nature of life.

According to the second law of thermodynamics, in a closed system, without an external input of energy, everything runs downhill; heat tends toward cold, motion toward stillness, order toward chaos. It is like having a house that is fully equipped and cleaned for rental, and then tenants move in and use all the facilities but never replace or maintain anything. Bit by bit, the dirty dishes pile up, the dust settles, newspapers are scattered, clothes are strewn, grime seals the windows; orange peels, chicken bones, apple cores appear at random until all the surfaces in the house are buried under the waste products of life. It is total disorganization. It is entropy.

"At first sight living beings, by their growth, development and ability to maintain their structures through successive generations, seem to contravene the second law of thermodynamics which causes the continual decay of the universe," writes François Jacob in his book *The Logic of Life*. "But though thermodynamics imposes a general direction on a system, it does not exclude local exceptions, nor forbid a counter-movement of certain components at the expense of their neighbors. It is the system as a whole that decays, not its individual parts. Because they receive energy from their surroundings in the form of food, living beings are able to preserve their low level of entropy throughout time. They can also, without breaking the laws of thermodynamics, continually produce the large specific molecules which characterize them."

With food, with energy, the body is like the house that is continually tended. Toxic wastes pile up in the bloodstream but the kidneys remove them; old blood cells die and fresh ones take their place; germs invade and the white cells engulf them; skin tears and fibroid cells are woven together to heal the wound. Everything is maintained in that exquisite balance called homeostasis. At the very center of all this is the DNA, the information-containing molecule that makes all the enzymes, hormones, and proteins that regulate all the functions of every cell in the body. But, as Jacob notes, ultimately there is no escape from the universal law: "Living or not, every system that functions tends to wear out, to fall into disrepair, to increase in entropy."

As Hart stared at the line on his graph paper after talking with Sacher, as he paced the floor and thought about what this correlation could possibly mean, as he argued with Dick Setlow about the implications, a picture began to form in his mind.

Reconstructing his thoughts at the time, he says: "One of the best accepted definitions of aging is that it is a loss of homeostasis, and one way to view the loss of homeostasis is as a loss of the information that the body needs to function at an optimum level. DNA is the information-controlling molecule, the command center for the cell. Our experiment has just shown that at least one form of repair correlates with maximum achievable life span and probably represents the inverse of the rates of accumulation of DNA damage. Could it be, then, that DNA repair is the modulator which maintains the stability of the information cellular systems and the homeostatic potential of that system? If that is so, then repair is one of the ways in which a living system cheats entropy. Because not only do living systems raise themselves in organization above the general decline in entropy of the universe, but they *maintain* themselves for X amount of time above that entropy. And one of the ways that they might do this is by the repair enzymes which the living cell contains in order to maintain the integrity of its information. This could be one of the mechanisms by which we are actually holding ourselves above the increase in entropy that we see in the universe as a whole."

Nineteen seventy-four was a big year in Hart's life. He married his technician, Terry Hoskins, and he and Setlow published their findings. "Correlation Between Deoxyribonucleic Acid Excision-Repair and Life-Span in a Number of Mammalian Species," in the June issue of *Proceedings of the National Academy of Sciences*. Although, as they pointed out, it could scarcely be argued that the UV damage from the sun was the cause of aging (with the notable exception of skin aging), it could be a model for how many things, both in the body and in the environment, caused continual wear and tear on the DNA. As they wrote in their paper: "The existence of different extents of excision-repair implies that cells proficient in such repair can remove more damage than cells deficient in repair. Hence, over a given period of time a mouse might accumulate in its cellular DNA more damage per unit of length than would a man. Such damage would result in a more rapid deterioration of the fidelity of transcription and translation and could account for the shortened life-span."

Years later, Nobel Laureate F. Macfarlane Burnet was to write in his book *Immunological Surveillance*: "The short lifespan of the mouse is ascribed essentially to the fact that its genes, coding for those DNA-handling enzymes, ensure that they are more error-prone than those that are coded for by the corresponding human genes. This basic contention must be regarded as the central thread running through my whole discussion of aging and of human diversity. It is one of those hypotheses that cannot be directly tested—though Hart and Setlow's experiment comes close to doing so. . . ."

Hart presented this work for the first time at the International Radiation Research meeting in Seattle, Washington, in 1973 along with the results of the second of his three experiments. In this study he and Richard Wilkins at Oak Ridge showed that not all the DNA in a cell was repaired. Some of the damage was "masked" by proteins that were attached to the DNA at certain points. Here the lesions remained, perhaps to cause trouble later in life. This paper, which was published in *Nature*, was considered highly controversial at the time, but, ten years later, formed the basis for a most surprising piece of research. At the radiation-research meeting, Austin Brues, the brilliant scientific administrator of Argonne, sent Hart a cryptic and perhaps prophetic message: "Fate has dealt a new hand. A leader has been chosen. Beware the slings and arrows of the pack."

From the beginning, Hart and Setlow's paper caused a tremendous stir. Many gerontologists were unconvinced that DNA damage and repair were involved in the aging process, while others thought the experiment held the answer to senescence and life-span extension: Simply find a way to increase DNA repair. But both men knew that DNA repair couldn't be the whole story and that a lot more work had to be done before their finding would be accepted. And in science, where there is nothing so ripe as a time whose idea has come, events were happening simultaneously in half a dozen labs that would not only bolster the work at Oak Ridge, but take the study of aging in a new direction.

Chapter Two

New Evidence

Opening up the June 1974 issue of *Proceedings of the National Academy of Sciences,* Arthur Schwartz was stunned by what he read. It's crazy, thought the young assistant professor at Temple University Medical School in Philadelphia. You think you're the only one in the world doing this work, and then someone comes along with basically the same idea. In a way the Hart-Setlow experiment was the flip side of his own. They were looking at DNA repair and he was looking at DNA damage, but for them to have related it to the life span of various species, even to the point of using cells from an elephant, was unbelievable, if not downright maddening.

A slightly built young man with a narrow face and close-set eyes, Schwartz seems the prototype of a reserved, serious, unemotional scientist. But just as his ear-to-ear grin belies his earnest manner, there is an intensity of feeling under the cool exterior. He has been infected more than once with the scientific fever that comes when one is on the verge of something momentous. The first time it happened, he was an undergraduate at Johns Hopkins, a premed major, headed straight for a career in medicine.

One of the researchers there was investigating the mechanism by which certain plant hormones stimulate cell division. The investigator was interested in photosynthesis, but Schwartz turned to other possibilities. If he could understand how hormones regulate cell growth in plants, he thought, it might offer a clue to how cell division goes awry in animals—in other words, how cancer originates. He began to spend more and more time in the plant researcher's lab. Suddenly a medical career seemed to him a lot less exciting than one in basic research, and he switched his major to biochemistry.

By the time he was in graduate school at Harvard, Schwartz had become a man possessed. It started innocently enough with an idea: If normal cells could be transformed into cancer cells, why couldn't the process be reversed? While still wondering how to pursue this in the laboratory, he heard about someone who had actually accomplished this feat. Normally mice will develop cancer if they are given cells from a tumor of another mouse. But a scientist at Temple University claimed to have treated mouse tumor cells with RNA from a normal mouse liver and found that the cancer cells retransformed into normal ones. To prove that the cells were no longer malignant, he injected them into mice and no tumors developed.

Seized by the desire to confirm this extraordinary claim, Schwartz approached Harold Amos in the microbiology department at Johns Hopkins, who he knew was interested in the idea, for permission to spend the summer trying to repeat the experiment. Then, in the early 1960s, the complexity of RNA, the nucleic acid cousin to DNA, was just being unraveled. It appeared that there might be several kinds of RNA in the cell. By far the largest amount was in the cytoplasm and formed the structural backbone of ribosomes, often called the "workbench" of the cell, since it is the site at which the amino acids are assembled for protein synthesis. But there was strong evidence for a messenger RNA, which shuttled the genetic information from the nucleus into the cytoplasm. The nucleic acid Schwartz succeeded in isolating was ribosomal RNA, which had no effect on the tumor cells. What they needed, said Amos, was a means for getting out the really active form of RNA, the messenger itself.

Leafing through *The New York Times* one day, Schwartz spotted a short report on the extraction of messenger RNA from mammalian cells. Looking up the reference, he found a recipe for the technique. It involved taking homogenized liver tissue, adding phenol, which is slightly soluble in water, and shaking it up in a test tube. After centrifugation, there was a water layer on top of the test tube and a phenol layer under it. The water layer was primarily ribosomal RNA, but the interface between the two layers contained messenger RNA.

Amos, according to Schwartz, was skeptical. Messenger RNA, he insisted, was just too unstable to survive the two-day extraction procedure. But Schwartz plunged ahead, making modifications that reduced the time involved to a few hours, and actually getting out some RNA from the phenol interface. He injected this extract into the mouse tumor cells in culture and then transplanted the cells into mice. As a control he did the same thing with the nonmessenger RNA that he had obtained with his earlier technique. "Sure enough," he says, "the mice which got the messenger RNA didn't get tumors. And the other mice did."

Schwartz could hardly believe the whole thing was happening. He had just started graduate school, and now his first original piece of research had mind-blowing results. "Amos really got excited," Schwartz recalls. "I decided I was going to switch to the microbiology department and work on this. It was an interesting idea, but it was a fairly difficult project," he says in his understated manner. Try as he would, Schwartz could not get it to work a second time. It began to look like a case of beginner's luck. Amos was probably right, he thought, the messenger RNA was inherently unstable and was being destroyed before it could have an effect.

"Drop the project," said Amos after a few months, when the prospects for repeating his original triumph seemed futile. Schwartz pleaded with him to continue it. He knew he could get it to work. Finally, after a year, he succeeded in getting out a fraction of RNA that had the magic touch. He duplicated his original results not once but several times. But then to his utter dismay, it failed again. "Amos kept saying he was going to take me off it and I kept talking him out of it," he says. "Finally the ax fell and I had to go off it. It was really depressing because it took two years off my life. It was a fascinating project, and I don't know, I still have some confidence it might be real.

"People don't understand that science is such a high-risk venture. The more important the venture, the greater the risk. Nothing ever goes smoothly. If you were totally cerebral, it would probably be the worst thing. You need to go from your gut a lot of the time. Many people in science just go with what is safe. That way they get the grant money. And the government thinks the same way. They're only interested in results. It makes me wonder what would have happened with Ehrlich and his 'magic bullet.' He called his compound 606 [Salvarsan, used to treat syphilis] because that was the number [of compounds] he had tried up to then. Would the government have given Ehrlich enough money to cover 605 failures? And this was the first successful chemotherapy."

After Schwartz got his Ph.D. on growth-promoting factors in tissue culture, he did postdoctoral research on cell fusion at Oxford University, working under Harry Eagle, developer of the tissue-culture medium that bears his name. There, Schwartz was in the grip of yet another idea to control cancer and hoped to use Eagle's tissue-culture system to test his hypothesis that steroids could be used to prevent tumors.

Schwartz had noted that the chemical structure of certain carcinogens closely resembled that of steroids. Perhaps, he thought, the body's own steroids and the cancer-causing agent might compete for the same site on the surface of a target cell. For any substance to affect a cell, it must first bind on to a receptor site, which, like Cinderella's glass slipper, is designed to fit only one substance. But receptors are not foolproof. A look-alike compound may squeeze in, filling the space, so that it becomes a "competitive inhibitor" of the natural substance. The antibacterial drug sulfanilamide is one such imposter, so closely resembling a certain growth factor required by bacteria that it tricks the microorganisms into incorporating their deadly enemy. If steroids could successfully compete in the same way with carcinogens for available receptors on human cells, the dream of a cancer preventative might be realized.

Because it bore a strong structural resemblance to steroids, Schwartz chose to work with dimethylbenzanthracene (DMBA), one of a huge class of chemicals called polycyclic hydrocarbons. These compounds, which are the products and by-products of better living through chemistry, are ubiquitous in the environment, occurring in everything from cigarette smoke to automobile exhaust.

Although the connection between cancer and environmental pollutants goes back to at least 1775, when Percival Pott, a London surgeon, singled out soot as the cause of scrotal cancer in English chimney sweeps, until recently, how such substances caused tumors was a complete mystery. Most chemicals do not attack the DNA, and yet the prevailing theory of cancer is that errors in the DNA, or somatic mutations, are the first step in the chain of events that culminates in the runaway cell growth of cancer.

Finally, in the early 1960s, the mystery was cleared up by a husband and wife team of scientists, James and Elizabeth Miller of the University of Wisconsin's McCardle Laboratory for Cancer Research. In a striking demonstration that nature and nurture are complementary rather than opposing forces, this husband-and-wife team of biochemists showed that carcinogenic substances from the outside environment had to be *activated* by enzymes inside the body to exert their malignant effect. This activation, which occurs during the metabolic breakdown of the compound, converts the inert chemical to a highly reactive form called an electrophile, literally a lover of electrons, which can now bind on to the DNA and cause mutations.

Various researchers in a number of laboratories continued to zero in on the metabolic pathway, or group of enzymes, responsible for this activation. This pathway, which is now known by various names, including "mixed function oxidases," "detoxification/activation," and "cytochrome P450," consists of a number of enzymes found in high concentrations in the liver. Since evolution generally equips the organism for survival rather than self-destruction, one has to assume that the enzymes evolved not to create cancer but to convert water-insoluble compounds into water-soluble forms that can be harmlessly excreted from the body. Unfortunately, in the process, intermediate products can be formed, which are highly reactive and unstable, and can wreak havoc on the DNA. Cancer viewed in this light is the fallout of normal functioning, a kind of legislative rider tacked on to a highly useful bill.

Schwartz believed that during this process of carcinogen metabolism, the steroids would exert their protective effect. But while running down this idea, he was diverted by an intriguing observation that years later would fit together with the steroid experiments in a most unexpected way. In his work with DMBA, Schwartz had noted that mouse and rat cells were highly efficient at detoxifying DMBA, but at an exorbitant cost—a high rate of cell mutation and death. Even at very low concentrations of the carcinogen, the rodent cells were extremely vulnerable.

There the observation might have stayed had not Harry Eagle walked into the lab with a batch of human cells and asked Schwartz if he would mind treating the cells with DMBA and seeing what happened to them. Schwartz ran the test and, to his complete surprise, nothing happened. Since there was always the remote possibility that he had forgotten to add the carcinogen, he repeated the experiment, and this time the conclusion was unmistakable: Human cells were virtually resistant to this powerfully toxic chemical. They did not activate the DMBA to its mutagenic form.

How very strange, he thought. Why should the cells of mice and rats be so much more sensitive to DMBA than those of humans? In most respects, the physiology of the mouse and of man is remarkably similar, or else one could never serve as the laboratory model for the other. And then, just as Hart did when he noticed the difference in the rate of spontaneous transformation between mouse and human cells, Schwartz wondered how the cells of animals on the evolutionary scale between rodents and humans would react. Was there a relationship between the life span of a species and the rate at which its cells activated carcinogens to their dangerous form? If it turned out that there was, it would tie together a number of ideas about mutation, cancer, and aging.

To do the experiment, Schwartz used a cell line, an immortal culture of transformed cells, in this case from hamsters. Known as V79 cells, they have the advantages of being easily cloned and containing a clear "marker" for mutation. On top of the hamster cells in the test tube, he layered normal fibroblast cells he had cultured from each of the animal species he was looking at. He now had created a kind of Jack-Sprat-and-wife situation. The animal fibroblasts, which he had irradiated with X-rays, could no longer divide but could still metabolize carcinogens. The V79 cells had lost the capacity to activate carcinogens, but they were superdividers. He then treated the fibroblasts with DMBA. As with most measurements of mutation, it had to be done obliquely, sort of like gauging the heat of a chili sauce by the amount of liquid drunk. If the enzymes present in the fibroblasts converted the DMBA to its reactive form, it would not affect the fibroblast cells that no longer divided, but it would cause mutant clones in the V79 cells, which could be easily detected by the mutation markers. Thus, the number of mutant clones per laboratory dish of V79 cells provided a measurement of the rate of carcinogen activation in each of the species tested.

This was a long, time-consuming procedure. There were interminable waits for lung and skin tissue of each of the animals: rat, guinea pig, rabbit, horse, elephant, and man; there was the inevitable fine tuning of the system, making certain that the rate of activation was real and not an artifact; there were the endless details of the experiment itself—mincing the tissue, irradiating the cells, layering them on the "tester" cells, identifying the dose of DMBA that would mutate but not kill the cells, and determining the number of mutant clones per laboratory dish.

The surprise for Schwartz had come much earlier when he had first observed the difference in activation between mouse and man. Now it was just a matter of holding his breath and praying that the correlation would hold up, that it would not turn out to be a dead end like the RNA experiment. Each time he added a new species, his heart was in his mouth. When the elephant tissue finally arrived, and he looked through the microscope to make sure the cells were all right, he had a sinking feeling in the pit of his stomach. What if the elephant turned out to be a good activator? Was it all going to fall through at the last minute? But his fears never materialized. There was a clear inverse correlation between the life span of a species and its ability to metabolize the DMBA to a form that could attack and damage the DNA. In othe words, animals with short life spans were highly vulnerable to the carcinogen, while long-lived animals were highly resistant. The cells from the elephant, which lives a maximum of 70 years, fell into place between the human at 110 years and the horse at 46 years; the rabbit followed at 13 years, the guinea pig at 7.4 years, and the rat at 3.5 years, just as though nature had drawn the line on the graph.

In keeping with his conservative style, Schwartz wrote a modest report of his findings in the "preliminary notes" section of *Experimental Cell Research*. But the implications were plain to him. His study had brought together aspects of aging, cancer, and mutation that lay at the forefront of knowledge in 1974. First, there was the fact that cancer was a disease of old age. The risk of developing cancer in a man sixty-five years old is fifty times that of a man of twenty-five. And the same age relationship holds true of most mammalian species that have been studied.

Second, Bruce Ames and his associates at the University of California, Berkeley, had clinched the case for somatic mutation in cancer when they showed that most carcinogens are mutagens. He devised a simple test, now the most widely used of its kind, for detecting potential carcinogens by measuring the rate of mutation in bacteria. About 85 percent of chemicals known to be carcinogenic in animals are mutagenic in the Ames test.

The third interconnecting event at that time was the publication of F. Macfarlane Burnet's book *Intrinsic Mutagenesis: A Genetic Approach to Ageing*. Although he won his Nobel Prize for immunology, Burnet was also known for his contribution to somatic mutation theory. He maintained that the greatest threat to the cell came not from outside sources, such as UV or X-ray, but from processes going on inside the body. Such an "intrinsic mutator," as he called it, might be an error-prone repair system, which, in the process of removing damage, would actually introduce it, like a careless typist correcting a manuscript. Eventually, he believed, the accumulation of "errors" took its toll in the form of cancer, arthritis, arteriosclerosis, and other age-associated diseases as well as the general overall decline.

It seemed to Schwartz that his experiment provided a connecting link between these three separate observations—cancer was age-related, carcinogens are mutagens, and somatic mutations might be the common denominator in cancer and aging. Hart and Setlow had shown a correlation between one form of DNA repair and the life span of various mammalian species. Now he had found a direct association between a metabolic system that activated carcinogens and length of life. Both were evidence of intrinsic systems that affected the rate at which somatic mutations became fixed in the cell and thus, presumably, the rate at which aging and cancer lay waste to the body.

For the first time in his life, he began to think like a gerontologist rather than a cancer researcher. Most scientists seeking the cause of cancer see the relationship between the disease and aging as coincidental, having more to do with the fact that the disease may develop silently for decades before making its appearance. Aging theorists, on the other hand, believe the connection is more causal than casual.

"Here you have an enzyme system that's activating a premutagen and a precarcinogen [DMBA] to a carcinogenic form, and that system is related to life span," he says. "You can't make the statement that this enzyme system *causes* aging and cancer, but it does seem to indicate a tie-in between the two. I think there's a reasonable chance that somatic mutations are playing a role in both. My gut feeling is that a lot of cancer is related to the aging process. In other words, cells become malignant for the same reasons that cells change with age. Most cancer researchers don't like to think this way. They like to think of cancer as a disease in its own right, like a cold, so that they can find a cure. Aging seems to them so diffuse that it might take a hundred years to understand, much less find a cure. But the reality of the situation may be that the best way to deal with cancer is by delaying the aging process."

In January 1976, Schwartz went to his first meeting in the field of gerontology. All too often the scientific conference is an exercise in frustration. Between the few tidbits of fresh data, there are often large servings of information grown stale from exposure at previous meetings or in published form. Still, these meetings provide a break in the routine, a chance to see and be seen, to keep up old relationships and make new ones, and offer even an occasional surprise or two. Conferences along with grant applications and peer review are considered part of the necessary evils of the scientific life.

The Gordon Research Conferences, sponsored by a number of organizations including the American Academy for the Advancement of Science, are the perfect antidote for the meeting-weary scientist. Held at scenic locations on either the East or West Coast, they are limited to one hundred or so invited participants who are housed dormitory-style. The participants eat their meals in a common dining hall and spend whole days together. The chairman of the conference, who is elected at the previous conference, produces and directs the show, chooses the theme, and selects the leaders for each of the sessions. Sessions are held in the morning and evening, with long afternoons free for recreation or for holding ad hoc meetings on topics of mutual interest. For many Gordon devotees, these informal get-togethers with one's colleagues are the high point of the conference. The media are barred from the conferences. Indeed, not a word of what goes on is recorded in any way, so that ideally, if not in practice, the conference becomes a testing ground for preliminary data, theories, and off-the-wall ideas.

The January 1976 Gordon Research Conference on aging, in Santa Barbara, California, was a strange and heady mix of domestic gerontologists; young, up-and-coming molecular biologists; biochemists who were not primarily in aging but had done exciting work in the field; and international stars in the biology of aging. Schwartz immediately felt a kinship with these people, who seemed to him more open, expansive, daring, and intellectually stimulating than those he had met in cancer research. There he met Ron Hart, who was also attending for the first time, and the two of them excitedly exchanged information on their related findings. They were soon joined by a vibrant young woman, Joan Smith-Sonneborn, a relative newcomer to the field.

Although the theme of the conference was "The Search for Molecular Mechanisms," Richard Adelman, the chairman, who was known for his studies on the effects of age on the induction of insulin and other hormones, had scheduled four sessions on "Regulation of Enzymes and Other Proteins."

Each day, as the presentations on physiology, cell biology, collagens, and protein biochemistry took place, a small but growing number of people began haunting the back room, talking, smoking, drinking coffee, occasionally returning to hear a particular talk, and then coming right back. It soon became apparent that there was a primary distinction between the group that stayed to hear the talks and those in the back room. The former was, for the most part, involved in the physiology of aging, in diet, hormones, enzymes, while the latter group was concerned in one way or another with DNA and the mechanisms of damage and repair.

By the third day, about twenty-five people milled about between sessions, growing increasingly restless. "This is ridiculous," said one of them quite loudly. "We're all bored with the talks and we're all dying to hear what each of us in this room has to say." Suddenly the room began buzzing like a hive of bees, as one person after another began talking. "We're crazy to sit around here doing nothing." "Why don't we get together and talk about the real work that's happening in aging?" "Why don't we hold a counterconference?" In a moment, the small band was galvanized, throwing out topics for discussion, looking for a blackboard, scrounging up scotch and gin. In a body they marched over to a guesthouse that had been set up for the attendees. Taking possession of a room about the size of a small office, they filled the available chairs, sat on the window sills, and lined the walls. Someone locked the door to assure that they wouldn't be disturbed, and the "Renegade Repair Conference," as it came to be known, was called to order.

Like a gang of rowdy schoolchildren when the teacher has left the room, everyone began talking at once. Some tried to pitch their voice above the babble of the crowd or pound the table, but to no avail. One person would holler over the general hubbub, and receive a few shouts of encouragement, but in short order the cry would go up, "Shut up now and let someone else talk." The questions flew like arrows in an Indian attack, deflecting the speaker from his theme and setting up local debates. When the tangent got too far afield, the next speaker would jump in. No one got to speak for more than five minutes. Concepts were set up and knocked down like so many bowling pins.

Despite the general clamor, there was a euphoria among the group, a self-intoxication, a conviction that each experiment reported in that little room was the hottest, the most relevant, the most interesting in the field, that this was what the Gordon Conference was designed for. Out of the chaos and excitement, radical ideas, insights, approaches were springing up, like the notion that hormones might act as signals switching the activity of genes on and off; that DNA damage might not only cause mutation but actually affect the winding of the double helix; that differentiation—the commitment of the cell to a specialized function—may play a dominant role in aging; that human syndromes that mimicked aspects of accelerating aging might provide clues to molecular and genetic mechanisms.

True to the rules of the Gordon Conference, there was no tape recorder or reporter to preserve the discussions or trap ideas swept aside in the heat of the moment. And when the conference was over, the biologists, the biochemists, and the DNA repair workers went their separate ways, drained but exhilarated, their minds buzzing with a cacophony of thoughts, images, impressions. But there was no doubt that a kind of cross-fertilization had taken root in their minds. A number of people present went on to publish papers embodying many of the concepts that emerged in half-baked form in that little room. Schwartz was not among them. He put aside his life-span-correlation work, having no way of taking it any further, and went back to his original idea of using steroids to protect against carcinogens; three years later, his results would drop, as Smith-Sonneborn put it, "with the impact of a neutron bomb."

"Not Why Do We Die,
But Why Do We Live So Long?"

When Ron Hart called George Sacher at Argonne National Laboratory in Illinois to ask him for life-span data on the animals in his DNA repair study, a channel opened between the two men that was to flow with powerful currents for eight years. Surrounded by books on animals, brain evolution, aging, mathematics, radiation biology, psychology, neurology, history of science, philosophy, physics, and astronomy, and by file drawers full of "biocards" with the statistics on the life span and physical characteristics of hundreds of animal species, Sacher was uniquely equipped not only to answer Hart's question, but to see, in the correlation that took shape as they spoke, a new dimension to the ideas he had been developing for the past two decades.

Sacher (pronounced Saysher) combined a nineteenth-century natural historian's approach to science—observing, describing, cataloging—with the most sophisticated statistical-mathematical analysis. Possessing an encyclopedic mind, he had a passion for fitting new facts into a grand scheme of how things worked, without ever losing sight of the limits of his knowledge. Even his demeanor seemed out of step with that of his colleagues. In an era marked by aggressive, power-seeking, often cutthroat competition, he was modest, self-effacing, courteous. I remember being struck by his genuine surprise and delight when, after discussing general aspects of gerontology, I inquired about his own research.

"George Sacher was always different," said Warren K. Sinclair, his friend and the former division chief of Argonne, in a memorial address shortly after Sacher's sudden death at the age of sixty-three in January 1981. He was "a theoretician rather than a practical man, a dreamer rather than an organizer, and a thinker and discussant rather than a hands-on performer in the laboratory." But Sinclair also noted Sacher's "complete disdain for the more mundane affairs of regular life or administration." That attitude, while not without its charm, is a luxury during hard times. And the qualities that enabled him to bring a wholeness of understanding may have in the end cost him dearly.

When he was a youngster growing up in Newark, New Jersey, his interest and curiosity in the world were boundless. "If they had had that word 'hyperactive' when I was a kid, that was what they would have called me," he once said. His druggist father hoped he, as the oldest of four sons, would follow him into the family business, but after a year at the Rutgers University College of Pharmacy, Sacher felt stifled. He transferred to the University of Chicago, an intellectual oasis from which he drew sustenance for the rest of his life. His first love was psychology, but true to his multifaceted and synthesizing nature, he studied everything that might bear on the workings of the mind, including physiology, genetics, biometrics, mathematics, and physics.

World War II interrupted his studies and changed the course of his life. While working as a civilian psychologist testing enlistees for the Army in Milwaukee, he began hearing rumors from his Chicago friends about a hush-hush project at the campus. He returned to the university in 1942, where his lightning ability to do complex mathematical computations was suddenly of great interest to certain people. His official title was "assistant mathematician" in "theoretical physics group, metallurgical laboratory, Manhattan Project"—but his real job was "human computer" for the developers of the first atomic reactor.

After the war, the metallurgical laboratory, where the bomb project had been carried out, was secreted in a woods outside the city and rechristened Argonne National Laboratory, which took its name from the forest in France. Sacher moved with it, continuing his studies on the long-term effects of atomic radiation. But even then his disdain for mundane affairs was getting him into trouble. Since he was now supervising Ph.D.s, his boss, Austin Brues, director of the biological and medical research division at Argonne, thought he should at least possess a bachelor's degree. Although he had completed all his course work in 1939, Sacher had balked at paying a $5 fee for "a piece of paper." Brues paid the fee himself and then helped Sacher obtain a fellowship to do graduate work in cell physiology.

These were hard times for Sacher, who was now married and had one child and another on the way. The fellowship paid $200 a month, which even in 1950 was barely survival level. Out of this sum came money for mortgage payments, food, books, transportation, and medical care. By the end of the month, Dorothea Sacher recalls, his watch and ring were usually in hock, not to be retrieved until payday. But again he spurned academic convention, refusing to hand in his doctoral thesis despite all appeals to do so, because he felt it wasn't good enough. Conservative in his politics, patriotic to the core, he seemed to take a perverse delight in going against convention. "It's *Mr.* Sacher, not Dr. Sacher," he would say with an unmistakable note of pride.

It was Sacher's particular genius to approach every problem in biology as though he were a diamond cutter, turning the raw material around and around, examining every possible facet before deciding where to cut in. In the late 1940s and early 1950s, when most of his colleagues in radiation toxicology were focusing on the acute, short-term, tumor-inducing effects of atomic radiation, he took the long view and asked, "What happened to the whole animal over its life span?" This perspective allowed him to look at data in a new way, and what he found changed the course of both radiation biology and gerontology.

He had been asked by the Atomic Energy Commission to review a project that had been aborted by the sudden death of the project director a few years after the war. Set up in conjunction with the National Cancer Institute (NCI) to determine the risks of low-level radiation to workers in the field, the program had been a large-scale, enormously expensive undertaking. Now the AEC wondered if the program was worth continuing.

The first problem, Sacher found, was that the laboratory data on animals went both ways. Looked at purely in terms of average survival time, the irradiated population clearly did worse. But if you did a statistical analysis, it turned out that there was so much variability in survival time that the differences between the irradiated animals and the controls were not statistically significant.

In puzzling this out, Sacher came across a striking mathematical observation that had been made in 1825 by an insurance actuary named Benjamin Gompertz. The rate at which people die off is not random, but fixed; in a given population the number of deaths doubles every seven years. Although well known in actuarial circles, the Gompertz curve had been largely ignored by biologists. Sacher, who was the first to apply this curve to animals, found that the same relationship between age and mortality held, except the doubling rate in mice was every one hundred days. When he replotted the laboratory data using the Gompertz analysis, the true relation between radiation and life span was revealed. Both the irradiated and the unirradiated mice followed the same curve, but the treated mice started with a higher death rate, and at any given age the rate remained higher; the bigger the dose, the more pronounced this effect. In other words, irradiation caused the mice to age faster and die younger.

"This discovery of the dose-related, life-shortening effect of radiation was the thing that got lots and lots of physicists interested in aging," says Harold Ducoff, who was among those influenced by this work. "For the first time, it gave you a tool to work with."

Sacher had hardly opened up the field of aging for a generation of scientists when he realized that he was headed in the wrong direction. "At that time I was working on life shortening in mice," he told me. "But the real problem, what we are actually being paid for, is to find out about life shortening in people. So I said the question is not why do we die, but why do we live as long as we do? What does a long-lived species do better than a short-lived species? Because if I don't know this about mice and men, how can I find any basis for understanding the lifetime effects on both mice and men?"

It seems such a simple thing on the face of it—to go from "Why do we die?" to "Why do we live so long?"—but it represented nothing less than a revolution in thinking. It was like becoming aware that the reason it was dark was because you were wearing a blindfold. "Scientists make boxes and then they can't get out of them," says Ron Hart. "It's like that puzzle where you have three rows of dots forming a box, and you have to connect them using four lines, without taking your pencil off the paper. The only way you can do it is by going outside the box. And that ability is what the game is all about."

The box that surrounded contemporary gerontology, in George Sacher's view, was the idea that we were born perfect and immortal and then something bad happened—bad hormones, or serums, or tissues, or genes. And like Pandora's, this box contained a multitude of ills. If anything was clear about growing old, it was that *everything changed with age.* Every function, every response, every reaction was slowly, silently being altered in some way until a breakdown was inevitable. Like an old car, the parts went in unpredictable fashion. Shore up one part, and a second was sure to go soon after. Looked at in this light, how was anyone to find an answer to aging? For every collapse of function, there could be a different underlying reason. Tens or even hundreds of thousands of genes might play a role in the slow rusting and sudden failures of aging. Unless some miracle root, or herb, or plant, or even some overall controlling substance in the body, existed, there appeared to be no way out of the aging box.

But there was one way out, Sacher thought. Since most animals in the wild were eaten by predators or felled by accidents long before senescence set in, there was no need for evolution to "invent" mechanisms designed for aging. On the other hand, there *was* a need for built-in longevity "factors" to ensure that animals lived long enough to reproduce themselves. Maybe this was what aging was all about, not the turning on of "aging" genes, but simply evolution equipping every organism from the simplest to the most complex with just enough of whatever proteins, hormones, or enzymes were required for that species to survive and reproduce in its ecological niche.

As he was to put it to me years later, "There is a fundamental, philosophical kind of conflict [in aging research], a dialectic, if you will. Most people believe that we could live indefinitely if it weren't for those aging genes that crept in. This is something that I think we have to reject. I'd say that on the contrary, we all have just about the mortality that our gene system, under natural selection, is able to assure for us." He saw this view as liberating rather than limiting. If he were right, then the number of factors involved in longevity, in contrast to those in aging, need not be large, but their influence would be far-reaching.

He began his search by asking what the "obvious constitutional characteristics" were that enabled human beings to live fifty times longer than a shrew and twice as long as their nearest relative, the chimp. Aristotle, an early gerontologist, noted that larger animals live longer than smaller ones. In 1908, Max Rubner, a German physiologist, offered a possible explanation for this phenomenon in the metabolic rate, which, he found, runs directly counter to body size. The smaller animal eats more food, runs around more, and burns up energy at a much faster rate than the slower-moving, slower-living, larger animal. The inverse correlation between metabolic rate and body size is so close for some species, ranging from cat to cow, that the total lifetime expenditure of energy per gram of body weight is approximately the same for each—about 200,000 calories. Indeed, by the end of their lifetimes, the machine-gun heart of the 3.5-year-old mouse and the cannon heart of the 70-year-old elephant will have beaten roughly the same number of times.

One reason for this correlation is purely physical. The smaller the animal, the larger its surface area is in proportion to its weight. This means a greater loss of heat from the body surface, and consequently a higher expenditure of calories per gram of body weight in order to maintain a constant body temperature. But there is intriguing evidence that metabolic rate may regulate not only body heat, but aging. More than sixty years ago, Raymond Pearl doubled and halved the life span of fruit flies solely by lowering or raising temperature in their environment. This became the basis for Pearl's "Rate of Living" theory, in which the life span of a species is fixed by the rate at which it expends energy. Or as one writer, Roland Fisher, poetically put it: "The length of our lives is inversely proportional to the height of our metabolic flames."

As is so often the case, the beauty of this idea was marred by the originator's own findings. Human beings not only fell wildly off the curve, they turned the whole notion upside down. Far from being slow metabolic burners, we humans are prodigious energy expenders, using up in our lifetime a whopping 800,000 calories per gram of body tissue. Nor was this the only discrepancy, for several other species of similar body weight and metabolism had markedly different life spans. To resolve this difficulty, a contemporary of Rubner, H. Friedenthal, added another factor to the hypothesis—big-brained animals live longer than the small-brained animals of comparable size. But his work fell into obscurity and no further research was done along these lines.

After poring over the available zoological literature, Sacher chose sixty-three species for which there were reliable data on brain weight and body weight. He found that a huge chunk, more than 80 percent of the variation in life span among species could be accounted for solely in the ratio of brain size to body size. In animals of a similar size, such as an opossum or a cetus monkey, the larger-brained monkey outlived the minibrained opossum forty years to five years. Without knowing it, he had stumbled upon Friedenthal's relationship.

For more than a century, physiologists had been impressed with what they called the "index of encephalization," which described a mathematical relationship between the brain and body. Since as one goes up the ladder of evolution, brain size increases in proportion to body size, there was an intuitive feeling that the index of encephalization predicted intelligence, says Sacher. This notion was almost rejected when anatomists made the humiliating discovery that dolphins and whales came a lot closer to man on the index than primates. But when the scientific community recovered from this insult and accepted the fact that a fish might be smarter than a chimp, the relationship was truer than ever. Now Sacher had shown that this well-established predictor of intelligence was just as good an indicator of longevity: Brainier animals lived longer.

"George was so impressed by this datum he essentially uncovered that he is noted in several places as the philosopher who claimed that the brain is the organ of longevity," says his colleague, Don Justesen. Sacher's first idea was that the brain was a kind of orchestral conductor for the body, cueing in each instrument, bringing it to the desired pitch and tempo, blending it with the overall sound. Any deviation or fluctuation from the norm undermines the general harmony, and if there are too many deviations, the result is a cacophonous breakdown, or, in terms of a living organism, death.

For the next two decades, he became a kind of twentieth-century Linnaeus. Like the great eighteenth-century Swedish botanist, who named and classified thousands of animals and plants in his *Systema Naturae*, Sacher traveled to zoos around the world, pored over museum records, trapped animals in the wild, and even turned his basement into a menagerie in his quest for the underlying structure of aging and longevity.

But soon after publishing his classic paper on "Relation of Lifespan to Brain Weight and Body Weight in Mammals" in 1959, he realized that if he were to make the case for longevity factors, he had to move beyond observation to experimentation. And for that he needed an animal model. After reviewing the field, he found, much to his surprise, that virtually all of his colleagues favored short-lived animals, mice or rats. This was understandable enough in view of the expenses involved in maintaining a colony, but why did they invariably choose a strain that was among the most rapidly aging of its own kind? Moving in the opposite direction, he was determined to find a rodent model for "success in living."

The ideal one turned out to be no farther than his own garage. Commonly known as the white-footed mouse, *Peromyscus leucopus* is an endearing-looking creature with large eyes and ears, a rounded body, and a white underbelly and feet that often seeks shelter during the winter months in suburban attics and garages. About the same size as the common house mouse *(Mus muscalis)*, granddaddy of all laboratory strains, the deer mouse lives a whopping two-and-a-half times longer than the house mouse, or more than eight years, compared to a maximum of three and a half.

Starting with specimens caught in traps set in the woodlots around Argonne, Sacher began his colony of *P. leucopus* with ten breeding pairs. At the same time, he began breeding randomly caught house mice, so that he could compare two wild-type populations. For more than two decades, despite an atmosphere at Argonne increasingly hostile to aging research and enormous cutbacks in his budgets, he maintained the colonies, cultivating and characterizing them, becoming one of the world's foremost authorities on these species.

It was pure chance that events begun by Sacher's collecting and breeding his deer-mouse colony in 1962 would intersect with those started by Hart's experiment on DNA repair so many years later. When Hart called in 1973 to ask about the life span of the various species he was looking at, Sacher was ready.

"Look, Ron," said Sacher, "people differ from rats in more than length of life. There are huge [species] differences. They diverged evolutionarily [from tree shrews] tens of millions of years ago. Let's take my two mice, *M. muscalis*, and *P. leucopus*, and see what the differences in DNA repair are between them."

For the fastidious Hart, Sacher's dwelling was a revelation. It was a combination museum, zoo, gallery, and workshop. The whole house—living room, dining room, kitchen, bedrooms, library, attic—was filled with the objects of his passion—living animals, skulls of animals found on nature walks, fossils of animals, prints of animals, books on animals. Lying everywhere were open folders on a particular subject or idea that would occupy him for the moment and then be forgotten while he moved on to something else. Downstairs in the only air-conditioned room in the house were flying squirrels, an agouti, tree shrews, hamsters, rabbits, and, of course, field mice.

"He was the ultimate egocentric person, doing science more for his own self-enlightenment than for anyone else," says Hart, who was both enchanted and astonished by what he found. "To George, his role in life was to understand how things worked. He would conceptualize an idea, using it as a framework, putting it together with hundreds of obscure facts in his mind, examining the whole concept mathematically, rigorously. He was the brightest man I've ever known in aging, a great scientist, a tremendous synthesizer, but he left it for other people to do the experimental work that would prove or disprove the concept."

The experiments worked out better than either man had dared or hoped. At Ohio State, Hart looked at DNA repair in the two mouse species, using two different methodologies. He and Sacher also did a Hayflick-type experiment and found that the cells of the short-lived house mouse went through ten divisions before dying out, while those of the deer mouse went through twenty doublings. Since human cells go through fifty to sixty divisions, there appeared to be a rough correlation between the life span of a species and the Hayflick limit—something later studies would confirm. Even more gratifying were the DNA repair experiments. Both techniques independently showed that the repair capacity for the deer mouse was 2.5 times greater than that of the house mouse—a ratio that almost exactly paralleled the difference between the life span of the two species. But the real excitement was yet to come, when the two men would be joined by a third.

In 1974, while Hart and Sacher were in the midst of their experiments, a symposium on DNA repair in Keystone, Colorado, attracted the big names in this field from all over the world. It was there that Hart met James Trosko, an expert in somatic mutation at Michigan State University. "Trosko?" asked Hart when they found themselves standing together on the ski slopes during a conference break. "Weren't you one of the first people to go into DNA repair?" Yes, he was, Trosko told him, and his link to repair was the same as Hart's—they had both done postdoctoral work with Richard Setlow at Oak Ridge. But while Hart was starting to put together a DNA repair laboratory at Ohio State that would become one of the largest in the country, Trosko, after a promising beginning, had been forced out of the very field that he had helped to pioneer.

His entry into DNA repair had come about quite abruptly in 1963 when, as a young postdoc, he stepped across the hall to listen to a noon seminar given by Setlow. He had been trying to understand how radiation caused chromosomes to break, but when Trosko heard Dick Setlow talk about his discovery of a DNA repair mechanism in bacteria, he decided on the spot to switch his area of study. Here was something that no one had ever dreamed about—that the cells of an organism actually contained genes and enzymes that repaired DNA.

"It's interesting to me as a student of science," he said years later, "that no one ever predicted this years earlier. We knew that genes existed from Mendel's work. We knew that genes could be damaged from H.J. Muller's studies with X-rays in the 20s; we knew that the gene was DNA from the experiment of Avery, McCarty, and MacLeod in the 40s, but even after we found out from Watson and Crick that the DNA was double-helixed, no one surmised what would happen to the DNA replication if the DNA was being damaged all the time. Nobody even gave it a thought. It strikes me that we must have believed that either somehow the DNA escaped being damaged, or if it did occur, it didn't make any difference."

As Trosko listened to Setlow describe how UV-sensitive bacteria that couldn't repair their DNA had a higher rate of mutations, he was struck almost visibly with the fact that what was true for microbes might also be true for man. Buttonholing Setlow after the talk, Trosko asked him, "Dick, have you looked at DNA repair in human cells?"

"No," he said, "we don't work with human cells."

"What do you think would happen if human beings couldn't repair UV damage to their DNA? Would they have more mutations?"

"I don't know," said Setlow. "But I would predict that humans are no different than bacteria."

"Do you think it would be worthwhile if I checked the literature to see if there are people who are UV-sensitive?"

"Maybe, but don't waste your time on it."

Setlow wasn't really too excited about the suggestion, Trosko recalls. "Dick was a biophysicist, working with naked DNA and bacteria. He couldn't care less about higher organisms' problems. But I was fascinated."

Trosko's hunch proved to be right. Looking through dermatology textbooks, he found that there were human syndromes in which the primary symptom was an extreme sensitivity to the ultraviolet rays of the sun. Could it be that these people lacked the ability to repair the DNA damage caused by sunlight? He realized he was getting ahead of himself. First he had to show that DNA repair occurred in man. Since no one in his laboratory at Oak Ridge was culturing human cells, he settled for Chinese hamster cells that were available. At least that was a mammalian cell, and if repair could be shown there, it would establish that the phenomenon was not just a curious, if interesting, property of bacteria.

Trosko knocked himself out for the better part of a year, bombarding the hamster cells with UV light, extracting the DNA, separating big pieces of DNA from little pieces of DNA, but he came up empty-handed. Even though he found that Chinese hamster cells formed thymine dimers in response to UV radiation, just as the bacterial cells did, they did not appear to remove the dimers. Trosko brought the negative results to Setlow, who just shrugged and said, "Well, I told you it wasn't interesting. It's not relevant to anything. It's only a bacterial story, and I wouldn't get too excited about it."

His blasé reaction took Trosko aback. "I think he was kind of disappointed," he says. "Because if I had shown that human cells repaired like bacteria, then Dick would have felt that his finding was of universal importance." Setlow vetoed publishing the results since they were negative. So Trosko tucked the data into his desk and began working on something else.

A self-styled "stubborn Hungarian" who clings tenaciously to his theories, he refused to give up on his idea. Science is a matter of asking the right questions, but often it is the simple and obvious ones that prove most elusive. Whatever the reason, it took Trosko a full year before he thought of

something that should have hit him at the outset: "My God, if Chinese
hamsters are not repairing damage to their DNA, how in the world do they
cope with the damage? How does their DNA continue to replicate? How
can they be different from bacteria?"

By this time, a newcomer to Oak Ridge, Jim Regan, had become expert
at growing human cells. At Setlow's suggestion, Trosko began working
with Regan to find out if human cells repair DNA damage. Earlier work by
William Carrier and his coworkers at Oak Ridge had shown excision repair
in cancerous human cells. But since cancer cells were abnormal by definition, the question of whether mammalian cells repaired their DNA was still
up for grabs. This time Trosko's efforts did not go unrewarded. He and his
colleagues showed that normal human cells, like those of bacteria, use excision repair to get rid of UV-induced thymine dimers.

While these experiments were going on, Jim Cleaver, an Oxford-trained
physicist who had gotten a job in the United States, came to Oak Ridge to
give a seminar on his research on UV light and DNA synthesis in mammalian cells. During a discussion with Cleaver in which both men shared ideas
about their work, Trosko mentioned the notion that had excited him when
he first heard about DNA repair—that there were human beings, like bacteria, who were UV-sensitive because they were deficient in DNA repair.

Soon after that visit, Trosko left Oak Ridge to take a research-and-
teaching job at Michigan State University in East Lansing. A handsome
man with piercing blue eyes who does everything with style and wit, he
hung a sign on his laboratory door:

DNA REPAIR SHOP
YOU NIX IT, WE FIX IT.
EXPERIENCED REPAIR MAN ON DUTY 24 HOURS A DAY.

And like anyone else in his business, he began applying for grants. Back at
Oak Ridge, Jim Regan finished up the experiments that he and Trosko had
started, and their joint paper on the work came out.

Like actors and writers, scientists are very concerned with star billing,
called "first authorship" in their trade. If the paper involves two costars
who have made their reputations in different fields, they may as well just
flip for first. The same is true if the work of two is so intertwined that one
comes to think of the collaborators' names as a single unit, like Comden
and Green, or Watson and Crick. On the other hand, if there are more
than three names on the paper, usually only the first name gets cited and

the rest become a kind of chorus line known collectively as "et al." With three names, the picture is more obscure. The first and third names are the most important with the middle name generally considered to have made the least contribution. Collaborations have been known to break up over problems of billing, and one investigator is reputed to negotiate the issue of first authorship with his potential collaborators before the first experiment is even carried out. Yet it is not just ego demands or assuring one's place in the pecking order that fuel such behavior, but also economics, since how much you publish, in what journals, and whether your name heads the list of authors, usually correlate with the rate of advancement in an academic career.

Trosko, who prides himself on a value system that puts ethical and humanitarian considerations above the quest for power and glory—a position that he believes has cost him dearly in his career—says of his years at Oak Ridge, "I started those experiments, but I left just before we finished. Because it took me a year to get set up here, Regan finished the work at Oak Ridge, and as a result, Dick Setlow thought he should be given senior authorship, and I had no problem with that. So it's 'Regan, Trosko, and Carrier' in that memorable paper showing for the first time that normal human cells could repair damage."

While at Michigan State, Trosko attempted to pursue the story of DNA repair in UV-sensitive people. But although he had identified several possible syndromes in which people might lack the ability to repair UV damage, he lacked the access to a large metropolitan medical center that could supply cells from patients with these very rare diseases. He abandoned the idea and began working on other projects.

One day in 1967 he received a call from Jim Cleaver, the British physicist whom he had met at Oak Ridge, who was now working at the University of California in San Francisco. After trying unsuccessfully for more than a year to create animal mutants that would lack DNA repair, Cleaver had seen an article on xeroderma pigmentosum (XP), a hereditary syndrome, in the *San Francisco Chronicle* in May 1966. People with XP are so sensitive to ultraviolet light that even slight exposure to sunlight causes skin tumors. Like Job covered with boils, the patient becomes riddled with cancers that usually metastasize, resulting in death at an early age. Recognizing that this syndrome had all the characteristics he was looking for in a repair-deficient animal model, Cleaver obtained some cells from an XP patient and within a year knew he had the right disease.

Cleaver had done the experiment Trosko had hoped to carry out. Now

Cleaver was asking him to collaborate on a follow-up study in which Trosko would measure the amount of excision repair both in normal human cells and in those of the XP patient, something Cleaver had done only indirectly. Trosko agreed to do the work and two papers were published on the relationship between xeroderma pigmentosum and a deficiency in DNA repair, the first by Cleaver, alone, in *Nature* and the second, by both men, in *Photochemistry and Photobiology*.

The two papers were a significant advance in both cancer research and DNA repair. In 1968, when they appeared, the theory that cancer was caused by viruses was riding high, backed by massive funds from the National Cancer Institute, and almost any other hypothesis received low priority. Now, for the first time, it was clear that genetic and environmental factors—sunlight and DNA-repair deficiency—could play a role in the development of cancer. The reports also underscored the importance of DNA repair in human health. Not only did humans repair their DNA, the studies said, but if they didn't they were in trouble.

The careers of the two men went in opposite directions. Cleaver had done a breakthrough experiment, published in the journal *Nature*, which is practically required reading for research scientists, and, because of it, became a major figure in molecular biology and cancer research. Trosko's contribution to the XP story, which appeared in a highly specialized journal with a small readership, was all but ignored. Added to his problems was the fact that he was caught in a kind of time lag when it came to getting grants.

His former employer, the Atomic Energy Commission, which had supported much of the original work on DNA repair, had moved on to other concerns, while his would-be supporter, the National Cancer Institute, caught up in the hunt for tumor viruses, had yet to see the relevance of DNA repair. The upshot was that from 1966, when he left Oak Ridge for Michigan State University, until 1971, he could not get the money he needed to do DNA repair studies in cancer. Even after switching to the area of mutagenesis, where the funding prospects looked brighter, he continued to look for a way back to his first love. That hope brought him to the Keystone, Colorado, symposium in 1974, where he met Ron Hart.

The mutual attraction between Hart and Trosko had the same roots as that between Hart and Sacher. "We realized," says Trosko, "that we shared the same philosophical holistic view of life. We tried to put things into bigger pictures. Ron found that extremely refreshing because most scientists are so narrow. That's what we saw in each other."

By the end of the conference, Trosko agreed to spend a semester the following spring working with Hart at Ohio State. Trosko still associates that time with the smell of pizza and other takeout foods they often consumed as they worked late into the night. Over the course of their many conversations, their ideas on aging, cancer, mutagenesis, and repair cross-fertilized, breeding vigorous hybrids.

Sacher came to visit once, bringing his two mouse species and the story of the work he and Hart had done. Sacher and Trosko quickly became friends and soon all three were comparing their ideas. Sacher provided his whole-animal perspective and his view of built-in processes that modulated the life span of each species. Hart contributed his thinking on DNA damage and repair, and their relation to carcinogenesis and aging. And Trosko provided a philosophic structure for thinking about aging as well as a concept that he had developed with his collaborator, Ernie Chu.

In 1972, at the age of thirty-five, Trosko had taken a year off to go to the University of Wisconsin, where he spent half his time doing cancer research and the other half helping to revise a book called *Bioethics—Bridge to the Future.* The author of that book, who served as a kind of mentor to Trosko, was Van Rensselaer Potter, a leading cancer researcher as well as a philosopher of science.

"Each one of us," says Trosko, "has a role model in life whose behavior, achievements, and values we try to emulate. For me that was Potter. He was so gracious, noble, humble, sincere, brilliant, and energetic that I thought such a person could not exist. Here was a man who literally turned me around and opened my eyes to new arenas."

Potter had helped to pioneer a way of perceiving biological phenomena as part of a "hierarchical-cybernetic" framework. In this point of view, living organisms are viewed as a hierarchy of organizational levels, from the atom to the whole animal. With humans, the hierarchy goes beyond the individual to the interaction between people and with the environment. Simply stated, the hierarchical principle says that the whole is always greater than the sum of its parts. The cell is more than a collection of molecules, the tissue more than a collection of cells, and so on. The reason for this is that when two subunits of a hierarchy are combined in a specific, organized way, properties emerge that could not be predicted from the two original components. For instance, when the gases oxygen and hydrogen are combined in a particular manner, a third substance arises that is totally different in almost every way—water.

Hierarchical levels interact with one another by means of the cybernetic principle. Coined by the creator of computer science, Norbert Wiener, cybernetics is Greek for pilot or helmsman. It refers to the way in which self-regulatory systems, whether electronic, mechanical, or biological, control the flow of information through feedback signals. When two people talk to each other, they create a feedback loop that keeps going as long as information is transmitted. As soon as one person stops talking or listening, the loop is broken. Feedback loops are what make the world go 'round. They exist within each level of hierarchical organization, such as between two cells, and between the levels, for example, between the cells and tissue.

"The minute that the information flow is blocked," says Trosko, "the hierarchy collapses. If your body stops making hormones, your organs fall apart. If suddenly people stopped talking to you, your identity and personality structure would break down. All living things are the result of a hierarchical principle of life. And that hierarchy can exist only because of the cybernetic flow of information, both positive and negative, between the various hierarchical levels.

Trosko, who sees aging and cancer as expressions of the breakdown in the hierarchical-cybernetic order of the body, believes that hard data extracted in the laboratory must be incorporated into this overall philosophic view like jigsaw pieces into a puzzle. This is what he tried to do that spring in 1975, when he worked with Hart.

At that time, he and Ernie Chu, who was at the University of Michigan, had identified three classes of genes, a triad of security systems for the DNA, which acted as fail-safe mechanisms, each class coming into play after the failure of the previous one. The first line of defense is protection. There are genes that shield the DNA against damage by environmental agents, such as the one for melanin—a protective barrier against ultraviolet light.

Since even the most well-constructed barriers can be breached, the second class of genes includes those involved in DNA repair. Successful repair of damage from ultraviolet light, X-ray, chemicals, heat, or other toxic substances means that the information stored in the DNA remains intact and no mutation takes place.

If the DNA is incorrectly repaired, or if the cell divides before it is repaired, the third defense team—the antipromotion genes—provides a final backup. These genes try to keep the mutated cell from growing into a tumor, possibly through the immune surveillance system—the body's search-and-destroy force—or through hormonal control, or through some other as yet undescribed regulatory mechanism. If this system fails, the single genetic error can be reproduced many times over with malignant results.

Most of the experiments Trosko and Hart started never got finished—it took seven weeks just to get the lab set up to do tissue culture—but they did finish two review articles, which incorporated the idea of a series of hierarchical/cybernetic control systems that might regulate the rate at which damage is accumulated, and thus the rate of cancer and aging.

Soon after Trosko left Ohio State at the end of the semester, Hart visited Sacher and they walked through the dense Argonne woods. Some of their best thinking had been done on these long strolls where they would often pause to scratch the structure of a chemical or a mathematical formula in the soft earth with a stick. Over the years they had become collaborators in the best sense of the word, their minds completely attuned to each other's thoughts, their speech a kind of shorthand of half-finished sentences.

Why should repair relate to life span? they asked themselves now. Why should there be other relationships, like the brain weight-body weight ratio and metabolic rate, that held between mammalian species? What was nature trying to tell about how life span was built into the system? Hart had been talking about Trosko's three-classes-of-genes idea and Sacher suddenly connected this to an idea he had formulated about two years earlier.

Although aging was obviously a tremendously complex phenomenon, Sacher believed that only a small number of genes might actually regulate life span. This he deduced from the fact that evolution became vastly accelerated at the start of the Pleistocene epoch. Brain, limbs, stance, and other anatomical features of man's early ancestors changed so rapidly at that point that if the entire history of life from a single cell to man were run as a movie, the last two million years would look like the frenetic antics of the Keystone Kops. During this time, as early man progressed from a stooped-over apelike creature to his present form, brain size tripled and longevity doubled. This unprecedented advance in evolution required a number of gene changes. The question was, How many? Too many changes in too short a time would mean a mutation overload in the genes that is incompatible with life. Using the best information available at that time, which placed the upper limit at one gene substitution for each one hundred generations, Sacher calculated that since the entire molding of man from his early ancestors is believed to have occurred in about one hundred thousand generations, this would mean that one thousand genes accomplished everything from walking upright to expanding the brain. Assuming that nine hundred of these mutations were needed to carry out all the anatomical changes, he argued, that would leave very few, perhaps a hundred genes in all, for the doubling of life span.

"Okay," said Hart now. "What might these life span genes do?" Like Trosko's three classes of genes, they might be involved in the protection and repair of DNA. What was the evidence for this?—Schwartz's work connecting life span and the enzymes that converted chemical carcinogens to their harmful form, his own work with Setlow on life span and UV repair, and now his last study with Sacher on the house mouse and the field mouse. These genes, and no doubt there were many others that were yet to be discovered, all had something in common—they helped to ensure that the information in the DNA, which coded for every one of the body's functions, remained intact and inviolate.

Sitting at their favorite picnic spot, where they could watch the white deer whose antlers were almost as tall as their bodies, they decided that the mechanisms coded for by these genes needed a name. After some deliberation, they came up with "longevity-assurance mechanisms." What it said was that there are built-in processes intended to keep us going for as long as possible, a literal design for living. The concept represented a total reversal of gerontological thought, shifting the emphasis from senescence to longevity, from aging genes to repair and protection genes. It was, in fact, the answer to Sacher's original question: What do longer-lived species do better than shorter-lived ones? They simply have a greater expression of these genetic mechanisms. (Even as they were formulating this idea, a priority fight was shaping up. The same key concept with almost the identical name, "longevity-determinant genes," would be put forth by Richard Cutler of the Gerontological Research Center in Baltimore at about the same time.)

Hart and Sacher formally announced their revolutionary conceptualization of aging, longevity, and death in a joint paper in 1978. In it they also introduced what they called the "two paradigms of aging," or two ways of approaching research in gerontology. The "ontogenic paradigm," which is used by the vast majority of researchers in the field, measures the changes in aging that occur in the cells and tissues over an individual's lifetime. Although it illuminates the differences between young and old cells, it fails to get at the root cause of age changes, they said.

For that, one must use the "evolutionary-comparative paradigm." This approach addresses the differences in aging rates between species as widely separated as mouse is from man, or as closely related as the house mouse and the field mouse. "Most specifically," they wrote, "the hypothesis is that the eventual fate of the organism, in terms of its rate of aging, disease susceptibilities and life span, is primarily determined by specific genetically determined constitutive [built-in] properties, both molecular and organizational, which can be measured in its youth prior to the onset of aging. The explanation for the longer life of one organism (species) compared to another is therefore sought by asking what it is that the longer-lived organism does better, by way of protection, stabilization, and repair of its essential molecules."

Since Weismann's time, they pointed out, gerontologists have been concerned with the "evolution of senescence," arguing over whether or not aging serves as an adaptive function. What gerontologists have not looked at is the evolution of longevity.

"When attention is focused on longevity," they wrote, "as assured by positive, genetically controlled mechanisms, rather than on aging as a process that the organism passively endures, this long controversy about how aging evolved is seen to be essentially meaningless. Aging did not evolve: What did evolve were the longevity-assurance systems that confer on each organism in the population the length of life and vigor requisite for its development and reproduction."

In 1976, after delivering a paper in Louisville, Kentucky, Sacher walked into the next room and sat down next to a friend, saying nothing. He seemed so distracted that the friend thought the speech had had a poor reception. Approaching George tentatively, he asked, "Well, how did it go?"

"Perfectly fine," said Sacher, his head still bent.

"Then what's the problem?"

"I just got a phone call."

"What's the matter? Did someone die?"

Finally, Sacher looked at his friend, an expression of sheer amazement covering his face. "They just called to tell me that I got the [Robert W.] Kleemeier Award."

"He was a very modest person about his work," says Dorothea Sacher, "and I think that he had been knocked down so often by his critics that he just couldn't believe that it could happen."

In a supreme irony, Sacher received one of the most prestigious awards given by the Gerontological Society, just after the national laboratory had decided it was no longer in its interest to do aging research. For the next five years it was an uphill battle for Sacher to keep his colony of field mice going. Undaunted, he continued to do some of the finest work in his career, for aging studies, paying mostly out of his own pocket and going through all his savings. He gave thirty-seven years of his life to Argonne, and in the end he felt that Argonne had let him down.

"The problem was that the mission of the Argonne National Laboratory changed," says Hart. "In the beginning, George's work was acceptable since it was on radiation and the effects of radiation, whether it related to mutation, cancer, heart disease, immunology, or aging. But later, the orientation shifted toward energy-related problems. But George's work didn't change. So he was caught between the devil and the deep blue sea."

The situation eased somewhat with the appointment of a new director: Sacher was able to continue seeking answers to aging questions, while carrying out research for Argonne on microwave energy and the effect of environmental agents on the body's functioning. In 1978, he reached a high point in his career with his election to the presidency of the Gerontological Society.

But a year later, everything came crashing down. On December 21, 1979, after learning that his budget had been cut from $100,000 to $50,000, he wrote his first memo to Douglas Grahn, director of the division of biological and medical research, indicating his wish to take an early retirement. The budget, he wrote, "is inadequate for any meaningful research program . . . and can only be regarded as an insult and an expression of disinterest in what I am doing and in my continuation on the DOE payroll." He then asked for specific things to be done, noting that he could rescind his retirement decision any time prior to March 31.

On December 27, Grahn responded by saying that he had accepted Sacher's request for early retirement with reluctance, especially since George had brought him to Argonne in the first place. He promised to try to restore the funding and ended by saying, "Let us hope this is a transient situation, because the Biological and Medical Research Division needs your help, as does the nation's programmatic work in chronic radiation toxicology."

In January 1980, Sacher formally submitted his resignation, effective March 31, to Walter Massey, director of Argonne. His association with Argonne had begun in September 1942 and he had come to the decision regretfully. But, he said, he had deep resentment for the "capricious and incompetent administration actions that made my situation intolerable."

Two weeks after his effective retirement date, the money came through with the express stipulation that Sacher head the program. Upon hearing the news, he burst out laughing. For the first time in his career he could call the shots. Argonne had no choice but to hire him back as consultant, and his price was going to be high. Although administrative rules forbade rehiring employees for one year after they had left, Argonne could provide office space, a secretary, phone, and incidental money. Sacher would spend two or three days working for free at Argonne, but he had just been appointed professor of human development and evolutionary biology at the University of Chicago and would get a percentage from the grants there as well. And in April 1981 he would be on Argonne's payroll again. "George figured he was in clover," says Dorothea Sacher. "After spending all that money on gerontology on his own, it was all going to pay off."

The following winter, after returning from a business trip on an icy day, he fell at the Chicago airport and broke his leg. His injury did not deter him from speaking at a symposium on theories of aging at the annual meeting of the American Association for the Advancement of Science, in Toronto on January 4, 1981. In great pain, and hobbled by crutches, Sacher gave a speech that was, prophetically, the summation of his life's work.

He began with a theme, integrating science, philosophy, and history, that he began playing with a year earlier—that scientists are very much creatures of their own time. Now it had matured into a statement that had the ringing certainty of the first four notes of Beethoven's Fifth.

Since August Weismann, he noted, there has been a century-long quest "to develop a satisfactory evolutionary theory of aging," but the effort has been frustrated by "the paradoxical and internally contradictory terms in which the problem is customarily formulated. The paradox lies in the attempt to reconcile the deteriorative, disruptive processes of aging, senescent disease, and death with the evolutionary concepts of adaptation and selection for increased fitness."

He proposed to offer a history of biological theory on aging, in which he would show how the very ways in which scientists have thought about these matters "arise from unverbalized preconceptions that have ancient roots in our cultural and religious traditions." In the twentieth century, Weismann's idea that aging had an adaptive role for the species was attacked most prominently by Peter Medawar, who shared the Nobel Prize for immunology with F. Macfarlane Burnet. The problem with this theory, Medawar pointed out, is that it "canters twice round the perimeter of a vicious circle. By assuming that the elders of his race are decrepit and worn out, he [Weismann] assumes all but a fraction of what he has set himself to prove. Nor can these dotard animals 'take the place of those which are sound' if natural selection is working, as he [Weismann] tells us, in just the opposite sense."

Medawar's own solution was to view evolution as an effort to postpone the age at which unfavorable traits were expressed. When an animal was past reproductive age, it had no more opportunities to pass on its genes and thus allow natural selection to take place. In other words, the postreproduc-

tive period of life became a "dustbin for the effects of deleterious genes."
Several years later, George C. Williams of Michigan State University added
a new wrinkle to this theory—the idea of pleiotropy (having more than
one effect). Genes that are helpful while the individual is maturing become
harmful later in life. So, for example, a gene that promotes calcification of
bones in youth might contribute to hardening of the arteries in middle age.
Aging in this view is a nasty by-product of genes designed for fitness.

The only difference between Weismann's theory and what Sacher
termed the "neo-Weismannian reformulations" of Peter Medawar and
George Williams was that for Weismann, senescence developed because it
was selectively adaptive, while for Medawar and Williams, it was selectively "neutral."

"The rejection by Medawar and Williams of an adaptive advantage for
senescence was not a scientific statement so much as it was an expression of
the repugnance that mid-twentieth-century man—imbued with the attitudes of liberal individualism—feels toward a conception that finds its justi-
fication in the nineteenth-century value system that stresses the duty of the
individual to serve an established social order," said Sacher. "It is interesting to note that there is no objective difference between the outcomes of
the nineteenth- and twentieth-century theories. A subjective difference is
that in the former theory the individual ages and dies for some reason,
while in the latter theory it is for no reason."

But Sacher believed that there were reasons for biologists' "strong at-
tachment to the hypothesis of senescent genes" that were far more profound than the prevailing zeitgeist. "I ask you to consider," he told his
colleagues, "the possibility that deep within all of us is the will to believe
that we are, in our essential natures, immortal, and that our mortality is due
to adventitious factors that can some day be removed. The story of the creation in the Book of Genesis beautifully embodies that belief and explains
our mortality, after the expulsion from the garden, as being due to the error
of original sin. Does this religious belief differ in any essential way from the
theory, enunciated by tough-minded biologists who surely consider themselves to be uninfluenced by revealed religion, that our biological natures
were originally immortal and only later became corrupted by the accumulation of senescence genes?"

Instead of negativistic aging-gene theories, what was needed, he said, was
"positive theory . . . based on the postulate that length of life is the basic
biological variable on which evolution operates." Referring to his own research on the correlation between longevity and certain anatomical and

physiological factors, he asked, "Why should there be a close correspondence between increased brain weight and life span?" One reason, he argued, is that over the course of evolution, as a species becomes brainier, the length of time that it takes its progeny to reach sexual maturity increases. At the same time, the number of offspring decreases. This shrinkage in reproductive rate "can only be paid back," by stretching out the reproductive span and, along with it, the life span.

He had a proposition for the audience. Sacher urged that the scientific establishment place their money, literally and figuratively, on the perspective given by his hypothesis. By betting on the senescent-gene theories, he said, one gains nothing. The problems involved in finding these unknown genes would be intimidating for the most dedicated scientist. But by betting on the longevity-assurance theory, one could gain everything. While the longevity-assurance theory denies the assumption of "essential immortality," and accepts that a maximum life span of about one hundred years is built into the human species, it "more than makes up for the loss of a delusive immortality by providing a basis for a feasible strategy to prolong human life by evolutionary natural means." This would mean first identifying the protective and repair mechanisms and then finding ways, such as genetic engineering, of turning up their volume in the somatic cells. The result might be an end to cancer, as well as providing the "key to the understanding and control of aging."

And then he ended with what, in retrospect, can only be considered a valedictory: "The biomedical research establishment in the United States is not yet ready for such a radical research strategy. The National Institute on Aging, which was set up within the National Institutes of Health, to break out of the commitment of the categorical institutes toward disease-oriented research, has instead been pulled into the disease-oriented modes of thought that prevail in Bethesda [Maryland]. Work on the diseases of age is important, but the National Institute on Aging was supposed to look beyond immediate social needs toward basic solutions. Although our hopes for innovative thought by the current research managers are fading, we can have confidence in the clearer vision of the rising generation of researchers. It is possible that someone within the sound of my voice today will open the path to our eventual understanding and control of genetic error and, therefore, of aging and age-related disease. I wish him or her Godspeed."

Sacher died three weeks later on January 24, when a blood clot from his fractured leg lodged in his pulmonary artery. Many thousands of words were written in memoriam, but none more moving than a letter sent by his wife to his many friends and colleagues: ". . . I have been trying to decide just what George would have said to you as a good-bye. I am sure it would include urging you to persevere with utmost enthusiasm in your own field, to give credit to everyone assisting in your investigations, thus encouraging younger scientists, to inspire students toward independent thought, to encourage them, too, to find a thinking place."

We were driving past Argonne one day, when Dorothea pointed toward the deep green woods and said in her quiet, humorous, laconic way, "George is there." I looked at her, puzzled. "I had George cremated and was wondering what to do with the ashes. Then I remembered the spot where he and Ron used to take their lunch into the woods and watch the white deer. And I knew that was the place. One of my Christian friends was shocked. 'How could you not give George a Christian burial?' she asked me. I said to her, 'But George was a free spirit.' "

Chapter Four

Biochemistry Rather Than Brains

It was an auspicious debut. The title of the 102-page paper, which represented three years of experiments and thought—"Reiterated DNA Sequence Classes throughout the Life-Span of the Mouse"—gave no indication of the radical ideas contained within its final third. With an audacity rarely seen in one's first contribution to a field, Richard Cutler not only offered a "working hypothesis of senescence" but on the basis of limited data, went on to make a series of predictions about aging and longevity that he expected to be borne out in future experiments.

The reaction to Cutler's 1972 paper was a big disappointment to him. Most scientists ignored it, and the few people who took the time to read it ridiculed it: "DNA repair a modulator of aging?; DNA 'protective processes' a determinant of longevity?" There was not a shred of evidence that DNA repair or any mysterious free-radical scavenging enzyme had anything to do with aging.

But one person did pay attention, George Sacher. "He was the only one who had read my paper and understood it," says Cutler. "And he was my key supporter." Beginning in friendship and collaboration spiced by an amiable competition, their relationship dissolved just a few years later with bitter recriminations and charges of plagiarism on both sides.

Cutler seems to me at times to have a split personality. At conferences, standing at the edge of a small group of his colleagues, listening rather than joining in, he appears aloof, guarded, coolly reserved. Other times, in more congenial settings, he is relaxed, ebullient, witty, and charming.

Now in his late forties, he feels himself at the crossroads of his life. For ten years he feels he has struggled under a cloud of contempt, ridicule, and ostracism from his peers. No stranger to struggle, on which he appears to thrive, he has known it all his life. Cutler grew up in a small religious community in rural Colorado, where his dream of a career in engineering or science seemed just that. Between them, his father and mother serviced the only high school in town—his father as the sole teacher for its fifty pupils and his mother as the school-bus driver. Even transferring to the 150-pupil high school in the neighboring town—where he was given a choice between typing and chemistry, the one science course offered, was of doubtful help. Finally, his father moved the family to Anaheim, California, in Cutler's senior year.

It was a move not just from one state to another, but from a tradition-bound world into a realm of unlimited possibilities. Cutler registered for a full range of courses and, most important of all, discovered the high-school machine shop, where he would launch his career in science. And like most everything he did, it would verge on the outrageous.

Not for Cutler the bookcase shelves or model boats. He designed and built a helicopter with jet engines in the tips of the blades. Meanwhile, his father, indifferent to his ambitions, had arranged for the high school to waive half the requirements so that his son could help him pump gas at the service station he ran. Still, Cutler managed to find time to work on his beloved helicopter, and when it was finished, he brought it to his backyard for its test flight.

The home-made whirlybird set up such a racket that neighbors called the police. A hometown newspaper ran a story on the incident, and a reporter in the neighboring town of Santa Ana picked it up, turning it into a feature story for the Sunday edition, pictures and all. Overnight, Cutler became a local hero, a junior version of Orville Wright.

The Santa Ana reporter, who had befriended him, advised him to start thinking about doing something with his life. With his help, Cutler got into Northrop Aeronautical Institute and from there went to Electronic Engineering Institute, both in Inglewood, California. Since he received little financial help from his family, he had to work during the day and attend classes at night. Nevertheless, he did so well that he was made an instructor after his first year, teaching himself algebra and trigonometry, even as he taught others these subjects. And then his life took another unexpected turn.

Recognizing the boy genius chronicled in the newspaper articles, and seeing in his helicopter design the wave of the future, the accountant at the electronic school approached four millionaires with the idea of setting up a helicopter company. In 1954, at the age of nineteen, Cutler found himself the director and chief design engineer of the Cutler Helicopter Corporation in Pasadena. He headed a staff of five, with a budget of several hundred thousand dollars, and collected a salary that included 20 percent of the action.

The vision behind the corporation was to build the "model-T" helicopter, a compact chopper for everyone's backyard. It would combine Cutler's wing-tip ramjets with a conventional engine to allow vertical takeoff flight and yet be very efficient in forward flight. But neither the corporation nor the helicopter ever really got off the ground.

When he wasn't at school trying to stuff his brain with engineering, flight technology, and math, Cutler was developing ramjets on the cutting edge of technology. The results were sometimes calamitous. One of the test stands was located at Van Nuys Airport. To the horror of everyone concerned, the test stand blew up, and its parts sliced through the airplanes like butcher knives through slabs of meat. The company was stuck with thousands of dollars of damage, and Cutler was lucky to escape with his life.

To add to the company's difficulties, one of the partners went bankrupt. Money began to run low, the investors were loath to sell any of their stock and lose their interest in the corporation, and certification from the CAA was still lacking. Arguments broke out among the members of the corporation. The coup de grace came when Howard Hughes developed a gas turbine helicopter engine and Cutler's ramjets were obsolete.

At the age of twenty-six, with degrees in both electronic engineering and physics, and having headed his own corporation, Cutler was out of a job. At the same time, he was going through a "philosophical crisis." The church no longer held the answer for him. He became an agnostic studying metaphysics, going to philosophical societies, listening to lectures on humanism. After extensive contemplation, he decided that the primary purpose of religion was to shield human beings from the terrifying awareness of their own mortality.

"I became impressed with how much misery and suffering are caused by the aging process and the knowledge that life is not infinite," he says. "I guess I was particularly aware at the time because I was very close to my grandmother and grandfather and could see the problems of growing old."

He vowed to go after the one thing that stood in the way of man's happiness—the lack of time to do all the things one wanted. "On just humanistic grounds, it seemed to me that understanding the biological basis of aging and longevity, and to prolong life if possible, were automatically good things."

Cutler had a plan of attack. Although he felt he would never be a top-notch physicist, he could borrow a trick from the greatest masters and look for the simple rules that governed complex phenomena. The movement of the planets, the trajectory of objects in motion, the relationship between matter and energy—all the phenomena that had stumped learned minds for centuries—turned out to be explicable by formulas that could be taught to high-school students. In biology, there were examples of this in Mendel's laws of genetics or the discovery that four substances in the DNA directed the formation of every living organism. "So I got to wondering," he says: "Was it the same story with aging? Aging looks so complex, it puts everybody off. But what if there were simple processes underlying it?"

Since there were no departments at that time in biogerontology, he decided to get his doctorate in the brand-new field of biophysics at the University of Houston. Applying his engineering talents to manipulating living organisms, Cutler turned out batches of *E. coli* bacteria that all divided at the same time as though they were on an assembly line. He had accomplished the first synchronization of large batches of bacteria, an important research tool.

Working with the synchronized cultures, he was able to isolate segments of the DNA of *E. coli*, map the position on the chromosome of certain genes that transcribed DNA to RNA, determine the direction the DNA took in replicating itself, and chart which genes turn on during the various stages of division. He even began exploring the idea of using the same technique to isolate genes from other organisms and transplant them into *E. coli* to make new substances—in effect, the beginning of genetic engineering.

He sent the two papers on his work to the *Journal of Molecular Biology*. Ole Maaloe, an eminent bacterial geneticist who edited the papers, found Cutler's results so incredible that he flew to Houston to satisfy himself that this young graduate student could actually do all the things he claimed. The papers were published and subsequently selected for inclusion in a volume entitled *Benchmark Papers in Microbiology*.

Having achieved a measure of prominence in the field of molecular biology, with postdoctoral offers pouring in from places like Rice and Stanford, Cutler proceeded to turn his back on it all. Crazy as it seemed to his friends who tried to argue him out of it, he was still hell-bent on the idea of going into gerontology. When Howard Curtis offered him a position in his lab at the Brookhaven National Laboratory, Cutler felt as though he had just gotten his big break.

In 1966, when Cutler went to Brookhaven, Curtis was a major figure in aging research, a pioneer in somatic mutation theory who helped provide laboratory evidence that the gradual accumulation of errors in the DNA caused the breakdown of functions in the body's cells and organs over time. In one of his most important experiments, he found that the rate of spontaneous mutation was inversely proportionate to life span in mice. Long-lived mice developed mutations much more slowly than short-lived mice, while mice with intermediate life spans had a mutation rate in between the other two. He was also one of the first gerontologists to do a species comparison—in this case, between guinea pigs and dogs—in which he uncovered the same relationship between length of life and the rate of spontaneous mutations that he had found in the mice. Curtis was Cutler's kind of scientist, a fellow seeker after basic laws, whose article on the "Biological Mechanisms Underlying the Aging Process" first stimulated his own thinking on the subject.

Cutler credits Curtis with turning him loose in the laboratory, giving him a couple of technicians and a postdoc worker, even though Cutler himself was still one, and allowing him to pursue his ideas to his heart's content. But he still felt somewhat disappointed. He had had fantasies of being taken under Curtis's wing, of sharing their views on aging, being offered guidance, perhaps collaborating. But instead, Curtis told him he had done his research completely on his own, and that was how Cutler was to do it.

Cutler's first idea was to use techniques he developed at the University of Houston for synchronizing *E. coli* to look at life span in the mouse. In doing so, he would ask some very fundamental questions.

The "central dogma," as Crick irreverently put it, of molecular biology states that the transfer of information contained in the genes is a one-way street—DNA to RNA to protein. Once information has passed into protein, like toothpaste from a tube, it can never go back again. The entire development from the fertilized egg to the sexually mature adult organism is governed by the pattern of this information transfer: which genes are switched on—that is, transcribed into RNA and the appropriate protein synthesized—and which are switched off. Presumably, development proceeds in orderly sequences like a choreographed ballet with various dancers making their appearance at designated times—a concept called "genetic programmed development."

A number of researchers had looked at the patterns of transcription from DNA to RNA during embryonic development. Now Cutler proposed to look at what happened to the transcription patterns after the organism was fully developed. Was the genetic program set at that point, with no further changes made? Did an "aging program" switch on at some point during development? Or was there another program designed for life maintenance that counteracted the damage which occurred to the DNA over the life span?

Contrary to the prevailing idea of the day, Cutler found that there were alterations in transcription after sexual maturity had been reached. But what these changes meant, whether they were part of the continued program of development, or development gone awry, he could not say.

After three years at Brookhaven, Cutler had still not submitted a single paper on his work on aging. Despite this, he was able to obtain an assistant professorship at the University of Texas in Dallas (UTD) on the basis of his earlier *E. coli* work. But he soon ran into trouble. Among the reasons he had selected the school was the fact that a group of people there were involved in DNA repair, which, he felt certain, played a role as a "life-maintenance mechanism." But as he succinctly puts it, "I never did convince them that DNA repair was important in aging, and they would have been much happier if I worked on *E. coli*." His difficulties were further compounded when none of the four grants he applied for were funded. At that point he met his first nongovernment benefactor, Don Yarborough, a venture capitalist who would later play a role in the private financing of aging research.

Soon after he started at UTD, Bernard Strehler, a prominent gerontologist at the University of Southern California, invited him to summarize the work he did at Brookhaven for a chapter in a volume Strehler was editing on *Advances in Gerontological Research*. The paper, which took Cutler a year to write, was his first on aging and, he still believes, the best.

His thesis was that senescence occurs not because of "aging genes" or as an evolutionary strategy for ridding the species of its frailest members, but as the result of "intrinsic pathology," caused by the unwanted side effects of existence itself, that is, of breathing, metabolizing, growing, and development. In biology it's called pleiotropy (having more than one effect), and according to Cutler, all living processes are probably pleiotropic in nature. For example, the good news about breathing oxygen is that it is a highly efficient means for the production of energy; the bad news is that oxygen generates noxious particles called free radicals as it breaks down in the body. Like George Williams, who first proposed a role for pleiotropy in aging, Cutler postulated that the genes themselves could be pleiotropic, with the good news being expressed during early development and the bad news appearing later in life.

But his most important idea in the 1972 paper, and one he believes may represent a breakthrough in thinking, was that "the evolution of increased life-span for mammals such as mice, guinea pig, dog, monkey and man is considered to be the result of an increase in repair and/or protective processes for a common spectrum of damaging agents, rather than an elimination of the original genes responsible for producing these agents."

Cutler, who has the words of evolutionary biologist Theodosius Dobzhansky hanging on his wall—"Nothing in biology makes sense except in the light of evolution"—says, "It hit me that the reason that different species have different aging rates had to do with the way that aging and longevity evolved. The chimpanzee has a life span that is half that of man. Yet even today many people think that if you really took care of the chimp, gave it vitamins, etc., that it would live as long as man. But that isn't true. The chimp really does age faster across the board in every aspect—tasting, hearing, seeing, hair growth, reproduction, strength. The chimp, the rhesus, the mouse all have the same processes that age us. They are not different in this regard. They don't have more severe aging processes. And at the same time, they are not made with inferior parts. The molecules, the cells, the way we are constructed are essentially identical to shorter-lived animals. So what makes the difference? It must be the maintenance processes, the things that regulate the rate at which mutations accumulate or proteins are cross-linked, that account for the difference. In other words, it is like a car that lasts longer than another car, not because it is made of stronger steel or has more nuts and bolts, but because it is better maintained—its oil is changed more often, it has more tune-ups. We simply have more mechanics, not better mechanics—that is, we have more of the same repair-protective mechanisms."

He had also suggested four types of experiments to test his hypothesis, including one to measure "the presence and relative efficiency of specific enzymatic DNA repair processes" in mammals such as the "mouse, guinea pig, dog, monkey, and man." In brief, it proposed the experiment actually carried out by Hart and Setlow two years later.

While preparing his manuscript, Cutler had scoured the gerontological literature, and few papers had excited his interest as much as Sacher's. "He was the first person to seriously ask the question, What might be the mechanism determining longevity among the different species?" he says. In one of Sacher's important early theoretical papers, "Systemic Versus Molecular Theories of Aging," he indicated the direction he believed gerontology should go in finding the answer. Since the striking difference between man and mouse was in their brain rather than in their biochemistry, which was "minor and without known physiochemical significance," Sacher gave his vote to looking for a systemic explanation of senescence. Cutler came to exactly the opposite conclusion: that it was precisely the small, subtle changes in biochemical processes that were responsible for the variation in life span between species.

Cutler found little experimental support for Sacher's idea that the brain was the "organ of longevity." "Brain size appears to have nothing to do with the physiology of aging or in governing aging rate," he says, "but appears instead to reflect the evolutionary pressure of why longevity evolved in the first place. In other words, one of the reasons man is so long-lived is to take advantage of his superior brain."

As Cutler tells the story, the issue was clearly drawn at the International Conference of Gerontology in Kiev in 1973. After Cutler's talk, Sacher praised his paper, saying "You might be right." They decided to collaborate on a series of experiments, using Sacher's house mouse and white-footed mouse, to test whether brain or biochemistry, Sacher or Cutler, or even both, held the key to longevity.

Over the next year, their relationship could not have been friendlier. Cutler visited Sacher at Argonne, worked on experiments using his mouse species, and even presented his ideas at a seminar that Sacher held on "Aging at the Molecular and Cellular Levels" for a group of Midwest dentists, who wished to keep abreast of the latest biomedical developments. They also coorganized a symposium on "Evolution of Mammalian Longevity and Aging" at the 1974 Gerontology Society meeting in Portland, Oregon.

"There's a young man who seems to have something on DNA repair that I think you might be interested in," Sacher told Cutler one day. "His name is Ron Hart. Why don't we invite him as a speaker for our symposium?" Cutler and Hart met for the first time at the gerontology meeting, and together with Sacher they spent some time discussing their ideas and work.

The controversy that was to sever all relations between Sacher and Cutler, and almost destroy the latter's career, began almost innocuously. At the Portland symposium they cochaired, Cutler says he presented for the first time new work that supported his original contention that a few simple processes may regulate the aging process.

He had been galvanized into action by several papers that his wife had discovered while culling the scientific literature. In comparing man and his closest relatives, chimpanzee and gorilla, biochemist Allan C. Wilson and molecular anthropologist Vincent M. Sarich at Berkeley had found there was only a 1 percent difference in their genetic makeup: that is, that man and the great apes were virtually identical—99 percent the same. Since this difference is so small, it implies that the variation between closely related species is more a matter of differences in gene activity—that is, in how much of a certain protein is made—than in the genes themselves.

Cutler believed this discovery confirmed an idea that he had first written about in his 1972 paper: "It appears that the basic cellular and physiological processes of these animals are very similar and that their substantial differences in lifespans are due to a relatively small number of genes." All evolution did in terms of fitness, then, was provide us with more of the same processes that repair the DNA and protect the cell against damage. Man and monkey essentially shared the same genetic equipment, with the only difference being a matter of fine tuning a little more of this, a little less of that. All the distinctions between the hairy ape swinging through the trees and his near-bald relative driving down an LA freeway could be traced to the timing and degree of expression of a few genes during embryonic development.

He then had the ingenious idea of estimating the life spans of man's apelike and hominid ancestors by using the animals' brain weight-body weight ratio, which Sacher had shown to be correlated with life span. In this way he was able to show that life span had doubled in a very short time; and based upon calculations others had done of how fast the molecular clock ticks, he estimated that of the total number of genes involved in the evolution of the entire body from ape to man, only 150 to 250, a handful of the entire genome, played a role in the evolution of longevity.

The "few-genes" theory of life span was a turning point in Cutler's life. These "longevity-determinant genes," as he dubbed them, could be the biological equivalent of the physical "laws" of gravity, motion, thermodynamics—simple principles that explained complex events. If longevity were really a matter of a few genes that regulated the cells' repair and protective processes, then extending life might not be as difficult as scientists believed it was. "I thought," he says, "there really could be a simple explanation for how longevity evolved. My idea that longevity is just more of the same could be true. I was not going to get out of the field, after all. I was going to see this thing through to the end." There was only one problem—Sacher maintained that he had advanced the same argument, that a few genes governed longevity, at an international meeting a year earlier.

During neither the symposium nor in the hotel-room discussion after the meeting did Sacher or Hart ever indicate that Sacher had done essentially

the same work, asserts Cutler. It was only on a Sunday night several
months later, when he had written his work up for publication and called
Sacher, that he learned that the two ships that had passed each other in the
night were about to crash.

"I said, 'George, you know that work I presented at the meeting? I just
want to check to be sure that I've got your up-to-date equations on the correlation between life span and brain and body weight.' I went over the correlation with him and everything looked pretty good. And then he said,
'By the way, I've got a chapter where I've also looked at the evolution of
longevity and it says the same thing. I just received a galley proof and I'll
send it to you.'

"This was the first time he even mentioned that he was working along
the same lines," Cutler insists. "I got the paper in a couple of days and I just
couldn't believe that he did this without telling me. And how could he be
surprised at what I had said? Here all this time, in the whole meeting at the
symposium, and when we talked with Ron Hart, he never said one word.
It was unbelievable. The meeting was in October and this was in December."

Although Cutler had originally planned to send his manuscript to Sacher
to proof, he decided that that would no longer be appropriate and instead
submitted it directly to Richard Setlow for inclusion in the *Proceedings of the
National Academy of Sciences*. Setlow approved the paper but in keeping
with the customary practice, told Cutler he was sending it out for review.
The reviewer was George Sacher.

Sacher tried to get Setlow to reject the paper, starting with his own negative review based on scientific objections. After Cutler had answered all his
objections to Setlow's satisfaction, Sacher then told Setlow that the paper
was an outright plagiarism. Hart suggested as a compromise that both men
coauthor the paper.

"I refused to do this," says Cutler, "because I felt very strongly that it
was my independent work, and that if I put Sacher's name on it because of
his long involvement with this, it would be identified as Sacher's work.
And I wouldn't get any credit for it."

At this point, Cutler feels, his scientific career began a downhill slide
from which he has yet to recover. The paper was finally published in the
November 1975 issue of *PNAS*, but not before he agreed to include an acknowledgment at the end that Sacher had independently come up with the
same conclusions. Subsequently, Sacher severed his relationship with Cutler. Coincidentally, Cutler's grants were turned down and tenure denied

him at the University of Texas. But worse than all of this, he asserts, was the usurpation of the theoretical structure he had been building for years.

"Over the next several months and years, Sacher not only claimed that the idea that a few genes might govern the aging rate was his originally; he plagiarized even the grand idea I had of which the 'few genes' was only a part in a paper he wrote with Hart in 1978," says Cutler. "This was that longevity might be determined by small changes in biochemical processes, rather than his idea that the brain was the organ of longevity. The minute Ron Hart's data came out showing that it looked as if it might be biochemical processes, Sacher threw the 'organ-of-longevity' idea out the window. And he never mentioned it again.

"He started creeping in and taking everything, so by the time he died, you could see in his last paper, published posthumously, that he was claiming everything of mine." According to Cutler, all his efforts to either reach Sacher and end "this bitter controversy" or to get a well-respected gerontologist to review the facts independently were unavailing. "In my whole life the idea of a few regulatory genes controlling longevity, my longevity-determinant hypothesis, was the best one I ever came up with. Then someone else claims that I plagiarized the data, and he doesn't even give me credit for the possibility that it might have been reached independently. The credit for that discovery has been taken away, and I have been accused of plagiarism. I am happy, however, that I did get recognition from the National Academy of Sciences in Germany, which gave me an award after I lectured there in May 1976."

Priority fights and plagiarism charges are the secret vice of the scientific life. While sometimes it is a matter of "great minds thinking alike," all too often the purity of independent thought has been contaminated by contact between the thinkers. Credit for the invention of the computer, for instance, has been claimed both by a team of scientists, John W. Maunchly and Dr. J. Presper, who built Eniac, forerunner of the modern thinking machines, during World War II, and by Dr. John Atanasoff, a physicist, who erected a much cruder model in the 1930s. The priority dispute might have been a classic case of scientific coincidence had it not been for the fact that Maunchly had actually met Atanasoff and corresponded with him several times before designing his own device. The same cloud hangs over the Cutler-Sacher controversy.

Sacher was dead by the time Cutler had related his version of the events to me. But Sacher did allude to the central dispute in a 1979 telephone interview with me: "This [the few-genes idea] is something I conjectured

about in the mid-70s. You'll probably hear that Cutler said the same thing.
Just remember that I said it a couple of years earlier. He will tell you he
knows it all."

The only other person who had any knowledge of what went on between Sacher and Cutler was Ron Hart. The following details are based on
his recollection of what Sacher told him at the time. In September 1973,
Cutler visited Sacher at Argonne and presented data with him at the seminar on aging for the dental group. According to Hart, Cutler became well
acquainted with Sacher's latest idea—that the evolution of longevity in man
and his primate antecedents probably did not involve more than a few hundred genes. This concept was included in the 1973 paper that Sacher gave
at the International Congress of Anthropological and Ethnological Sciences
in Chicago, held August 28 to September 9, just prior to Cutler's arrival.
The dental symposium went off well and the two men drove to the airport,
sharing ideas on their projects for future research.

Over the next year their friendship continued. They talked often on the
telephone about their upcoming joint symposium for the Gerontology Society meeting in Portland.

The turnout at the symposium was larger than anyone had anticipated,
says Hart. The lecture room was rather small and filled to capacity. Hart
and Sacher gave their presentations, followed by Cutler. By this time, the
room had become uncomfortably hot. Although speakers were supposed
to keep to a twenty-five-minute presentation, with ten minutes for questions, Cutler, who chaired the session and served as timekeeper, declined to
observe the limit. Over the next hour or so, he presented a mountain of
material, while the audience became noticeably restless. In such a situation,
says Hart, he cannot remember if the "few-genes" theory "was one of the
many ideas he tossed out or not." Later Sacher, Hart, Cutler, and several
other interested scientists gathered for drinks and conversation in a hotel
room, and he doesn't recall whether or not the subject arose during the
general discussion. "Neither man published his presentations and, therefore, I'm afraid that this detail may be lost forever," Hart says. (Cutler al-
leges that this is not the case, that he and Sacher agreed to write up their
presentations for a forthcoming book to be edited by Cutler. In this book,
published in 1976, Cutler does state his "few-genes" theory. However,
Sacher's speech at the 1973 international congress in Chicago also appeared
as part of a volume published in 1975.)

Several months after the Portland meeting, Hart received a phone call
from an extremely agitated Sacher. He had just received for review from

Setlow a paper written by Cutler. In it, he said, were whole sections that were very close, although not verbatim, to the paper he had presented at the 1973 International Congress on Anthropological and Ethnological Sciences. Cutler was now planning to present these ideas as his own in *PNAS*. Sacher could barely contain feelings of anger, betrayal, hurt, disappointment, and sheer disbelief. Here was a friend and colleague, a man he had taken into his own home, worked with in the laboratory, given opportunities to present his work at meetings, even tried to help in getting a job, who suddenly and unaccountably had turned on him. There was no way, he insisted to Hart, that Cutler had worked out this idea independently. He had even used his own equations to arrive at the answer. Cutler had learned of this work while staying with Sacher and again at the dental symposium. It was a clear case of plagiarism. Sacher had, quite simply, been "ripped off." And not only his ideas but his trust and friendship as well.

With Sacher dead, it is impossible to get to the bottom of this controversy or even to get a complete version of his side. While Cutler had a chance to learn about Sacher's ideas on the evolution of longevity, the reverse is also true. In an outline, which Cutler sent Sacher in May 1973, of the lectures he planned to present at the dental symposium, he wrote that the rapid evolution of mammals suggests that "only a few different regulatory factors are governing the rate of expression of mammalian aging processes." In fact, as Cutler points out with amusement, Peter Medawar beat them all to the punch in 1946 in an essay on "Old Age and Death" when he wrote: "One of the most useful lessons to be learnt from the natural historian's studies of animal longevity is that the life span varies greatly in length between quite closely related types of organism. What can this mean, if not that the aging process in the individual as a whole is geared by one or two limiting or 'master' factors?"

As to Cutler's contention that Sacher abandoned his own scientific territory of the brain and homeostatic mechanisms and little by little moved into Cutler's turf of molecular mechanisms, the issues are extremely complex. Both men looked at the same problem, mammalian aging, from the same perspective—evolution—and arrived at the same conclusion: "longevity-determinant genes" to use Cutler's phrase, or "longevity-assurance processes" to use Sacher and Hart's term, regulate the rate at which we grow old and die.

In 1976, Cutler got the job that he had wanted for years, a position on the staff of the National Institute on Aging's Gerontology Research Center in Baltimore. Freed for the first time from the tyranny of writing grants, he was able to pursue aging research exclusively, with a full complement of technicians, students, and postdocs working with him.

On a limited budget with no guarantees of lifelong employment, a scientist must be as canny as a small-scale stock investor, forever on the lookout for the highest yield from the smallest outlay of cash. Cutler is a master at this game, devising straightforward easy-to-do experiments which, if successful, pay off with far-reaching implications. He now proposed to test his idea that the basis of longevity in mammals was simply a greater endowment of repair/protective processes. In doing so he chose to work with one of the most interesting enzymes discovered in the twentieth century. Its target in the cell is a species of one of the most notorious molecular malefactors—the free radical. So widespread and so destructive are its effects that an entire theory of aging bears its name.

The creator of the Free Radical Theory of Aging is a soft-spoken, gentle, midwesterner who has been fighting the good fight for more than thirty years. Denham Harman is a scientist for all seasons, holding both a Ph.D. in chemistry from Berkeley and an M.D. from Stanford. A former research chemist for Shell Oil, he is a professor both in the departments of medicine and biochemistry at the University of Nebraska, where he indefatigably conducts his life-extending research on mice; carries on an active medical practice; functions as founding father and prime mover of the American Aging Association (AGE), which holds annual meetings on biomedical aging research; and churns out contributions to the scientific literature, most of which are entitled "The Free Radical Theory of Aging," followed by subtitles such as "Nutritional Implications" or "Origin of Life, Evolution, and Aging."

One of the most dedicated of the small brotherhood of scientists who seek a solution to aging, Harman first had his interest kindled by an article in the December 1945 issue of *Ladies' Home Journal*, called "Tomorrow You Will be Younger." The piece dealt mainly with the work of a Kiev physician, Dr. Alexander A. Bogomolets, who claimed to have developed a serum that rejuvenated connective tissue, uplifting sagging skin, and firming flabby tissue. Eleven years later, while at the radiation laboratory in Berkeley, Harman published his own version of why we age and suggested a possible treatment.

As an industrial chemist, Harman knew that free-radical reactions take place continuously in the presence of oxygen, causing butter to become rancid, iron to rust. A free radical is simply an unpaired electron, a single in the molecular world of couples, an atomic particle on the make, constantly cruising for a partner. Oxygen molecules actually contain two such unpaired electrons. They satisfy their need for coupling by pulling off electrons from other molecules, a process known as oxidation/reduction. The molecule receiving electrons is said to be "reduced," while the molecule donating electrons is "oxidized." Since oxygen enters our body with every breath we take, Harman reasoned that the same process that had been observed in inanimate matter had to be taking place in our cells all the time as the oxygen is metabolized.

Most biochemical reactions in the body are clear-cut, moving along well-defined pathways. An enzyme catalyzes a reaction; a product is produced; and other enzymes transform that product into something the body can use, or else break it down into components that can be harmlessly excreted. Free-radical reactions, on the other hand, are one-way, irreversible, "junk" producers. The water and carbon exhaust produced by the combustible engine, for example, can never be returned to gasoline and oxygen. Worse still, the reactions are self-generative—a chain reaction occurs, where every time a molecule loses an electron, it becomes a new electron-seeking free radical. The result is like a youth gang on a rampage, looting stores, turning other youths into lawless marauders, leaving chaos and wreckage in their wake.

Harman knew that free-radical reactions played a major role in the well-documented effects of radiation—mutation, cancer, and life-shortening. A free-radical mechanism had already been shown to aid in the destruction of hemoglobin. Might not the process of oxidation/reduction in the body, he reasoned, create myriads of these highly reactive bits of molecules with their one-way, irreversible, scattershot effect? And might not the accumulation of this damage be a primary cause, if not *the* cause, of aging and the associated diseases of senescence? In the fall of 1954, based on the scantiest of supporting evidence (almost nothing was then known about free-radical chemistry in the body), he published his first paper proclaiming his theory. A few years later, he offered his first empirical results to substantiate his contention. When he fed several antioxidants that neutralized the effects of free radicals, he was able to increase the average life expectancy, but not the maximum life span, of mice by as much as 30 percent.

Meanwhile, as Harman continued his dietary manipulations, extending and refining his theory, another scientist, Irwin Fridovich, at Duke University, was making some very puzzling observations about a common enzyme in the body's tissue, xanthine oxidase. For no clear reason, the enzyme caused a free-radical chain reaction. He had also discovered that a certain tissue extract, a piece of tissue from which the water has been separated out, would remove this free-radical activity entirely. When he and his associates put together all the pieces, they realized that the effects they saw with xanthine oxidase were due to the enzyme's generating a free radical. Since the radical contained one more electron than oxygen, they called it superoxide. This was the first conclusive evidence that free-radical production took place in living bodies as well as in inanimate matter. Much of the oxygen that we breathe is harmlessly reduced to water but a small percentage of the oxidation/reduction process leads to the formation of intermediate substances like the superoxide radical. The message was clear: The breathing of oxygen is hazardous to your health.

But, Fridovich and his colleagues found that in the crossover to oxygen breathing, evolution had equipped respiring organisms with a secret weapon against the devastating superoxide radical. The tissue extract that removed the superoxide activity contained an enzyme that acted as a go-between, mopping up the extra electrons. In 1968, Joseph McCord, a student of Fridovich, isolated the active ingredient, superoxide dismutase (SOD), which turned out to be the first of a family of similar enzymes. It was a momentous discovery, the first proof that the body manufactured its very own antioxidant, a built-in preservative that extended the shelf life of our cells.

Ten years later, when Cutler was casting about for a means of testing his theory, SOD seemed the perfect candidate. Clearly, if oxygen was highly toxic, then SOD, which protects against oxygen's adverse effects, should be higher in longer-lived species. All he had to do was compare SOD activity in a number of different species to get the answer. The experiment was simplicity itself, clear-cut in its implications, and easy to do—so easy in fact that he could turn the entire project over to a young student, Julie Tolmasoff. The technique, which had been devised by Fridovich, involved using a xanthine oxidase-containing mixture to generate free radicals and a compound called cytochrome C, which detects their presence. The greater the production of superoxide radicals, the faster the rate at which the cytochrome C oxidizes and changes color. Adding a tissue extract containing SOD will slow the oxidation reaction in direct proportion to the amount of enzyme present.

Tolmasoff, Cutler, and a Visiting Fellow, Tetsuya Ono, measured tissue extracts from the liver, brain, and heart of fourteen mammals, two of which were the house mouse and field mouse, and of a dozen primate species ranging from the tree shrew, which lives a maximum of twelve years, to man, which they estimated at ninety-five years. But much to their dismay, there was absolutely no correlation between the level of SOD activity and maximum life span. Many of the species had approximately the same level of the enzyme. And while it was exceptionally high in man, the longest-lived mammal, it was also very high in the much shorter-lived lemur and marmoset. Mouse, as might be expected, had very low values of SOD, but then so did the gorilla, which lived almost fifteen times as long. Furthermore, Fridovich himself, who had looked at various mouse strains with different life spans, had also come up empty-handed.

Cutler pondered these strange results for some time without being able to make sense of them. It went against all logic. Nature, as a rule, is frugal, not extravagant. Why would animals manufacture amounts of SOD far in excess of anything they would need over their lifetime? He could only conclude that if longevity did evolve, greater production of SOD was not one of the routes it took.

In a flash of insight, he realized he had been looking in the wrong direction. The main function of SOD appeared to be to protect against by-products of oxygen. This meant that the amount required by an animal should be related to its total energy consumption over its lifetime. The needs of a mouse, which burns up oxygen as though it were going out of style, were going to be very different from the slow-breathing, lumbering elephant. Feeling as if he was holding the winning ticket at the daily double, he pulled out all his data and redid the calculations, this time looking at SOD level as a function of the amount of energy consumed per gram of tissue over an animal's lifetime. And there it was. "Everything came out in a line that was just so neat," he says. "And then I really got excited. Because when you have twelve different species all come out in a linear correlation of about 98 percent, that's incredible. It had to be right. There had to be something there."

Cutler was jubilant. It looked as if he had been right all along. Aging *was* a by-product of metabolism, longevity *did* evolve, regulatory processes *were* important. It was a great moment, the first direct proof of his theory. Not only did it show that he was on the right track, bearing out the predictions he had first made in 1972, but it pointed the way toward a means of carrying out the goal he had sought since his helicopter days. For Cutler, as for a handful of gerontologists, understanding the biological basis of aging is not enough; one must intervene, wresting time from the grip of age. "What it said," Cutler pointed out, "was that while aging was very complex, the processes regulating it might be very simple. In other words, you may have a thousand different metabolic processes producing toxic superoxide radicals, but you need only one enzyme to clear it up."

He felt he was only just beginning his life's work. But, ironically, the very experiment that appeared to be the springboard for promising strategies of life extension would also serve to launch a new round of problems in his career.

Chapter Five

A Supergene for Aging?

Roy Walford was waiting for the mice to die off. Unlike most life-span experiments, this was not a test of a particular diet, exercise regimen, drug, chemical, or vitamin; in fact, he was not disturbing the animals in any way. The mice—more than one thousand in all—were simply living six to a cage, eating standard Purina laboratory chow, waking and sleeping, growing old and dying. And Walford was waiting—counting the dead mice, seeing what they died from, doing the statistical analyses. The entire study, which took more than three years to complete, could not have been further from the kind of rapid, sure-fire experiment in which the answer comes almost as easily as the question, and yet it was the most important one that the California researcher had ever undertaken. It would provide the first demonstration of his "supergene" theory, bring together the two fields —immunology and gerontology—in which he had achieved prominence, and be the highlight of his scientific career.

"Man has occasionally postponed death, but he has never wholly prevented it. A great opening into which few have entered exists in the biological sciences. . . . Certainly man cannot call himself supreme when his most profound intellects die of natural and simple causes." Walford was seventeen years old when he wrote these words for his high-school senior newspaper. It was his manifesto, "The Conquest of the Future," and Marx himself could not have ended with a more ringing challenge: "Fools of conservatism, let not the stagnant imaginations be shackled by blind precedent; for then you shall defy the overstatement: 'There was the door to which I found no key; there was the veil through which I might not see.' "

From the age of eleven, when he first heard a radio broadcast of Christopher Marlowe's *Faustus* (who made a pact with the devil for twenty-four extra years of life), Walford had made a pact with himself. He would outdo the devil at his own game and extend life far beyond a mere quarter century—without surrendering his soul. Like Faust, his two great drives are to know and to experience. He has been a Las Vegas gambler, a radical anarchist, impresario for a guerrilla theater, underground journalist, poet, short-story writer, scuba diver, wrestling champion, top man on a hand-balancing team, and classical pianist. He has crisscrossed the world, explored many fields, developed many talents. Time is his enemy and what he needs most.

He moves easily among the different subcultures that make up his world. In the hierarchical world of science, where professional reprisals are apt to be taken against nonconformist views or behavior, Walford can show up at a scientific convention wearing a black motorcycle jacket and boots, and his colleagues not only accept him, they shower him with honors. When a Young Turk graduate student who was having trouble with his colleagues asked him, "Why is it that you get away with dressing and acting the way you do, and other people can't?" Walford just shrugged and said, "They think of me as an eccentric and that makes anything possible."

But it also helps that he plays the science game well. At the age of sixty, he has more than two hundred journal articles to his credit and four books, one of them, *Maximum Life Span,* written for the layman. His experiments are unassailable, he publishes in the right journals, and his results are impressive. At a recent gerontology meeting, Richard Weindruch presented work that he and Walford were doing on life extension in mice. After two scientists complained that the experimental conditions were not rigorous enough, gerontologist David Harrison of the Jackson Laboratory in Bar Harbor, Maine, rose to his defense, pointing out that they must be doing something right since "even the controls were fantastically long-lived."

With his shaved head, Spock-like ears, penetrating blue eyes, Fu Manchu mustache, and supercool manner, Walford can be intimidating even to his colleagues. "Actually, what he is hiding under that exotic exterior is that he's really a nice, warm guy," says Kathleen Hall, his friend and collaborator at UCLA.

In Venice, California, an eclectic collection of erotic, mystical, primitive, and modern art, Indian wall hangings, rugs, photographs, political posters, statues, and unclassifiable objects fills the cavernous space of his two-story-high apartment. Inescapable are the images of death. Sharing space on a small desk, with his Kleemeier Award for Outstanding Research in Aging, is a statue of the skull-faced voodoo god of death surrounded by his minions with devil horns. Even Walford's choice of pathology as a medical speciality seems one more reflection of his obsession. Watching over the whole room is a huge, stuffed animal. "The Teddy Bear God," says Walford playfully.

He was not always this hip and loose, he says. The only child of a retired naval officer living in San Diego, he had a conventional upbringing, but his far-ranging interests were apparent early on. "Wonder boy of the senior A class," his high-school paper called him in a feature story when he had racked up a total of thirty-nine A's. Among his interests recorded in the story are mathematics, natural philosophy, jitterbugging, playing Chopin and Beethoven on the piano, portraying the villain in the senior play, and collecting books "by authors with original ideas."

Upon finishing high school, he felt pulled in two directions. On one side was his first love, philosophy; on the other, gerontology. He opted for philosophy, and following such distinguished practitioners as Descartes, Bertrand Russell, and Alfred Lord Whitehead, he began by studying advanced math. For Walford, math and physics are not only a means to understanding the laws of the universe, they are the gateway to another reality. He calls it "mathematical mysticism"—where calculus, cosmology, and consciousness intersect at a point inaccessible by means of our five senses.

World War II interrupted his studies. Inducted into the Army, he was sent back to Cal Tech with the option of studying either civil engineering or medicine. Since the latter opened the way to future gerontological research, he chose that, but he says somewhat wistfully, "If the war hadn't come along, I might have gone into metaphysics. I never really have resolved that. It was kind of resolved for me. Maybe I'll go back to it when I finish my work in life-span extension."

In 1968 he went to Paris to work with Jean Dausset, a pioneer immunologist who would later win a Nobel Prize. This was the time when all of France was in an upheaval as students and workers were united in an uprising that threatened to topple the de Gaulle government. Walford was a part of it all, doing research in immunology during the day, joining the rioters at night, and writing dispatches for a countercultural newspaper in Los Angeles.

As though science were imitating life, the 1960s were for immunology a time of both tremendous activity and confusion. Recent insights and discoveries were toppling old conceptions; for example, the idea that the immune system of the body "learns" to adapt to new challenges from the outside—that is, it makes antibodies to substances such as industrial pollutants by using that substance as a blueprint. Now that molecular biology had shown that genetic information could only be transferred from the DNA to the protein and never directly from protein to protein, i.e., a man-made chemical to an antibody, this kind of "learned response" was seen to be impossible. Some other explanation had to be sought.

Walford was also a part of the "New Immunology," as one of its founders, F. Macfarlane Burnet, dubbed this revolution in progress. For the past decade he had been doing experiments in both gerontology and immunology, hoping that at some point the parallel lines of research would converge. With a combination of luck, instinct, and an uncanny ability to be at the right place at the right time, it all came together for Walford in a way that was as unexpected as it was gratifying.

Alexis Carrel may have sent a generation of tissue culturists and gerontologists on the wrong path, but for Walford, he inadvertently pointed out the right direction. When Walford started his research in the late 1950s, the immortality of cells, once they were freed from the confines of the body, was a given. Therefore, the answer to aging had to lie in the interaction between the cells, rather than in something inside them. And this left only two possibilities, the neuroendocrine system and the immune system. Walford chose the latter.

In the body imperial, the immune system is charged with the mission of internal security. It is an exquisite detector of foreign material, more efficient than the most zealous border guard. Through its antibodies and white blood cells, it searches out and neutralizes invaders, including viruses, bacteria, and bacterial toxins; fifth columnists such as abnormal cells; and foreign tissues—skin grafts or organ transplants.

The soldiers of the immunological army, the antibodies, are the most diverse group imaginable. Each antibody is directed against a specific alien, called an antigen. Indeed, just how such a staggering variety of antibodies, running into the millions, could be encoded into the genes has until recently been a major mystery, leading one group of tongue-in-cheek immunologists to attribute the whole affair to GOD, or a Generator of Diversity.

The antibody obeys the Socratic injunction to "know thyself," and will not under normal circumstances attack its own tissue. "Antibody formation is thus not just a mere defense reaction against infectious disease," write Gunther Stent and Richard Calendar in *Molecular Genetics*, "but is a phenomenon of rather wide biological significance: a mechanism for the recognition of nonself." The problem is that the immune system's finely tuned abilities of differentiating friend from foe can go awry. A common instance of this is allergy to such harmless substances as plant pollen and molds. Far more sinister is the autoimmune reaction in which the antibodies turn on the "self-substance"—the body's own tissue—treating it as a foreign invader. The result may be an autoimmune disease, such as rheumatoid arthritis or systemic lupus erythematosus.

As we age, the immune system disintegrates in two directions, both of which spell disaster for the body. First, the internal security function becomes less effective, so that it no longer efficiently wards off disease-carrying virus and bacteria or potentially cancerous cells. Second "the ability to distinguish between self and nonself becomes blurred," says Walford. "Aging is a kind of self-rejection process. You begin reacting against yourself, as though you were a foreign kidney or a foreign heart."

Immune rejection even looks like aging, and nowhere is this more graphically illustrated than in the "graft-versus-host reaction." Rejection can go both ways. Not only can an animal or person reject a transplanted graft, but the graft can turn on its host. This can happen in the laboratory, for example, when cells from an adult mouse are injected into a fetal mouse that has not yet developed "immunological competence"—the ability to react against foreign material—or it may occur clinically when a leukemia patient is given a bone marrow transplant. Within a few days the recipient shows gross and microscopic signs of accelerated aging, including loss of hair, failure to thrive, vascular and kidney disease, and a foreshortened life span. As Walford wrote in his 1969 classic *The Immunologic Theory of Aging,* as organisms age, "loss of adequate self-recognition occurs, and in higher animals this sets up minor-grade, long-term graft-versus-host reactions resulting in aging. Terminal aging . . . is an explosive loss in self-recognition."

Throughout the late 1950s and early 1960s, as Walford was carrying forward simultaneous but independent research projects in gerontology and immunology, momentous events were occurring in the latter field. Much of the impetus came from recent developments in organ transplantation. While surgeons had made great strides technically, a successful transplant remained elusive. The immune system's compulsion to fight off foreign elements had to be overcome.

Why animals should reject tissues from a member of their own species had long been a mystery. Then in the late 1930s and early 1940s, Peter Gorer, at Guy's Hospital in London, and George Snell, at the Jackson Laboratory in Bar Harbor, Maine, carried out experiments, first independently and later together, that led to the discovery of histocompatibility antigens, protein markers on the surface of mouse cells. Tissues could be exchanged between mice if both individuals had the same surface antigens; too great a difference and the tissue would be rejected. The experiments had been made possible by Snell's "invention" of congenic mice—the inbreeding of mice to such an extent that only a few mutations in a single genetic region kept them from being identical. Snell and others subsequently showed that the histocompatibility antigens were clustered together on one segment of chromosome 17 on the mouse.

In the late 1950s, Jean Dausset, who was studying the antibodies produced by patients who had received many blood transfusions, found the first evidence in humans of a histocompatibility antigen, which he named MAC. Over the next few years, researchers in Europe and the United States, including Walford, began identifying other tissue antigens that might or might not be related to one another, and naming them as fast as they discovered them. So much was happening so fast that it was like trying to get a clear picture from overlapping exposures. Finally, in 1965, D. Bernard Amos of Duke University called all the researchers together to pool their antigens, nomenclature, ideas, and information.

It was a grand group of eight: Dausset from France, Ruggero Ceppellini from Italy, Jon Van Rood from the Netherlands, Kissmeyer-Nielsen from Denmark, and Amos, Paul Terraski, Rose Payne, and Walford from the United States. They were the founding fathers (and mother) of the International Histocompatibility Workshop, which still meets on an irregular basis every two to three years. From the outset the workshops were an anomaly in the world of science. "There were no elected officers, no society, no secretary, no minutes, no nothing," says Walford, who believes its anarchistic structure could serve as a model for small-group interaction. "It controlled the whole field," says Walford. "If you were not invited to the workshops, you were automatically two years behind everything that was going on. It wasn't planned that way, it just came about."

Mainly through their efforts, it became clear that all the human histocompatibility antigens were located at one small segment of chromosome 6 that corresponded to chromosome 17 of the mouse. Both these loci are now known to be part of a complicated network of closely linked genes, perhaps several hundred in all, which make up the Major Histocompatibility Complex (MHC). Histocompatibility antigens, which are found on the surface of almost every cell in the body, are as unique to an individual as his profile. Tissue matching has turned out to be almost as important to the success of organ transplants as blood typing in transfusions. But like the perfect marriage, the perfect tissue match is unattainable (except, of course, with identical twins).

Meanwhile, Walford, who returned to Los Angeles in 1969, continued his search for an answer to aging. There are only two methods of life-span extension that have been proved under controlled scientific conditions. One of them is by lowering body temperature. Putting life on ice is an old idea. Experiments going back over fifty years showed that decreasing body temperature increased life span. But most of the research had been done with insects, such as water fleas and fruit flies. When Walford came across a report that fence lizards, vertebrates with backbones and vital organs, lived twice as long in the New England climate than they did in Florida, he was intrigued. Lizards are poikilothermic, literally heat-variable; that is, their temperature fluctuates with the surrounding environment. Did the cooler temperatures up north account for the Yankee lizards' living longer than their southern counterparts?

The simplest way to test the idea, he decided, was to use another poikilothermic vertebrate, fish, in which lowering body temperature was simply a matter of cooling the water. The problem with fish, however, is that their life spans are far too long for quick answers. After a long search, Walford located the "shortest-lived, evolutionarily advanced cold-blooded vertebrate in the world," the Annual fish of South America, which lives about a year to a year and a half. That a large number of this species inhabit the shallow ponds on the outskirts of Buenos Aires gave Walford an excuse to hop on a plane, don fishing gear, and net specimens of the pinky-size Argentine pearlfish, *Cynolebias bellotti.*

Back at UCLA, he and his associate, Robert Liu, experimented with the tiny fish with some surprising results. First, they found that lowering its temperature just a few degrees lengthened life span by as much as 200 percent. But the benefit was mainly seen in the second half of life. Second, the simplest explanation—that lowered temperature slowed the metabolic rate—did not appear to hold. The cold fish actually grew faster, and although some enzyme reaction rates decreased, others speeded up. Whatever happened, he believed, was far more complicated and probably involved a complete metabolic reorganization.

One thing was not in doubt: Cooling down slowed aging. Indeed, purely on thermodynamic principles, investigators at Northwestern University have calculated that lowering body temperature 7 degrees would increase our own life span to a maximum of 200 years, while plunging it still further to 87.8 degrees Fahrenheit could extend survival to 280 years. But the question—as always—was how to apply this to human beings. With mechanisms such as shivering and sweating, we homeotherms are programmed to maintain internal core temperature under conditions ranging from the arctic to the tropical. Just lowering ambient temperature would merely add to one's misery, while doing nothing for life span. Resetting core temperature would mean resetting the body's thermostat, located in the hypothalamus of the brain—a tall order, requiring science-fictionesque solutions like implanting devices into the hypothalamus that could be warmed or cooled from the outside.

But drugs can also affect the hypothalamus. And the most promising ones that Walford and Liu found were the tranquilizer chlorpromazine and THC, the active ingredient of marihuana. The latter drug appeared to be so effective and relatively nontoxic in the first experiments on animals that Walford was almost ready to go public with the news. "I got so excited when it worked," he says, "I was going to go on TV and say that grass was the answer to long life. But then we found that it only works temporarily. The animals become tolerant to the effect and their temperature doesn't go down so far. So after two or three times, the mice are stoned but they are not hypothermic."

His next idea was biofeedback: Think cool, pick up the lowered body temperature with a sensing device, feed this information back to the conscious brain by means of an external signal such as a beep or light, and voilà! It works with blood pressure, heartbeat, and a host of other physiologic functions that are not ordinarily subject to voluntary control, so why not body temperature? The only drawback is that for biofeedback to be effective, it must be virtually immediate. After death, when metabolism has come to a standstill, the body temperature still goes down only one degree per hour, Walford points out. "So even if you get your head in the right place, it would take an hour before you got the feedback."

With drugs and biofeedback out, Walford wondered if there weren't some other way. The Yogis of India were reputed to be able to lower their body temperature through trance and meditation and they were also known, perhaps not coincidentally, for their long lives. If he could substantiate that they could regulate their body temperature, it would show that hypothermia in human beings was at least possible.

If he got his political and scientific selves together in France, then he combined his mystical and gerontological pursuits in India. For the next eight months he wandered the country, exploring cosmic consciousness with Indian sages, checking out left-wing activity among the Dalet Pathers for the underground press, and trying to convince the Yogis to let him monitor their rectal temperatures. Oddly enough, the most famous Yogis, the gurus with the largest following, both native and American, proved the most disappointing, and Walford realized that he would have to forsake the ashrams for the mountains, caves, and forests where the Saddhus lived. With an Indian monk as guide and interpreter, he tramped the foothills of the Himalayas. Dressed in a loincloth, like the holy men, he showed them his book, *The Immunologic Theory of Aging,* and explained to them what he wanted. "Involved in heavy spiritual and isolation trips, with daylong periods of meditation, they were receptive once they realized that I was also on a serious quest," he wrote later in *Maximum Life Span.*

The Yogis could lower their temperature about half a degree or more through meditation and trance. But even more important, Walford located a few holy men whose *normal* body temperature was an astoundingly cool 94 to 95 degrees, and unlike the Galápagos tortoise, it was not achieved at the price of sluggishness and lethargy. This proved that hypothermia was possible in warm-blooded humans and even lent some credence to the Yogis' claim of extreme long life. But clearly the yogic discipline and lifestyle, with its "heavy spiritual and isolation trips," was not ready to be mass marketed as an aging cure.

The Indian experience did suggest that something else was going on that might be just as important as the hypothermia and far more promising. Because the hypothermia induced by meditation and trance is transitory, the naturally supercool Yogis must have been doing it by some method other than an alternate state of consciousness. Walford suspected that diet, or, rather, the lack of it, might be the cause. The hypothermic Yogis were found among people who inhabited the Himalayan caves and forests and lived on a bare subsistence diet. This tied in nicely with the one other known method of life extension: caloric restriction.

Undernutrition has been gerontology's one real success story. Since 1935, when a Cornell nutritionist, Clive McCay, doubled the average life span of rats by severely restricting their food intake after weaning, researchers have been routinely retarding aging and prolonging life in a variety of species with similar results. The regimen also cuts cancer incidence way down. But the most important aspect of McCay's work was not that it changed the average life span of a rodent, which has occurred throughout human history as living conditions have improved and childhood diseases been eliminated. McCay was able to extend maximum achievable life span, the age attained by the oldest survivor of a population, suggesting that something fundamental to the aging process was at work. What it might be is anybody's guess and there have been many. In fact, so ubiquitous is the finding that either food restriction, or every-other-day fasting, slows aging and stretches out the life span, that most aging theorists strive to accommodate this phenomenon in the framework of their overall hypothesis.

Walford knew that food-restricted mice often have temperatures two to three degrees lower than animals who are fed all the time. And unlike temperature reduction, underfeeding exerts its greatest effect in the first half of life. When he and his UCLA colleagues added caloric restriction to temperature reduction, they were able to increase the life span of the Annual fish by a whopping 300 percent.

By 1974, Walford had found that his three main areas of research—diet restriction, temperature reduction, and the major histocompatibility system—were related as the spokes of a wheel to the hub, with the immune system the hub. Diet-restricted mice have a better immune function for a longer period of time than their normally fed counterparts. And autoimmunity, the down side of the immune function, is practically nil in both underfed and hypothermic animals.

But the most interesting aspect of his work and the one that tied it all together was the major histocompatability system. Back in 1969, Walford had the germ of an idea that has since grown into one of the most powerful concepts in gerontology. In one of those insights that characterize the creative scientist, he turned a common observation inside out, focusing on the "chaff" rather than the wheat. Ever since Hayflick had clearly established that normal cells stop dividing in culture and that transformed (potentially cancerous) cells do not, gerontologists routinely discarded cancerous cells, both from their laboratory dishes and their thinking, as having anything to do with the aging process.

But, Walford pointed out in his book *Immunologic Theory of Aging*, they may have gotten things backwards: "Cancer cells, just as normal cells, take in nutriment, respire, excrete, divide, multiply. They perform nearly all the functions of a normal cell. Most of their biochemical mechanisms are like those of normal cells. And the information-containing molecules of transformed cells and cancer cells do not 'run out of program,' do not experience a 'mean time to failure,' and do not succumb to any other kind of metaphor! A perfectly legitimate form of living matter, the cancer cell has learned something the normal cell doesn't know, or has forgotten something the normal cell might well forget."

In that book he also noted that different strains of mice that share the same histocompatibility gene have a longer life span and develop fewer tumors than other mouse strains. A year later in a paper in *Lancet*, he added more evidence for his belief that the H-2 system, as the major histocompatibility system in mice is called, might play a role in regulating aging and longevity. Two years later he put these observations together, with the lesson to be learned from the cancer cells, to form what he called "one promising new route of attack." In 1972, in an introduction to a special issue, Immunology and Aging, in *Gerontologia*, he wrote:

"According to Hayflick's well-known studies, a normal cell line possesses only a finite lifespan; however, we know that a 'transformed' cell line is probably immortal. Transformation can be brought about by viruses, especially by oncogenic [cancer-causing] viruses. These contain from 7 to 50 genes, but only a small fraction thereof (as few as 1 or 2 genes in some instances) are required to bring about 'transformation.' Furthermore, transformation is not necessarily equivalent to malignancy, although it is one step in that direction. The point is, current knowledge about viruses and 'transformation' suggests that the 'programming' of senescence and clonal death may be alterable by genetic manipulation involving only a few genes—by way of speculative example, it might be those genes determining the mutation rate of histocompatibility genes."

In 1974, in *Federation Proceedings*, he stated the concept even more forcefully and gave it a name—the "limited gene theory of aging." Thus, starting out from a completely different point and taking an entirely different path, he had arrived at the same place as Cutler and Sacher—the idea of a few master genes regulating longevity and perhaps mortality itself. Walford's unique contribution was to nominate the major histocompatibility system as a prime candidate for those genes. "A limited gene theory . . . as corollary to an immunologic theory could thus unite a great many observations," he wrote, including the fact that histocompatibility genes controlled many aspects of the immune function, that they were associated with certain diseases of accelerating aging such as systemic lupus erythematosus, and that there was some indication in both mice and man that they were linked to life span.

"Roy has this idea that if you want change to happen in science, *you* have to make it happen," says his associate Kathleen Hall. "You have to write about it and talk it up and then everyone starts testing it. And because they are thinking about it, very often it starts to come out the way that you said." When I asked Walford to elaborate on this idea, he smiled like a magician who has something up his sleeve and said, "If you wish to change reality, you must first make it. For instance, you say 'DNA repair,' and all over the world, enzymes start repairing DNA." For whatever the reason—creating reality or sheer hubris—in 1974 Walford first promulgated the hypothesis that histocompatibility genes play a leading role in aging and then proceeded to test it.

The Jackson Laboratory, a private biological-research institution in Bar Harbor, Maine, is a center for world supply of what might be called the "custom-bred" mouse. There are mice that develop diabetes, mice with neurological problems, autoimmune mice, obese mice, leukemic mice, and even "nude" mice—rodents whose lack of an immune function allows them to accept all kinds of transplanted tissue including feathers. It is also the place where almost forty years ago, George Snell began breeding his congenic mice, which are now the primary model for histocompatibility research. So it was only natural that Walford and his coworker George Smith should turn to Snell and the Jackson Lab for the particular strains of mice needed to carry out their experiment.

For their study, Smith and Walford used congenic mice on three "backgrounds." Like people, mice share certain "racial" characteristics that distinguish them from other groups. For instance, there are the C57 mice, which are all black and have a completely different genetic makeup than the A mice, which are white. Congenic mice that are made of a C57 black background are as identical as two peas in a pod except for differences in the one genetic region to be studied—in this case, the short segment of the seventeenth chromosome carrying the major histocompatibility complex (MHC). In all, the California researchers used fourteen congenic strains, seven on the C57 background, four on the A background, and three on another background, called C3h.

The rest of the experiment consisted of waiting for the mice to die off, plotting survival curves for each of the strains, and seeing what diseases they died from. If the MHC—which was the only variable between the strains of each "race"—had little effect on aging, then the life spans of all the mice on a given background should be virtually the same. But if the MHC was a primary regulator of senescence, the survival rates between each of the congenic strains should vary significantly.

By the spring of 1977 they had their answer. While the C57 black mice, as a whole, had the longest life span and the C3h mice the shortest, each of the strains on each of the backgrounds had a characteristic life span. Both the mean life expectancy and the age of the oldest survivors—considered to be the most accurate measurement of life span—were as different between one strain and the next as might be expected between unrelated strains of mice on the same background. In their paper in *Nature*, in 1977, "Influence of the Main Histocompatibility Complex on Ageing in Mice," Smith and Walford refer for the first time to the MHC as a "super-gene" system, which they define as a "cluster of genes influencing the same category of functions." They also referred to the MHC as the "master genetic control" for the immune function and concluded that the data from their experiment "strongly suggest that the MHC may be one of the principal genetic systems involved in controlling lifespan."

Almost two decades earlier, following the red herring of Carrel's immortal cells, Walford had begun work simultaneously in immunology, gerontology, and the obscure area of histocompatibility antigens. Now the three separate strands had been braided together by his study.

A connoisseur of experience, Walford ranks his MHC life-span study right up there with, say, hitchhiking across Africa or traveling with the Living Theatre. "Since it was a four-year experiment, it isn't the kind of thing where you yell 'Eureka.' But I think it is the best single and most satisfying experiment that I have ever done."

If the MHC were a supergene for aging, what vital functions did it command? In an expanded version of their congenic-mice study using nineteen different strains on three backgrounds, Smith and Walford found that histocompatibility genes were also associated with the rate of cancer development among the mice and the age at which it first appeared. Walford and his colleague Patricia Meredith then looked at the rise and fall of the immune system with age. The longer-lived strains, they found, showed higher levels of immune function for a longer period of time. With the third study of these mice, he added a new strand to the intricate braid of aging research—DNA repair.

Hart and Setlow had looked at DNA repair and life span among species as widely varied as shrew and mouse. Sacher and Hart had narrowed the gap to two rodents, *Mus mucus* and *Peromyscus leucopus*, two different species of mice. Volker Paffenholz, a German researcher, removed the species barrier and looked at three inbred mouse strains: the CBA mice, which lived an average of 900 days; the C3h, which lived 600 days; and the NZB with 300 days. Again the efficiency of DNA repair fell into line with life span. This study was of particular interest to Walford because of its immunologic implications. The short-lived NZB mice are highly prone to autoimmune disease, while the long-lived CBA strain enjoys one of the best-functioning immune systems and the lowest incidence of autoanti-bodies in the mouse family.

However, it was not Paffenholz's experiment that inspired Walford, but, rather, another study showing an association between xeroderma pigmen-tosum (XP) and the major histocompatibility complex. Since XP is a disor-der of DNA repair, perhaps there was some relationship between repair and the MHC, he thought. He already had the congenic mice, he had es-tablished their life spans, and now all he had to do was look at how well each of these strains repaired DNA damage. Ironically, it turned out that the alleged relationship between the histocompatibility antigens and XP did not hold up, but Walford's study did.

He and Kathy Bergmann, a technician at UCLA, selected long- and short-lived strains from two backgrounds and compared how well the cells from these animals performed repair of DNA after damage with ultraviolet light and bleomycin, a chemical agent that causes breaks in the DNA strands. In their preliminary studies they found that the longer-lived strains on both backgrounds were better at both forms of DNA repair than their shorter-lived congenic partners. "Our study," they wrote in *Tissue Anti-gens,* "provides the first direct evidence that genes linked to and perhaps within the MHC may exert an influence upon certain DNA excision repair mechanisms."

Why should there be a connection between DNA repair and the gene of the MHC? The question is one that intrigues Walford and appeals to him on a metaphorical level. "The immune system is involved with recognition, and recognition of self and nonself is under MHC regulation. Well, you have to recognize something to repair it, so maybe the MHC also controls DNA repair," he says.

The study was a preliminary one, lacked sophistication, and required more extensive work by someone trained in DNA repair. But neverthe-less, the implications for aging research were rapidly becoming exciting. Now it appeared as though there were a vital connection between life span, immune function, and DNA repair, and all were controlled by one small segment of one chromosome spanning a few hundred genes at most.

DNA repair was especially interesting to Walford because it opened up yet another avenue for life extension. Hypothermia was unworkable for humans, caloric restriction unappetizing to most, but if it were possible to induce higher repair levels without introducing more errors into the system, then life prolongation might be achieved painlessly. Of course, this would depend upon whether DNA repair was fundamental to the aging process. And that would not be proven until someone showed that increasing DNA repair could push the life span of an organism well beyond its set limit. By the time Walford had completed his DNA repair study, that had already been accomplished.

Chapter Six

"Life Extension Is In"

Joan Smith-Sonneborn was stumped. Alone in her office, she moved aside the old Diet Pepsi bottles, piles of manuscripts, journals, and reprints, and spread out the data sheets. Walking to the front of her desk, where the plaque "A neat desk is a sign of a sick mind" greeted all visitors, she stared at the numbers upside down. They made just about as much sense this way. Involuntarily, she glanced at the large photograph of Tracy Sonneborn, her former mentor at Indiana University, talking with great expression, his hands in blurry movement. He had discovered that the microscopic, single-celled paramecia were actually mortal and aged like multicellular organisms. Now it was up to her to explore the implications of this work for aging and longevity of human cells.

The problem was obvious. She was bombarding the paramecia with ultraviolet light, which was supposed to shorten their life span. Then the plan was to repeat the experiment, inducing DNA repair of the UV damage. If the theory was correct, the life span of the cells should return to normal. But the range of life spans for the UV-damaged cells was all over the place. Obviously some of the critters were able to repair their DNA without waiting for her intervention, while others were not. And until she started getting consistent life spans, she couldn't proceed with the experiment.

To make matters worse, she also had to answer to Ron Hart, who had suggested the experiment more than a year ago at the January 1976 Gordon Research Conference on Aging at Santa Barbara. Every time they talked on the phone, she had to tell him, "I can't do it." Although he'd always say something encouraging, she could still feel his disappointment. Now it was practically Gordon Conference time again. Hart in his usual way would come striding over, give her a big kiss, talk nonstop about his latest projects, and then, inevitably, ask how things were going. She had to come up with something.

Her mother named her for Joan of Arc, believing she was destined for greatness. Half German, half Irish, Smith-Sonneborn has always felt torn between opposing forces—the pursuit of learning and the pursuit of pleasure; hedonism and stoicism; the need to work all night and the wish to dance till dawn. The necessity of choosing between them was apparent by the time she was thirteen. In her freshman year at her high school in upstate New York, two upcoming events attracted her—the science fair and the cheerleader trials. She signed up for cheerleading practice and at the same time sent away for a packet of information about an experiment on fruit flies. As fate would have it, the scientific material arrived before pom-pom practice started. She began learning about the care and feeding of drosophila, acquired a hand-held UV lamp, and did her first experiments in genetic mutation. By the time spring rolled around, the cheerleading trials had been held without her, and she had won first prize in the science fair for the entire region.

Pushing her, encouraging her, nagging her was her mother. (Her father had died when she was three.) "She was a Jewish mother in every sense of the word, without being Jewish. She was absolutely insane and delightful," says Smith-Sonneborn. "And she had chutzpah."

Throughout her sophomore year she continued her fruit fly experiments, and, at the science fair that year, won a scholarship to the summer-student program in biology at the Jackson Laboratory in Bar Harbor, Maine.

Arriving at High Seas, the white Georgian mansion built by a sea captain for his bride, Joan felt she had stepped into a dream—the marble fireplaces, broad verandas, paneled ceilings were all set high on a bluff overlooking Frenchman's Bay. Here, with twenty-five students from across the country, she would spend the next three months.

They were a brilliant, fun-loving group, drawn from high schools and universities around the country, and among their number was Howard Temin, who would later win the Nobel Prize for his work in molecular biology. They ate together, shared household chores, collaborated on experiments, taught one another, and on Tuesday nights all turned out for softball. Alongside staff scientists at the Jackson Laboratory, they did hands-on science: tumor transplants, pseudopregnancy studies in mice, behavior studies in dogs. The work was arduous, and more satisfying than anything she had ever done.

In some ways her experience at High Seas and the Jackson Laboratory was to color forever her view of science. On one hand, it revealed the excitement, the enthusiasm, the sense of sharing that could come from working closely with like-minded colleagues. On the other, it ruined her completely for the kind of dry, desiccated, "academic" science found all to often in high school and college. Joan Smith found herself champing at the bit during her science classes in high school and at Bryn Mawr, while outside the classroom walls, biology was being dismantled and reassembled by molecular geneticists.

The attitudes toward science at Bryn Mawr seemed to her as medieval as its Gothic buildings. At the Jackson Lab the message was: "You are not too young to use your heads and be creative. You can do experiments. Let your full potential be expressed." At Bryn Mawr she was criticized for being "overly enthusiastic." Scientists were supposed to be detached, she was told. She was here to learn from scholars; later she could think for herself.

In her junior year, she learned that her mother had cancer. Dropping out of Bryn Mawr, she transferred to Russell Sage College in Troy, New York, and moved her mother to nearby Roswell Park Memorial Hospital, one of the finest cancer clinics in the country. There she witnessed the steep decline of this once dynamic and vigorous woman. She had been torn between going into medicine or doing research, but now pacing the hospital corridors, she thought, "My mother is dying, and the doctors with all their knowledge can do nothing. Doctors are technicians. They can only carry out orders from the front line, which is research. If I want to do anything, I have got to be on that line."

She returned to Bryn Mawr in her senior year, and Bob Connor, a professor who befriended her, told her, "A lot of the faculty don't like you. But I think you've got something. And I'm going to help you." He had gotten his graduate degree in biochemistry at Indiana University, a place where her "psyche would fit in very well." He introduced her to his former mentor, W. J. (Vim) Van Wagtendonk, who offered her a research assistantship and a chance to do studies on paramecia.

"When I went to Indiana University," says Smith-Sonneborn, "I was like a duck flapping its wings on dry land. They put me in the water and I swam."

Suddenly her enthusiasm was seen not as a sign of intellectual immaturity, but as the passion of the true scientist. Her questions were welcomed, her suggestions were considered, her opinions were sought. She was no longer a student, but a colleague.

Indiana University had long been a mecca for some of the country's leading biologists. In 1957, when Smith-Sonneborn arrived, the scientific giants on the faculty included H. J. Muller, the father of modern genetic mutation studies; Robert Briggs, a leader in developmental biology; and Tracy Sonneborn, a pioneer in paramecia genetics. No sooner did Joan hear Sonneborn talk to a small group of his students than she felt that she had to be one of them. She decided to do a dual program with both parameciologists as her mentors. From Sonneborn she learned not only science, but a way with students that she would later adopt as her own. "Tracy's students didn't love him," she says, "they adored him. It was his mind, his binding love of science and ideas, but, more than that, his ability to nurture the talent in each of his disciples. When he criticized us, he did it in a way that made us understand much more deeply. He tended us, watered us, and made us grow like flowers."

From the moment she looked through the microscope and saw the tiny, slipper-shaped paramecia surrounded by thousands of beating, hairlike cilia, deftly avoiding one another as they moved through the water, she was enchanted. Here, truly, was Blake's vision, except that the world was in a single drop of water rather than a grain of sand.

The amazing variety of microscopic shapes and forms has probably delighted researchers since Leuwenhoek first found that clear water teemed with life. In the early days of protozoology, most work in the field was confined to observation—describing and drawing new species. Anything beyond this was out of the question. The phylum of protozoa is so diverse and stretches out across such a vast distance of evolutionary time that comparing one species to another can be like comparing a fish to a man. In the twentieth century as biology became more mechanism oriented, the study of protozoa became even less appealing. They did not mate like fruit flies, and therefore had "no genetics." Nor were gerontologists interested. August Weismann had pointed out that multicellular organisms divided their cells between a germ line and a somatic line, with the former carrying on the generations. He believed the one-celled animals were comparable to the germ line and therefore immortal. L. L. Woodruff, an early worker in the field, confirmed this idea, even naming one species *Paramecia methuselah* after following the cells in culture for twenty-five years.

———

The modern history of one-celled protozoa both for biology and gerontology starts with the work of Tracy Sonneborn. In 1936, much to everyone's surprise, he showed that along with birds and bees, paramecia do it. In the microscopic version of sex, two cells swim together, establish a link between their half-moon-shaped gullets, and exchange their DNA, forming a new generation in the process.

In the early 1950s Sonneborn found that paramecia had a second reproduction trick up their sleeve that explained their seeming immortality and one of Woodruff's most puzzling observations. The older scientist had found that the doubling rates of paramecia would unaccountably vary. The cells would trundle along at their usual pace and then slow down for a day or two before resuming their regular rate of division. He viewed this depression in fission rates as a curiosity having little significance. But Sonneborn uncovered its true nature.

Just as Hayflick was to find later with human cells in tissue culture, he discovered that paramecia "age" and die out. Although it is difficult to think of an individual paramecium, since it is always dividing itself into two, the daughter cells are merely clones of the original one, an extension of it into space. The aging "clock" starts ticking from the time of fertilization of the parent cell, and each daughter cell of the clone keeps time along with it. Thus, if the original cell has a division potential of almost two hundred times, a cell that is formed after the hundredth fission has a division potential only half as long.

But paramecia have a sexual option that is not open to most animal life: They can do it all by themselves. The paramecium in effect splits itself into two sex cells, which each have half the number of the original set of chromosomes. Then it fuses these two cells together in the same way that a sperm and egg are fused together in higher animal reproduction. Sonneborn discovered that this process of autogamy, or self-fertilization, was what actually took place when the fission rate of the cells appeared to be slowing down. *Paramecia methuselah* was no more than a succession of clones that had undergone repeated autogamy.

Weismann and Woodruff had both been taken in by the tiny organism. Paramecia had far more in common with multicellular animals than they realized. Not only were they not immortal; they, too, carried within the confines of a single cell both a germ line and a somatic line. The germ line was contained in a tiny micronucleus and the somatic line in a larger macronucleus. The macronucleus controlled the cell's metabolic functions, while the micronucleus regulated division.

By isolating the cells, Sonneborn was able to tell a paramecium's "age." He would take a newborn cell—one that had just gone through mating or autogamy—place it in a depression tray, which looks something like an old-fashioned inkwell, and let it sit there. When he came into the lab twenty-four hours later, there would be sixteen cells in the tray, indicating that the cell had doubled four times. He then moved one of these cells into a second tray. Twenty-four hours later, there would be sixteen cells in the new tray, indicating four more doublings. The original cell was now eight divisions old. Day after day he would move one cell to a new tray, until one day he would look under the microscope and the tray was empty. That particular line of cells was now considered dead. The life span of a cell line was about 190 divisions. If, however, a cell went through autogamy or mating, then a cell line was born, with a new built-in life span of 190 divisions.

What Sonneborn established, in fact, was that the biological clock ticked as inexorably for these one-celled creatures as it did for man. Although through the process of autogamy, the paramecia could seemingly divide forever, this was like saying that the micronucleus, their germ line, could give rise to the next generation in the same way that the union of sperm and egg (our germ lines) gives rise to the next generation. "In that sense," says Joan Smith-Sonneborn, "they are immortal and we are immortal."

The paramecia also passed through three well-defined stages of life. First came immaturity, when they were not yet able to mate; second was the mature stage, when they were capable of mating; and third was senescence, when the probability that they could produce a viable offspring declined dramatically.

A year after Sonneborn discovered autogamy and the finite life span of paramecia, he made an important contribution to the somatic mutation theory of aging. The older the paramecia, as calculated by division time, the more mutations it accumulated. When he and his coworker Myrtle Schneller looked at "young" paramecia less than forty fissions old, there were no mutations. By the time the cells had reached the end of their life span, after almost two hundred fissions, their chromosomes were riddled with chromosomal damage.

Tracy Sonneborn had brought the study of paramecia out of the dark ages, where it was an "interesting curiosity," and placed it squarely in basic biology. The minute creatures had "genetics"; they could be crossed and mutated like fruit flies; they aged, reproduced, died. And having a life span of no more than forty days, the paramecia revealed their secrets in a very short time. At the same time, paramecia, like human cells, are *eucaryotes*, that is, containing a separate nucleus surrounded by a membrane. (Bacteria are *procaryotes* and do not have a walled-off nucleus.) The protozoa, according to Sonneborn, "represent the evolutionary link between the procaryote bacteria and multicellular organisms." What's more, paramecia interact with one another, something Herbert S. Jennings, Sonneborn's major professor at Johns Hopkins, had shown, just as nerve, endocrine, and other cells in our bodies do. As Smith-Sonneborn puts it: "When you find something that is the same between this unicellular organism and a multicellular one, you know you are onto something very basic. Paramecia tell you what the big things are."

When Sonneborn published his paper on "The Relation of Autogamy to Senescence and Rejuvenescence in *Paramecium aurelia*" in the *Journal of Protozoology* in 1954, the timing could not have been worse. Less than a year earlier, Watson and Crick had published their historic paper, and biology was off and running in the direction of DNA. Virus and bacteria became the model systems for the infant field of molecular biology, and interest in paramecia faded away.

By the time Joan Smith came to Indiana University in 1957, the campus was one of the few places where protozoology was still alive and well. The big story in Sonneborn's lab then was the "killer" paramecium. It appeared that not all paramecia were content to swim along peacefully, minding their own business. Certain strains preyed on other strains. Sonneborn named the aggressive ones "killers," and their victims "sensitives." The interesting thing was that when he mated the two kinds of paramecia, they did not obey the "rules" of Mendelian genetics. Since the cells had exchanged their DNA, both should have turned killers or both sensitives, depending upon which trait was dominant. Instead, the killers stayed killers and the sensitives remained sensitive. Paramecia can also be made to exchange their cytoplasm across a bridge that is formed between the two mating cells. When this occurred between a killer and a sensitive, all the cells turned into killers. There was only one explanation: The nucleus alone did not control inheritance; rather, it was a combination of both nucleus and the cytoplasm, which had to be exchanged during mating. Components from both the cytoplasm and the nucleus were required for the killer trait to be expressed.

This was not the first time that Sonneborn and his associate had turned up evidence that the expression of a physical trait required the dual action of nucleus and cytoplasm, but it met with the same intense resistance that the earlier research had. The concept that the nucleus alone did not determine the traits of the next cell generation contradicted principles of heredity that seemed inviolate. The nucleus, not the cytoplasm, contained the chromosomes, the genes, the DNA. Theoretically, nothing more should be required. Indeed, the idea that inheritance could be anything but a one-way street, that anything outside the nucleus could play a role, smacked of earlier, discredited, pre-Darwinian ideas of evolution.

The only way to convince the skeptics of a cytoplasmic factor was to isolate it. And one of Sonneborn's graduate students, Johnny Preer, did that. Observing that X-rays inactivate the killer trait, Preer calculated that the target of the radiation was large enough to be seen under the microscope. With great excitement, he flattened a killer paramecium, stained it, and looked under the scope. There was the most incredible sight—hundreds of minute particles. To his great relief, when he did the same procedure with a sensitive cell, he found nothing. These were named "kappa particles" and they were the first tangible proof that Sonneborn's theory that cytoplasm played a role in inheritance had been correct.

In subsequent experiments, Sonneborn found the kappa particles in the cytoplasm had to be transferred along with the kappa gene in the nucleus in order for the killer trait to make its appearance. If two cells exchanged their DNA but not their cytoplasm, so that only the gene was passed on, the killer trait was not expressed.

In the face of such overwhelming evidence, the scientific community gave way to Sonneborn's contention that the cytoplasm was involved in heredity, but, for the most part, they tried to circumscribe its importance. Although this might be true for paramecia, surely it was not applicable to higher life forms. But for Joan Smith, who was given the task of characterizing and purifying the kappa particle for her Ph.D. thesis, viewing inheritance as a kind of contract between the nucleus and the cytoplasm became second nature and was to have a profound effect on her thinking about aging, longevity, and immortality.

One day toward the end of her stay at Indiana, looking out the window of the lab, she saw a tall young man approaching, encumbered with luggage. "There's the man I'm going to marry," she mused. It was David Sonneborn, returning home for Christmas vacation from Brandeis University. Since Smith had expressed an interest in postdoc work with molecular biologist Julie Marmur at Brandeis, Tracy urged her to speak to his son. She did and, by the end of the afternoon, made up her mind to go. By the following June, she had finished her thesis and had returned to Indiana to get her doctorate and marry David Sonneborn.

After a two-year sojourn at Berkeley, where she did postdoctoral work in bacterial genetics with Nobel Prize–winning physicist Don Glaser, the couple went to the University of Wisconsin, where David Sonneborn had been offered a faculty position.

At Wisconsin she entered the blackest period of her life. She had hoped to do research and teach there, but nepotism rules on the campus forbade hiring of both mates in the same department. Although she was hired as a research associate in someone else's laboratory, the only way she could teach was on a volunteer basis. Her opinions were not taken seriously, her comments were ignored. Despite the obstacles, she was able to continue doing research. The head of the laboratory allowed her to hire students and write grant proposals. But because she wasn't a faculty member, she couldn't put her name on a proposal as principal investigator, even if she was the sole author. "Women are still doing this," she says. "I know how it feels. It feels like giving up a baby for adoption."

With her self-confidence at an all-time low, she experienced a stress of a completely different kind: the birth of her first son, Mark. "I loved having children," she says. "I loved everything about it, the way my body felt. The thing that attracts me to science is that it's an outlet for creativity. And there's nothing more creative than having a child. And yet, my drive in science was also strong. It was constant conflict: Do I leave the baby and go into the laboratory or do I stay home and let the science go?"

Two years later when her second son, Matthew, was born, and she was trying to devote herself equally to the care of her children and her science, she started having what seemed like recurrent flu episodes. One day David Sonneborn came home late from the laboratory and found her burning with fever and writhing in pain. He took her to the hospital, where the doctors discovered that she had an inflamed gallbladder.

That crisis, in which she was convinced she was going to die, proved to be a turning point. Once she had recovered, she began exercising three days a week and slowly reclaimed her old self—in mind, body, and energy level. It was then, in the late 1960s, that she began her first experiment in aging.

With Tracy Sonneborn, she had been content, even eager, to follow his bent and do basic science, wallowing, as she put it, in asking questions and getting answers. This was partly a reaction to her mother's death, a turning away from anything to do with doctors and disease. But after the grief and pain and guilt she had felt over her failure to save her mother had abated, she felt ready to tackle death itself.

She began by thinking about a puzzling characteristic of paramecia that had been noted by Richard Kimball, a pioneer in mutagenesis assays—laboratory techniques for measuring the rate of a mutation in a cell. Unlike most life forms, he had found that paramecia seemed virtually immune to X-rays, absorbing huge doses and just swimming away. Scientists abhor anomalies. Why, Smith-Sonneborn asked herself over and over, didn't the X-rays kill the paramecia? Why didn't they shorten their life span? It came to her in a word: repair. There were no mutations because the X-ray damage had been repaired. Aging isn't just damage and it isn't just repair; it's the *balance* between the two that is going to determine the outcome. Then she stopped and thought, okay, "Now how do I test this?" She didn't have much experience working with X-rays, but she knew a great deal about UV light.

The next day she strode into the laboratory and announced to her little group that she was starting a new experiment. They would UV-irradiate the paramecia and see what happens to mutation and repair as the cells age. She had come full circle from her high-school days, using UV light to induce DNA damage and then doing mutagenesis assays, only the paramecia had replaced the drosophila.

In the experiment she looked at several variables: the age of the cells, dose of UV, and two kinds of UV repair systems used by the paramecia—excision repair, and photoreactivation. By counting the number of cells that survived after UV-irradiation, she found that as the cells aged they became increasingly sensitive to high doses. On the other hand, their ability to repair damage declined. This was far more dramatic with excision repair, which decreased as the cells aged, at all doses tested. Photoreactivation repair remained stable for a long time in older cells but then fell off abruptly at the advanced age of 140 fissions. Just as she had theorized, aging was related to both damage and repair, and how well a cell handled damage appeared to hinge on the balance between the twin forces of destruction and reconstruction.

This study, she realized, could launch her entry into the field. She wanted that paper published more than anything in the world. But Walter Plaut, whose laboratory she was using, was on sabbatical in Chile, in an area rendered incommunicable by an earthquake, and she required his permission before she could send the manuscript out. Finally, with the help of a ham-radio operator, she tracked him down. Over the crackling noise of the short-wave transmission, she got permission to appear as the sole author.

The results of her study, Smith-Sonneborn noted in *Radiation Research*, suggested a possible explanation for Kimball's results. His failure to induce a shortened life span in X-irradiated paramecia may have been a reflection of the highly efficient repair system in young cells. But far more important was the implication for aging. If paramecia bore any relation to higher-order cells such as those in our own bodies, then it appeared that DNA repair had a significant role to play in aging. In April 1971, several years before experiments by Ron Hart and Dick Setlow were to bear her out, she wrote, "The prediction that aging is correlated with loss in the capacity to repair DNA is consistent with the data. According to this model, senescence then, or the increased probability of cell death after division would be correlated with the time when the DNA damage present exceeds the capacity of the cells to repair this damage."

In 1971 she went to her first real meeting in aging. It was ostensibly a National Institute on Aging conference in tissue culture given by the Jones Science Center in Lake Placid, New York, but for many people who attended, it launched the true beginning of the gerontology community. If disaster is a sure-fire method for promoting camaraderie, the conference could not have gotten off to a better start. Upon arrival, the participants found the accommodations appalling. They voted to go to a nearby hotel, share rooms, and prepare all their own meals. Soon they became a kind of commune, cooking, eating, sailing, partying, and always talking, talking, talking. The friendships that sprang up that week were to remain throughout the years.

Here for the first time, she had a chance to test the reactions of her fellow scientists toward using protozoa as a model system for cellular aging. They were mostly negative. In the whole group, only Hayflick seemed to grasp what she was saying, although he, too, was openly skeptical of the relevance of paramecia for human cells. Still, the parallels between his work and that of Tracy Sonneborn's were striking. As Sonneborn had shown that paramecia had a finite life span, Hayflick had revealed the life and death of human cells. Both had pioneered in systems that looked at individual cells. "Hayflick broke the ice by saying that his model system of cellular aging was relevant to aging of the whole organism. So he was also paving the way for the model system of protozoa," she says. "Not intentionally, surely."

She had gone to the meeting to learn the tissue-culture technique in human cells, but she returned even more convinced of the superiority of her system as a model of aging. Paramecia probably mimic human cells in life more than human cells in culture do, she thought. With them she would have the best of both worlds, an *in vivo, in vitro* system.

If her fellow scientists failed to understand or appreciate her model system, she believed, it was only through ignorance. After all, protozoology and paramecia genetics had been pushed into the backwaters of science. Clearly her job was to educate, proselytize, and popularize the paramecia system as a model for human aging. A decade later, when Tracy Sonneborn was dying of cancer, she told me, her eyes brimming with tears, "Tracy is like my father and I am like his daughter. And what gives me chills is that he was out there publishing, talking twenty-five years ago, but people weren't ready to receive it. And now when its time has come, he can't do it any more. I am one person who can. So, you see, *I am part of Tracy's immortality.*"

In 1971 Smith-Sonneborn, who was now divorced, hired a moving van and, with her two young boys, headed west for the University of Wyoming in Laramie. Ironically, Madison, Wisconsin, a hotbed of radical political activism in the 1960s, had been a source of oppression for her, and Laramie, a town celebrated for its macho-cowboy traditions, was the setting for her liberation. She unpacked the paramecia from her bag, acquired a dissecting microscope, bought test tubes, hung pictures on the wall, turned up the country-western music on her radio, and set Michael Klass, the graduate student she had brought from Wisconsin, to work. At first, it was only the two of them, but soon work-study students began wandering in "filling up the unoccupied space." Her department chairman, who was strongly supportive, hurried to supply the things she needed, and his wife, the victim of the university's nepotism rule that you cannot work directly for your husband, became her editor. And the work and the papers started to flow.

"I quickly developed an enormous affection for Wyoming," she says. "I really didn't have any colleagues then who had similar interests. If I had harebrained ideas, there was nobody around to tell me they were wrong. And so I would go forth in pursuit. I also found that if you stay active in research in a place like this, when you communicate with the rest of your colleagues, they're apt to think you're very creative. Because while you've been apart from them, they've all been talking to one another, and the kinds of things you're thinking about are not the sorts of things they're thinking about."

For these reasons, it was all the more surprising when, two years later, she went to a two-day workshop chaired by Hayflick at a marine-biology station in San Diego and found that someone was thinking along the very same lines. At first, she could not have been more bored. Again and again she would walk away from the endless talk and progression of slides onto a veranda. In the distance, hang gliders were soaring off cliffs over the majestic Pacific surf. Toward evening, she began to note that she was not alone, that every time she was out on the porch, someone else was there, too.

Pacing the terrace, Ron Hart had other things on his mind besides the meeting. He was waiting anxiously for a phone call to come in from his lab on the life-span-shortening effects of UV light on human cells. Pouring himself some coffee, he sat down at one of the tables and was soon joined by a very attractive young woman, who he realized had given that morning's talk on ultraviolet light and paramecia. As she recalls it, she opened the conversation by asking, "Why are you cutting the talks?"

"I don't think they're relevant."

"What do you think is relevant?" she asked, looking at him intensely. "DNA repair."

She flashed a radiant smile: "Oh, my God, that is music to my ears."

"You might as well forget about it, because nobody will listen," he said. "Nobody cares."

"Yeah," she said, echoing his tone. "We can make that one step worse. I work with paramecia and nobody cares about that either."

Partners in frustration, they immediately felt a kinship. That evening they went to dinner and talked for hours about aging, DNA mutation, and repair, with Smith-Sonneborn getting in an occasional word. Of that meeting she says: "Even though I had published a paper predicting a role for DNA repair in life span in 1971, he had so developed and expanded the notions of mutation and repair that I could never in any way claim to have developed this idea. My notions were still very naive. He really knew excision repair. He really knew strand-break repair. He really knew carcinogenesis and repair. Where I had the seeds of an idea even before he had published it, he had whole fields in bloom."

She left the meeting thinking how incredible it was that there was someone else who thought the same way. She did not see him again until the 1976 Gordon Conference on Aging in Santa Barbara, the one that would be remembered as the Renegade Repair Conference. Again, as self-exiles from the main talks, pacing and smoking outside the conference room, they picked up the thread of their conversation where they had left it over a year ago.

Hart began to tell her about a very interesting experiment he had done at Oak Ridge with Dick Setlow. Using a species of molly fish that reproduce asexually and are all genetically identical, they had removed tissue from one fish, UV-irradiated it, causing DNA damage, and transplanted the tissue into a recipient fish. All the fish that received the irradiated, DNA-damaged tissue developed cancer. They then irradiated the tissue of a second group of fish, but this time provided photoreactivating light so that the DNA damage was repaired. None of the second group developed tumors. According to Hart, this was the first direct proof that cancer was induced by DNA damage, that a particular form of DNA damage was responsible for UV-light-induced cancers, and that DNA repair of UV damage could prevent the malignant outcome.

Could she, he wondered, carry out a similar experiment with her paramecia, where she would treat them with ultraviolet light, shorten their life span, and then photoreactivate and bring them back to normal? If she could show this, it would make the case for DNA damage in aging and life span.

She told him about the experiment she had done in 1971 and, as Smith-Sonneborn recalls, Hart began telling everyone in earshot about her "marvelous experiment." Listening to him describe it, she realized that he had jumped the gun. "Oh, no," she said. "You misunderstood. I didn't look at longevity."

He gave her a long, hard look and said, "Well, then, do it now."

"Okay," she agreed. "It sounds good and I'll try it."

Exhilarated, she returned to Laramie, and her lab geared up for a life-span experiment. In contrast to her 1971 experiment in which she just looked at cells at different ages, this was a massive effort requiring isolating single cells every day for forty days and checking to make sure that the paramecia hadn't sneaked through autogamy, which would start a new generation and reset the aging clock back to zero.

Since the experimental design was to examine the role of DNA damage and repair in life span, the first step was to pin down the life-shortening effects of UV light. A self-confessed "lab rat," she worked alongside her students, isolating cells, bombarding them with UV light, and wrapping the trays in tin foil so that no photoreactivating light could reach them. In the days that followed, the group fed the trays and moved one cell from each well into a fresh depression with food, noting, on the isolation sheet, every time there was no longer a living cell in a compartment. Each column represented a single cell followed in isolation from its birth, after mating, until its death. The number of divisions it had passed through in this time was its life span.

It had taken much money and many man-hours to do just this part of the experiment, and now as Smith-Sonneborn sat at her desk staring glumly at the isolation sheets from all the groups tested, both experimental and control, she wondered if it had been worth it. The life spans of the UV-irradiated groups were so variable that they could not be significantly distinguished from the control group. Obviously, in spite of their precautions, the cells were repairing their DNA. If the experiment was to work, she had to find some way to prevent repair. And she had better do it damn soon. It was over a year and a half since Hart had first suggested the experiment, and she couldn't bear facing him at the next Gordon Conference without any results.

"When in doubt," she thought, "go back to the beginning." Going to her files, she pulled out the original paper by Richard Kimball, on induction of mutations in paramecia, that had stimulated her five years earlier. Thunderstruck, she realized that buried amidst the prosaic details of "materials and methods" was the answer. The cells, he wrote, were most refractory to repair at the point where they started to synthesize DNA. And that, she knew from her own studies, was one-and-a-half hours after cell division. "That's it! That's it," she yelled in triumph. "I just have to irradiate them at that time and then I'll keep them in the dark. They won't be able to photoreactivate and they won't be able to do excision repair. They'll be stuck with the damage. Now I'll get my life span."

By the time she went to the Gordon Conference, she knew she had the answer. Her heart was pounding so hard in anticipation of telling Hart that she was certain he could hear it across the room. He greeted her warmly and then turned to the woman sitting next to him, Audrey Muggleton-Harris, a fellow protozoologist. "Audrey," he said, putting his arm around her shoulders, "there's an experiment you could do with your amoebae." In front of Smith-Sonneborn, he proceeded to outline *her experiment*. She watched him in anger and disbelief, feeling her face redden. "I'll show you, you dirty bastard," she thought, and walked out of the room without saying a word.

Hart's staged scene had the intended effect. Although he apologized that evening, Smith-Sonneborn spent the night plotting out the next steps in her experiment. By the time she returned home, she knew how to proceed.

Three months after the Gordon Conference, she called Hart. For some minutes, she went through the inevitable small talk and then, without missing a beat, said: "By the way, I got some results on life span and the effects of UV and photoreactivation [PR]."

"Really?" he said, his voice rising in excitement. "What are they?"

"Guess what? Sure enough, UV shortened life span and photoreactivation brought them back to normal, just like we predicted. But then something else very weird is going on."

"My God. What's that?"

"The group that got ultraviolet light and photoreactivation is living *longer* than the control group."

"Joan, I'm taking you up on your offer to give a seminar at the university."

"Stay where you are. It could be just a fluke. It's only the first experiment. I know I got the system working. And it sure looks promising. But now I've got to do all kinds of controls. I have to get genetically marked cells, and it's going to be a long haul. So just hang in there. But I know we've got something going."

Three weeks later, Hart flew to Laramie. Although progress outdoors was at a snail's pace, inside Smith-Sonneborn's lab life proceeded as usual. Surveying the coffee-cup litter, the jean-clad students, the array of cartoons, photos, and posters on the walls, Hart sighed. "This is not a lab, Joan," he said. "It's a home." Finally, amidst many interruptions by her students and Hart's own schedule, they managed to review the data together. "It looks really good," he told her. "But I want you to plot it another way." Rapidly he drew a graph. She should put her percent survival along the vertical axis and her fission age along the horizontal axis, "and then we'll see what's happening," he said.

It was not until Hart had gone home and her students had left for Christmas vacation that she finally had a chance to graph the results of her second experiment. She had UV-irradiated the cells, allowed them to photoreactivate, and then put them through a second cycle of irradiation and repair. Her eyes traced the invisible line connecting the dots on the graphs and she began to quiver.

As Roy Walford likes to point out, to say that you have accelerated aging because you reduced the life span is invalid. If this were true, hitting an animal over the head could be considered an aging mechanism. But accomplishing the opposite is unassailable. Therefore, he says, the key experiment in aging to is to extend the life span.

If ever there was a key experiment, this was it. The treated group lived more than sixty days as compared with the control group's life span of forty days, an amazing 50 percent extension of life span. The greatest effect was at the tail end of life, which was stretched out by a whopping 296 percent. Although people have been looking for elixirs of life since biblical times, very few maximum life extenders have been found. Drastic diet restriction is one. Antioxidants, as Denham Harman and others have shown, will extend life expectancy—that is, a greater percentage of a population will live out a normal life span—but not the maximum life span, the age of the oldest survivor. And now the induction of greater DNA repair appeared to be a third, extending both mean and maximum survival. On the most profound level, the last approach was the most attractive because it said that the means for preventing disease, maintaining health, and prolonging life lie within each and every one of us.

Here she was alone with this knowledge. There was no one to share it with. Her lab people had dispersed for the Christmas vacation and Hart was back in Ohio. She went into the bedroom where her two young sons were playing, and brought them into her room. She said, "I want to show you the most exciting thing in the world. Look at how that line is extended out. My God, have you ever seen anything like it?"

The boys looked at her as though she had gone mad, mumbled something about how it was nice, and returned to their game. For one insane moment she thought of calling every student and getting them to return at once. And then she called Hart: "I plotted the data the way you told me to. And you would die. The cells that got two treatments of UV and PR are living 50 percent longer than the controls." Her voice was low, but throbbing with excitement. "Life extension is in. It's so clear."

Eight months later, in August 1978, after she and her staff had worked double time in repeating it several times and setting up rigorous controls with genetically marked cells, she was ready to publish. By now she had worked out a scenario to explain the unexpected increase in life span. DNA damage from UV light, she believed, stimulated a reserve repair system. But at the same time, she had provided the paramecium with photoreactivating light so that it now had at its disposal both the reserve repair system and photoreactivation—far more than it needed to take care of the UV-induced dimers. Nature being a tidy housewife, the cell put the excess repair enzymes to work, cleaning up the damage that had accumulated in the DNA with age.

She likened what was happening to a ship sending out a distress signal. Another ship, hearing the SOS signal, starts out to help the ship in danger. By the time it arrives, it finds that the first ship has already repaired the problem, so the captain of the second ship says, "While we're here, do you have any other problems we can help you with?" The rescue crew then patches up all the accumulated wear and tear on the first vessel until it is far better off than it was before the emergency.

She based this comparison on the fact that dramatic increases in life span were seen only in aged cells. In addition, the UV/PR treatment appeared to have a rejuvenating effect so that treated aged cells acted like much younger cells in their resistance to high doses of UV radiation.

The impact of these observations was not lost on Smith-Sonneborn. She believed in her system. As Tracy had always told her, the important things are conserved throughout evolution, from one-celled protozoa to sixty-trillion-cell human beings. So the lessons were that inevitable accumulations of damage to the cell might be erased; that cancer, heart disease, and other age-associated diseases might be prevented or delayed; that aging might not only be arrested but be reversed.

At Smith-Sonneborn's invitation, Jim Trosko gave a lecture at the University of Wyoming in 1979. His idea that errors in repair were the price we paid for species survival made her jump to her feet. If this were the case, he contended, if errors in DNA were built into the system to ensure that mutations would take place and evolution could proceed, then try as we might, we may never be able to do anything about cancer, aging, and death. "I do not accept the inevitability of cancer, aging, and death!" she yelled. Perhaps there was a sound scientific case to be made for the certainty of mortality, but until all the facts were in, she was holding out for life extension stretched to its very limit.

Even the conclusion to her paper "DNA Repair and Longevity Assurance in *Paramecium tetraurelia*" (*Science*, March 16, 1979) contained an affirmation and enthusiasm that would have made her Bryn Mawr teachers blanch. "Accordingly, age damage can be reversed or delayed," she wrote. "An understanding of the molecular mechanisms underlying this biological result could illuminate other means to activate the repair system. If higher organisms have maintained a reserve repair capacity, activation should lead to reduction in mutagenesis and degenerative diseases in higher organisms.

The results provide a new approach for regulation and reduction of mutation frequency: the activation of a reserve repair or protection process."

Her first formal presentation was at the Japanese Medical Association in Japan. The reception could not have been better, but for Smith-Sonneborn, the true test would come at the January 1979 Gordon Research Conference.

Chapter Seven

Bringing It All Together

It was January 1979. In Laramie, Wyoming, Joan Smith-Sonneborn was keenly anticipating sharing with her colleagues the incredible results of her life-extension experiment; in Baltimore, Dick Cutler was looking forward, with the same excitement, to presenting his evidence that an enzyme, superoxide dismutase, was a potential regulator of life span; in Columbus, Ohio, Ron Hart was putting together a chart that would illustrate the various processes that protected and repaired DNA, and the consequences to the cell if these mechanisms failed; in Los Angeles, Roy Walford was strengthening his earlier work linking DNA repair, life span, and the immune function; in Downers Grove, Illinois, George Sacher was preparing an overview of the evolution of longevity; and in Philadelphia, Arthur Schwartz was getting ready to take the conference by surprise.

Some would call the 1979 Gordon Conference on Aging the worst they had ever attended, while others would remember it as the culmination of the most exciting work in gerontology in the past decade. Those who didn't like it criticized the papers as "preliminary, speculative, theoretical"; those who liked it said that was what Gordon Conferences were all about. It was designed to bring together all the information on the molecular and cell biology of aging that had been generated in various labs, but it ended by further dividing the gerontological community.

Chairman of the conference was a large, athletic-looking, genial man, George Martin. An M.D.-pathologist and a genetic researcher at the University of Washington in Seattle, Martin studies aging in both microcosm and macrocosm, from cells in culture to the whole organism. One aspect of his work deals with what nature's experiments can tell us about the aging process.

A number of diseases due to genetic defects do not express their full ef-

129

fects at birth. Called abiotrophic, or delayed-onset disorders, they include Down's syndrome, in which virtually all the victims have senile dementia by their forties; progeria, whose bald and wizened sufferers look like octogenarians by the time they reach puberty; and Werner's syndrome, where a single gene mutation can cause an afflicted teenager to have loss and graying of hair, cataracts, skin atrophy, osteoporosis, hardening of the arteries, diabetes, and tumors of the connective tissue. "Aging itself," Martin points out, "is an abiotrophic degenerative disorder."

The question that Martin posed was, How many of these genetically based diseases had traits that could be characterized as accelerated aging? Since these were caused by mutations either on the level of a single gene or involving an entire chromosome, he might be able to make a crude estimate of how many genes were involved in senescence.

To carry out his analysis, he used a bible for students of human genetics, Victor McKusick's catalog *Mendelian Inheritance in Man,* which is based on a computer registry of human genetic disorders. The fourth edition, published in 1975, listed 2,336 genetic disorders. Of these, Martin found that 162, or 6.9 percent, showed age-related traits. "If one considers that the upper limit of genetic loci is 100,000 genes, that is, genes that carry information which is transcribed into RNA—there's a lot more DNA than there are known genes—then that means about 6,900 different genes may be playing a role in modulating the aging rate," he said. Although the prospect of dealing with almost 7,000 "aging" genes seems intimidating, Martin believes that only about 70 major genes may be *"regularly* important in modulating the rate of aging," a number far closer to that estimated by Cutler and Sacher. Like them, Martin also speculates that the genes involved are of a regulatory nature; that is, instead of directly coding for the production of proteins and enzymes, they control how much of a gene product is produced.

A fascinating aspect of his work is that there is some evidence that the cells of people with these diseases age faster. In Martin's own lab, he had found that cells from patients with Werner's go through many fewer divisions in tissue culture than do cells from normal people. This appears to be also true of people with Down's and progeria, although the reports on these syndromes from various labs have been conflicting.

The excitement was palpable as the participants in the 1979 Gordon Conference greeted each other. They had come out of the closet, so to speak. At the very same spot where the Renegade Repair Conference had been held behind closed doors, the ideas that had been expressed in embryonic form on DNA repair and gene expression and differentiation were now commanding attention. Instead of hypotheses tossed around like tufts of milkweed, there were data, evidence, experimental results. For five days speaker after speaker presented findings, many of them for the first time, that tended to strongly support a molecular view of aging.

The time had come, Martin believed, to see how all these disparate pieces of research fit together. Hart attempted to do just that on the second day. For several years he had been working on a schematic model that would depict the multistep nature of aging. He had worked out the first one several years earlier with Jim Trosko during his stay at OSU. Next he had constructed a more elaborate model with his student, Doug Brash, and finally, he had created a third-generation schematogram incorporating all the work that had been done up to that time.

In his model, Hart attempted to place DNA, aging, and longevity in a systems-theory framework. In this view, the human body, like any technologically advanced machine, can be viewed as an interlocking system of component parts. The components form an entity that is greater than the sum of its parts. For instance, a speaker, an amplifier, a receiver, and turntable can do little by themselves, but together they make music. Components are composed of interconnected parts, or subcomponents, like the woofers and tweeters of the speaker. The components of our body are our organ systems, such as the circulatory, respiratory, excretory, and digestive systems. These in turn are composed of organs, which consist of tissues, which are a collection of cells, which are made of molecules, that are formed of atoms. Each of these levels can be viewed as a subcomponent of the overall system or as a system in itself. Unlike a stereo system, however, the parts of a living system form a hierarchy of levels of systems and components: atom, molecule, cell, tissue, organ, organ system, organism. Aging, like an invading army laying siege to a city, can ravage the system on any level up and down the hierarchy.

Gordon Conferences enjoy immunity from the press, but the gist of Hart's talk, as revealed in later public statements, was as follows:

Man is composed, as Weismann noted, of germ and soma, the cells that carry the seeds of the next generation, and the cells of the rest of the body. All the cells are subject to aging and DNA damage. DNA damage comes both from the outside environment and from within the body: from free radicals formed during the process of oxygen metabolism; ionizing radiation; ultraviolet light; chemicals both man-made and natural; plants such as the aflatoxin-producing fungus; and even internal body temperature—one thousand damage sites per cell per day has been estimated as the cost of living at 98.6 degrees Fahrenheit. Many of these agents, such as ultraviolet light and ionizing radiation, have been shown to shorten life span, accelerate aging, and cause cancer.

So ubiquitous is the occurrence of DNA damage that had we no defenses against it, we would be riddled with cancer in our infancy. Using separate approaches, Richard Peto of Cambridge University, and Sacher and Hart estimated the chances of a spontaneous tumor arising in the cells of various species of mammals over their lifetime. The risk increased several thousand-fold as one progressed from the tiny, short-lived shrew to man. In other words, we have five thousand times more cells than a mouse and live fifty times longer. Therefore, the risk of damage to each of our cells over our lifetime is $50 \times 5,000$, or $250,000$ times greater for us than for a mouse. If we had no more protection than a mouse, we would have a tumor shortly after birth. But fortunately for us, nature is not a socialist, for as the species evolved, so did the means for preserving and maintaining our capital—the genetic material.

DNA has been likened to a chemical blueprint, a memory bank, a master plan, the library of the genes, a genetic program, but none of these terms begins to do it justice. "It is not just an information-containing molecule," notes Hart. "It's an information-containing molecule that produces its own enzymes for maintaining its own integrity." In other words, it not only codes for the proteins, enzymes, and hormones we need to function; it makes the enzymes that guard, protect, and repair that code. In the cellular society, it is the executive, legislative, and judicial branches rolled into one.

As with any system involved with its own security and maintenance, the first level of protection is prevention. It must maintain vigilance against attack at all times. To protect itself, the cell produces its own antioxidant enzymes, which, like garbage collectors, "scavenge" the toxic by-products of oxygen radicals. One of these scavenging enzymes is superoxide dismutase, which Dick Cutler had now shown was related to the life span of various mammalian species. Others were the enzymes involved in the metabolism of chemical compounds. Schwartz had shown that the ability to break down chemicals in a manner that did not release harmful end products that bound to the DNA also correlated with life span.

If an agent broke through the defenses and attacked the DNA, the cell had highly efficient means for dealing with the damage. There are many different kinds of damage, such as thymine dimers, breaks in the DNA strands, and gaps in the base sequences. At the same time, there are many repair processes to deal with each form of damage. Hart and Setlow had shown that with at least one form of DNA repair, the better the ability of a species to remove DNA damage, the longer its life span.

Most of the time, the repair is error free. The damage is removed, the DNA is restored, and the threat to the cell is over. But at least one form of repair is error prone. In certain situations, it appears that, faced with a choice between extinction and mutation, the cell chooses the latter. Called SOS repair because it represents an emergency response for the cell, it has been found only in bacteria, but there is some evidence that it might occur in human cells as well. Even without SOS repair, mistakes can spontaneously occur.

The other problem is one of timing. Say you have a railroad maintenance crew that is racing to repair the track before the train rolls over it. What happens if the crew loses the race? Is the train derailed? Lawrence Loeb of Washington State University has been considering this question. What happens to the fidelity of the genetic material when damage that is unrepaired or misrepaired is replicated? In laboratory experiments, he found that with some types of damage, the repair polymerases simply continue copying past the damage, randomly putting in the wrong bases as they go. This would be comparable to the railroad crew's failing to match up the ties correctly as they rushed through their job. There are some grounds for believing that mutations could accumulate until the message in the DNA becomes garbled. As with marriage, the consequences of infidelity could be ruinous.

Once the error in the DNA has been passed on in cell division, it becomes fixed in the genetic message. It is now a mutation, and the repair enzymes no longer recognize it. Mutations may be silent or expressed. Since less than 6 percent of the DNA in a given cell is actively involved in making gene products, the vast majority of mutations will not be expressed. But a silent mutation can be a time bomb for the cells. It can go off, for example, when cells are stimulated to divide during wound healing. Silent mutations that accumulate in the egg cell and are turned on during fertilization may be partly responsible for the escalation in birth defects and for spontaneous abortions as maternal age rises.

Mutations are very, very rare events but they can be promoted. Cancer is believed to be a clonogenic disease, the result of a mutation propagated many times over. The same thing may be true of heart disease. Seattle researcher Earl Benditt has evidence suggesting that arteriosclerotic plaques, the stigmata of the aging population in developed countries, may result from the proliferation of a single mutated cell.

If a mutation occurs in a structural gene—that is, one which codes for a particular product—the result is an altered protein. If it occurs in a regulatory gene, which oversees the operation of a structural gene, the outcome may be even more detrimental to the cell. Genes are like on-off signals. When a gene is turned on, the protein it codes for is synthesized; when it is repressed, or turned off, the protein is no longer made. A mutation in a regulatory gene may turn on a gene repressed since the time of embryonic development, causing the manufacture of an inappropriate protein, or it may turn off a gene that codes for a substance needed by the cell. The derepression of certain genes has been found in both cancer and aging cells.

The effect of damage on a cell probably depends upon whether or not it is mitotic or postmitotic, that is, dividing or nondividing. Mitotic cells include blood, skin, the lining of the intestine. Postmitotic cells include those that never divide, such as nerve cells, or that do so very slowly or under certain conditions, such as cells of the liver, heart, and smooth muscle. In the postmitotic, or nondividing cell, mutations, which are by definition changes in the genetic code that are passed on to the daughter cell, cannot occur. But DNA damage can and does build up over time. There are forms of DNA damage that do not change the genetic code, per se, but can attach themselves to the DNA molecule and alter gene expression, affecting which genes turn off and which turn on.

Once the unrepaired damage has become fixed in the DNA, the body still has ways of dealing with it. One of these ways is through the system of hormones. Hormones are the chemical messengers of the body, providing communication between cells and organ systems. The DNA codes for hormones, but they, in turn, can affect the DNA. During embryological development, hormones signal genes when to turn on and when to turn off. As the embryo moves through the various stages of organ and limb development, cells become differentiated, die, or reproduce in response to hormonal cues. Later on in the life cycle, particularly during puberty and menopause, hormonal changes cause widespread effects. For instance, they may unmask silent mutations, allowing them to become expressed. Such events may help explain the statistical upsurge in cancers that occur during these life stages.

Hormones, it appears, may also have beneficial effects on life span. Vincent Cristofalo of the Wistar Institute in Philadelphia has shown that certain hormones can to some extent push out the Hayflick limit. When he gave hydrocortisone and related hormones to humans cells in culture, they went through 70 population doublings rather than the usual average of 50, an extension of about 40 percent. This means that if DNA damage is responsible for stopping DNA replication, then hormones can overcome this effect at least for a limited time. However, Hart warns, since some hormones enhance the probability of cancer, the price of extending cell division may be to increase the production of mutations.

Even if the damaging agent is not stopped before it can attack the DNA, or is not repaired or is misrepaired, or is passed on during cell replication, and is expressed or promoted in response to a hormone, the body has still another weapon at its disposal—the immune defense system. According to the theory of immune surveillance developed by Lewis Thomas and F. Macfarlane Burnet, the body seeks out and destroys cancerous cells. There is some indication that the DNA of immune cells might be less able to repair than other cells of the body. The aging of the immune system—the body's primary defense against disease—might then contribute to overall aging.

Walford demonstrated a link between the immune system, repair capability, and life span in closely related strains of mice that differed only in the genes of the major histocompatibility complex. Longer-lived strains had fewer tumors, less autoimmune disease, better-functioning immune systems, and better repair than the shorter-lived strains.

Finally, somewhat along the lines of George Martin's human syndromes of accelerated aging, there were genetic disorders, linked to defects in DNA repair, that showed some aspects of speeded-up senescence. About half a dozen of these have been identified, including xeroderma pigmentosum, and Down's syndrome. Repair deficiency has also been linked to cancer, birth defects, high blood pressure, neurological malfunctioning, lymphatic leukemia, arthritis, and arteriosclerosis.

"Now you see how this is all starting to come together," says Hart. "The inability to repair genetic damage appears to be correlated with carcinogenesis, life span, tendency to autoimmune disease, tendency to arthritis, another age-related disease, and perhaps even with arteriosclerosis."

But, Hart emphasizes, "No single syndrome uniformly and proportionately mimics all aspects of aging, and no single damaging agent uniformly and proportionately brings forth in time all facets of aging." What this means is that no single form of genetic damage is the sole cause of aging, but, rather, that aging "is the summation, the total ability of all these systems operating in concert with one another, maintaining the longevity assurance of a system, the stability of a system."

The decrements in aging may be very small but, like rips in a seam, they add up until one day the fabric is in tatters. Richard Adelman of Temple University in Philadelphia, for example, has shown that the time it takes the body to release insulin in response to sugar goes up with age. Between the gene that codes for insulin and the manufacture of this hormone, dozens of enzymes must come into play. Slight alterations in any one of these steps—and different enzymes may be affected in different people—are enough to slow production down. In the same way, the rate of response of an immune cell to a bacterial toxin, or the firing of a neuron in response to a signal, declines. As different cells decline at different rates in different ways, stress builds up in the tissues and organs for which these cells are the building blocks. At some point, collapse is inevitable.

Weismann asked the question, How is it possible for a perfect germ cell to give rise to an imperfect soma? But, said Hart, the question can be turned around. Can an imperfect germ cell give rise to a perfect soma? The answer is, it can't. In the evolutionary scheme of things, a kind of balance must be struck between stability and change. If the germ cell is riddled with imperfections, the species will not survive. If the germ cell is perfect and impervious to mutation, the species will remain fixed for all time and will be ill-equipped to adapt to changes in its environment.

In other words, it appears that the needs of the individual and the needs of the species to survive may be at odds. From the individual human perspective, having a perfect repair system that maintains the DNA molecule in a pristine, unblemished state would be ideal, while for the survival of the species as a whole, a totally efficient repair system would be a disaster. "If, indeed, aging and various degenerative disease processes relate back to alterations in the ability of a system to maintain the homeostasis of its information molecule," says Hart, "and if that ability is unstable by necessity because it is required for evolution within the species, the dilemma of the soma may be the solution of the germ cell.

"It seems to me," Hart concluded at the conference, "that we in the late 1970s stand at essentially the same place in the understanding of degenerative diseases that Pasteur and Koch did a century ago in the understanding of infectious disease. As our forefathers looked at these microorganisms called bacteria and fungi, we the scientists of today view a whole different concept, the idea that changes in the information content and flow of a system may be related to degenerative disease processes. This whole idea of alterations in genetic information flow and content resulting in disease is just as radical as the notion of invisible germs causing man to run a high temperature. And as it took fifty years of accumulation of data before Koch and Pasteur could develop their conceptualized schemes, so it has taken us fifty years of understanding the data from pioneers such as H. J. Muller before we could start conceptualizing how the fidelity of DNA is maintained relative to aging and degenerative diseases. And as it took another twenty-five to fifty years to understand their control, indeed it may take us twenty-five to fifty years to control degenerative processes. But that is the way of science, and at least we can see that we have made phenomenal progress."

It was a stirring speech, and as Smith-Sonneborn was to say later: "Ron's systems approach was magnificent and people were very excited about it. But the sad part was that right after he spoke, Art Schwartz gave his stuff. So that while Ron's speech was the culmination of his thinking about the beautiful interactions of repair at every level, this dark horse, Schwartz, got up and dropped a neutron bomb."

Schwartz is about the last man from whom one would expect surprises. Unassuming both in personality and physique, he tends to get lost among the more colorful, individualist, extroverted, aging researchers. Nor did the title of his speech, "Comparative Metabolic Activation of Chemical Carcinogens Producing DNA Damage Within the Mammals," indicate that it would be anything more than an elaboration of the work he had first presented three years earlier at the Gordon Conference in Santa Barbara. Everyone sat back expecting a continuation of the theme that had just been sounded in Hart's presentation. But like a man who has remained poker-faced through an intense gambling session, Schwartz produced a wild card with the most unlikely name—dehydroepiandrosterone (DHEA).

To most of the cell biologists and molecular biologists present, DHEA was far from a household word. It was, Schwartz admitted, an enigma even to those who worked with it. Although it was the largest steroid substance secreted by the adrenal gland in the body, nobody knew what it did, why it was there, or even if it was a hormone. By a combination of mistaken assumptions, serendipitous publications by other people, and his own foresight and intuition, he had managed to become the prince in the story of this Cinderella compound.

His interest in the substance had begun five years earlier, around the time he had started the study comparing life span and metabolic activation of carcinogens. At that point he was captivated by the idea that steroids, because they chemically resembled certain carcinogens, might compete with them for receptors on the cell surface. If they were successful competitors, they could protect the cell from the carcinogen. Casting about for a candidate with which to begin testing his idea, he began combing the literature and came across a most interesting study.

A group of London researchers, headed by R. D. Bulbrook of the Imperial Cancer Research Fund, started a prospective study in 1961 of five thousand healthy women on the island of Guernsey. Nine years later they had found that most of the women who developed breast cancer had abnormally low levels of DHEA in their urine, and in some cases the appearance of these low levels preceded the disease by nine years. Could it be that the reverse was true, Schwartz wondered, that high levels of DHEA protected against breast cancer? If so, this would be the first study he could think of that implied a possible protective role for a bodily substance in cancer. What better compound with which to start his experiment.

Ordinarily, if one adds powerful carcinogens like aflatoxin or DMBA to animal cells in culture, one sees a high rate of cell death, mutation, and transformation. But when Schwartz added DHEA along with one of these carcinogens, it protected the cells against all three of these effects. Schwartz's first reaction was shock. He and his coworkers could scarcely believe their own results. Was it really possible that he had guessed right, that steroids could prevent cancer?

He next tried some DHEA analogues, compounds that differed only slightly in molecular structure, but much to his surprise, none of them worked. It now seemed likely that he had been wrong about the idea that steroids protected the cell against cancer by competing with carcinogenic chemicals. It had to be something about DHEA in particular, and he had been lucky enough to stumble on the right compound. He turned up two very interesting pieces of data. One was that the amount of DHEA present in the body peaked around twenty-five to thirty years of age and then went down with the passing years until, at around age seventy, it was only about 5 percent to 10 percent of its peak value. The other thing he found sent him scurrying back to the laboratory.

Several investigators had shown that DHEA was a potent inhibitor of an enzyme called glucose 6 phosphate dehydrogenase (G6PDH). Clinically, the absence of this enzyme causes no problems except for an extreme sensitivity to the fava bean. But G6PDH is also the first enzyme in one of the two metabolic pathways, or series of breakdown steps, that the body employs to utilize glucose. Ordinarily, glucose is broken down in a chemical pathway that provides energy for the body's needs—the "energy-yielding pathways." But there is a second metabolic route for glucose, known as the "biosynthetic pathway," which is used in the manufacture of fatty acids as well as nucleic acids (RNA and DNA). If DHEA blocked G6PDH, then it blocked the primary enzyme in the pathway for making fat and new cells.

Schwartz put two and two together. One of the substances on this pathway was needed to activate carcinogenic compounds to their mutagenic and carcinogenic form. If DHEA inhibited a substance which could unleash the toxic potential of certain compounds, that could explain its antimutagenic and anticancer effect on the cells.

He tested his theory and it worked: DHEA was able to block the activation of two highly potent carcinogenic chemicals, DMBA and aflatoxin B. He published this finding in 1975, just about the same time he completed his study showing a correlation between life span and the metabolic activation of carcinogens. He was now almost certain that DHEA worked by preventing carcinogenic activation. If this were so, then perhaps DHEA might not only have an anticancer effect, but it might also be antiaging.

The problem was he had no idea how to test this in animals, the dosages to use, or even how it should be administered. But then good fortune, which seemed to be following him around, appeared in the guise of yet another paper; this was by Terence T. Yen, a biochemist at Eli Lilly and Company. Yen had made a most astounding discovery: DHEA had a profound antiobesity effect and it acted not in the usual way, by suppressing appetite, but by directly affecting the metabolism.

In his experiment, Yen used a mouse strain that carried a gene for obesity. Obese mice grow to twice the size of their normal counterparts. Like the fat woman who claims she eats like a bird, these mice attain their huge bulk by eating only little more than the average mouse. In some unknown way they are much more efficient at converting food into fat.

Generally, virtual starvation is required to get the weight of such corpulent mice down to normal levels. But when Yen gave them three injections of DHEA a week, he was able to prevent obesity without decreasing their food intake. And the effect was reversible. When he removed the steroid, they gained weight at the usual rate. The most probable explanation for the effect, he believed, was that the DHEA was pushing more of the glucose toward the energy-yielding pathway and away from the biosynthetic, fat-producing pathway. The DHEA was changing the metabolism and in doing so, provided a rationale for the fat woman with the birdlike appetite as well as for the lucky few who can feast without fear.

Schwartz could scarcely contain his excitement. Things were coalescing in ways he had never dreamed. As a cancer researcher, he immediately saw a connection between the antiobesity effect of DHEA reported by Yen and the anticancer effect he had found with DHEA. Among the most important experiments in the whole cancer literature, he believed, were ones conducted in the 1940s and 1950s that showed that food-restricted animals got far fewer cancers, including tumors of the breast, liver, and lung, and leukemia. Perhaps the same mechanism that worked to prevent cancer in underfed animals was operating in the DHEA-treated ones. As further proof, obese mice had a higher rate of cancer and developed it at a much younger age than mice of the same strain that did not have the obesity gene. Obesity in humans is also associated with higher rates of breast and uterine cancer. Finally, there was the tie-in with aging: Cancer was an age-related disease; food restriction extended life as well as protected against cancer; and his own study had shown a correlation between carcinogen activation, cancer, and life span.

After calling Yen and working out the details of DHEA treatment, he began his first *in vivo* experiments. Since Bulbrook's study had shown a link between DHEA levels and breast cancer, Schwartz chose to work with a strain of mice called C3H, in which 70 percent of the females have breast cancer by the time they reach sixteen months of age.

Eight months later, he knew he was onto something: The control mice "were getting cancer left and right," while there were no tumors in the DHEA-treated animals. But that wasn't the half of it. While the controls, who were now approaching one year, had graying and coarsening of hair, the coats of the treated animals were sleek and black. It was obvious to the most casual observer that they looked much younger. In fact, thought Schwartz, they looked exactly like mice that had been diet-restricted.

Now the question of what DHEA was doing in the body took on added mystery. Obviously, the prevention of carcinogen activation was not the answer here, because the mammary cancer in these animals was caused not by chemicals but by an inherited tumor virus. How on earth could DHEA be preventing a virally induced cancer?

A few months later, Schwartz was attending a meeting of the American Cancer Society in New Orleans when a researcher from the National Cancer Institute, Michael Sporn, showed slides of rat breast tissue that had been treated with vitamin-A-related compounds called retinoids, which had been found to have anticancer activity. To Schwartz's amazement, they looked exactly like the pattern he had seen with the breast tissue of his

DHEA-treated mice. "My God," he thought, looking at the fine reticulations of tissue undistorted by the presence of cancer, "could DHEA be working like retinoid compounds to inhibit cancer promotion?"

The evolution of a normal cell into a tumor is a complicated process involving a number of steps. A popular theory at that time, which has since been modified, was that cancer required two primary stages, initiation and promotion. The first stage, initiation, takes place when the DNA of a cell is mutated either by a chemical carcinogen, virus, or other DNA-damaging agent, such as radiation. By itself, this stage is not sufficient to produce cancer. That requires a second stage, promotion, which enables the mutated cell to proliferate.

For example, a low dose of DMBA, a chemical carcinogen, applied to the skin of a mouse, will be enough to cause initiation but not clinical cancer. However, if a few weeks or months later, a substance called crotin oil, which is not a carcinogen but is a cell-division stimulator, is put on the skin at the same place as the DMBA, the animal will get ten to fifteen tumors. The crotin oil is a cocarcinogen, or tumor promoter. Many substances including such common ingredients of daily life as caffeine and saccharin, are believed to work in this way. Hormones, such as estrogen, may act via promotion. Even something beneficial, like wound healing, may promote cancer because it stimulates cell division. In fact, cancer can be induced in the laboratory simply by applying a carcinogen to the skin of an animal, cutting the skin, and then suturing the wound. In a short time, tumors will appear all along the site of the wound. Promoters of any kind can work on any cell that has been initiated by any cause, be it viral or chemical, or radiation.

There were chemicals known to have antipromotion activity and perhaps DHEA was one of them. To test this idea, Schwartz injected mice with DHEA at the same time he applied a tumor promoter to their skin. Ordinarily, a thickening of the mouse epidermis could be seen in a few days, and cells taken from these animals showed a two- to threefold increase in division rate. But, he found, with just one injection of DHEA, he could completely counteract the effects of the promoter. In subsequent experiments they were even able to take human white blood cells, add the Epstein-Barr virus, which has been implicated in a form of cancer called Burkitt's lymphoma, and prevent runaway growth of these cells with DHEA.

Now the plot of the DHEA story was beginning to thicken impressively. It certainly appeared that the compound prevented activation of carcinogens *in vitro*. But what was far more important and what may actually be happening in the body, Schwartz now believed, was that it displayed impressive antipromotion activity. In fact, it occurred to Schwartz, who was beginning to experience the satisfaction a detective feels when all the clues begin pointing in the same direction, antitumor activity is just what one would expect with an agent that has the same effect on the body as diet restriction. Undernutrition is a well-known antitumor promoter. If a rodent that has been underfed is injected with a carcinogen under the skin and put back on a full diet, it will go on to develop cancer. But if fully fed rodents are given the same carcinogen, and then, about a month later, placed on a severely restricted diet, cancer does not develop.

If it were true that DHEA worked in the body like undernutrition, the implications were mind-boggling. Diet restriction was known to (1) vastly reduce the incidence of tumors, (2) delay the onset of age-related diseases such as arteriosclerosis and autoimmune disorders, and (3) extend life span beyond that accomplished by any other feasible means. But undernutrition required lifelong self-abnegation, while DHEA produced the same effects with none of the pain. In fact, it allowed the animal to eat as much as it wanted without gaining weight. For that attribute alone, it seemed heaven-sent.

Schwartz is not given to speculation. But at this point even he began to have some very provocative thoughts. The DHEA-treated mice seemed to be aging at a much slower rate than the control animals. And his preliminary data showed that the compound might be extending life by 25 percent to 30 percent. It was not certain that the compound declined with age naturally in the mouse, but it was beyond doubt that it did in humans, reaching its peak of activity at the time of sexual maturity and then continuously receding with age, in a manner that corresponded with the loss of vitality and disease resistance. What if, as some gerontologists believe, aging was not an evolutionary accident but was built into the genes because it was beneficial to the species? Then the decline of DHEA might be some sort of rapid-aging mechanism that came into play during postreproduction. If that were the case, the effect of its replacement in humans might be far more dramatic than that seen with mice.

An antiobesity, anticancer, antiaging drug? It seemed incredible, yet there were all those observations, his own and those of others. It had to work. It had to be right. But although DHEA was a naturally occurring substance and, in tests on animals, appeared to be completely nontoxic, there were several obstacles to its use as a drug. First, almost nothing was known about DHEA, whether it was a hormone, a precursor of hormones, or the breakdown product of hormones. No one even knew what use the body had for this substance. According to New York biochemist Norman Applezweig, who did pioneering work on the compound, "DHEA is not only the largest secretory product of the adrenal gland, it is also the most abundant steroid in human plasma." It is found almost everywhere in the body including the testes, the ovary, the placenta, the lungs, and the brain. Large amounts of it are found in the urine, where it was first isolated in 1934. Yet as one researcher concluded after an exhaustive review of DHEA, the "hormone" appears to have "no biological significance except [for] excretion."

Second, there was the baffling fact that 99 percent of DHEA in human blood contained a sulfate group as part of its structure, and this sulfated form of DHEA was totally inactive. It neither inhibited G6PDH nor worked as an antipromoter. Only the 1 percent that was in the form of free DHEA was active. But then Schwartz came across some publications suggesting that the real form of DHEA in the blood may not be DHEA sulfate, but a bizarre compound called a sulfatide. There is really no precedent for this type of substance in the body. A synthetic form of the sulfatide compound, the researchers found, was an even more potent inhibitor of G6PDH than the free form of DHEA. Schwartz brought in a chemist to make the sulfatide and, to his great excitement, it worked. The synthetic substance not only blocked G6PDH *in vitro,* it was a powerful antitumor promoter in the mouse. But the sulfatide proved to be highly labile, rapidly breaking down into the sulfate form. This, Schwartz realized, could be the reason why scientists had failed to find the DHEA sulfatide in the blood. It had already broken down into the sulfate form by the time they had extracted it.

The problem was that even if the DHEA sulfatide was the true form in the blood and worked well in tests, its inherent instability would prevent it from having any shelf life if it were given as a drug. Furthermore, the doses necessary for anticancer and antiobesity activity would be something like 300 milligrams per day for a human being, far too high for a steroid that might presumably be taken, like a vitamin supplement, for life. Although no side effects had been picked up on animal tests, the compound was known to be involved in the synthesis of male and female sex hormones in the body, so the potential for trouble was there.

But perhaps the biggest barrier to DHEA as a drug was not scientific, but financial and political. Developing drugs is an extremely long and costly proposition, requiring about seven to ten years on average and an expenditure at that time of about $54 million. For any drug company to pick up the tab, there must be the promise of a pot of gold at the end of the rainbow. In Europe DHEA is packaged in dosages ranging from 10 to 50 milligrams and is sold over the counter for the treatment of menopause, emotional instability, depression, and stress. Still, the fact that it was already available in drug form was not what stood in the way of its development. Use patents for DHEA could still be obtained that would make the required research and testing worthwhile. What did stand in the way was Schwartz's naiveté. He had written and talked about the anticancer effect of the compound in 1975 and then failed to file for a patent within a year. Under the terms of a U.S. patent, no company could now hold exclusive rights to the compound. And he had made this mistake not once, but also with a related steroid called epiandrosterone, which his laboratory found had twice the G6PDH-inhibiting activity of DHEA and was even more protective against carcinogenic damage.

By the 1979 Gordon Conference, Schwartz was a chastened man. He spoke about DHEA but not about the fact that his laboratory had developed a drug based on epiandrosterone that was fifty times more potent than naturally occurring DHEA and that so far seemed to be free of side effects. This meant that the dose used could be far lower, perhaps a few milligrams per day. With the potential for a true drug in hand, he was not about to take any chances. Even later when he began to include reports of this synthetic compound in his talks on DHEA, Schwartz was careful never to reveal its chemical nature. An undertone of secrecy began to slip into his presentations, a forerunner of things to come at aging conferences as the research of more and more investigators neared the clinical testing stage.

For now, the story of DHEA was enough to electrify the Gordon Conference audience. According to Smith-Sonneborn, "Schwartz just showed this skinny, little, beautiful mouse with shiny fur that had the DHEA and a big, fat, obese, ugly mouse with his fur sticking out all over the place, ridden with tumors, that hadn't gotten DHEA. And as unbelievable as it sounded, DHEA was antitumorigenic, antiobesity, and the mouse looked younger."

Some of the reaction even surprised Schwartz. He was looking forward to stimulating interaction with his colleagues, but after the speech, he found himself being borne away by people who were not scientists and who usually were not invited to Gordon Conferences. Two of them were from drug companies, and the third was Don Yarborough, a founding father of the newly formed Fund for Integrative Biomedical Research (FIBER), which was to play a generative role in aging studies in the coming years.

Schwartz's report came on the heels of Hart's presentation and served to point up the divisions within the field. For the first time, all the work which supported a correlation between DNA repair-protective processes and life span had been brought together, including that of Hart, Sacher, Cutler, Walford, Smith-Sonneborn, and Schwartz himself. "As a result of the conference," Dave Harrison, of the Jackson Laboratory, was to say later, "the somatic mutation theory was on its way up again. I personally take the mutation theory with a grain of salt. But I couldn't help being intrigued, as everyone else was, with the fabulous correlations of Ron Hart and the others. You just don't see correlations like that in science. If it was my work, I think I would have been tempted to move the line over." (Although a number of scientists characterized his work as buttressing somatic mutation theory, Hart believed his own research pointed in another direction, one that would receive increasing support in the years to come.) But there was the bald fact of DHEA itself. Since it appeared to work as an antipromoting and antimutagenic substance that protected the DNA and prevented normal genes from being expressed, Hart saw it as an additional patch in the intricate quilt of the development of cancer and aging. But others believed that insofar as it fit into any scheme of things, it was closer to the idea of "extrinsic" causes of aging, advanced by Caleb ("Tuck") Finch of the University of Southern California.

In Finch's view, although aging was ultimately written into the genes, it was "read out" at the level of the hormones, particularly those secreted by the adrenal and pituitary glands. He rejected the idea that aging was intrinsic; experiments in his lab and elsewhere showed that the effects of age could be overcome by certain hormones or brain chemicals, or by stimulating the brain electrically. In his own work on the reproductive system, he had gotten old ovaries to function again by transplanting them to young animals. Furthermore, by stimulating the hypothalamus electrically or with drugs, he was able to get menopausal female rats to resume their reproductive cycle, or as he so colorfully put it, by going to the brain, he was able to "jump-start" the ovaries. Senescence, as he saw it, was controlled by a "brain clock," located, most likely, in the hypothalamus-pituitary area.

Lending credence to this idea were some of the most intriguing and provocative experiments in gerontology. A number of laboratories had shown that old animals could be made young again simply by removing the pituitary gland and giving them hormone replacements in the water. The signs of their remarkable rejuvenation included an increased immune function, more youthful collagen, and the fur growth of a young animal. Donner Denckla, the foremost proponent of this approach in the United States, claimed that the beneficial effects were due to the removal of a mysterious hormone, which he christened DECO, for decreasing oxygen consumption. This hormone, which, he says, begins to do its dirty work at about age twenty-one, appears to prevent the thyroid-gland hormones from reaching their target cells.

During the period of rapid growth in childhood, Denckla points out, we consume massive amounts of oxygen, and if we were not able to rapidly dissipate heat, we would cook ourselves to death. DECO, he believes, helps us keep our cool by blocking the action of thyroid hormones that raise our metabolic rate. But since the thyroid is also needed for the regulation of such life-sustaining functions as metabolism, protein synthesis, cell division, wound healing, the cardiovascular system, maximum aerobic capacity, and immune activity, the continued release of DECO, once we have reached maturity, slowly but surely does us in.

In Denckla's hands the results of removing the pituitary, and presumably DECO along with it, were dramatic. In actual measurements of twenty-two different parameters, including the immune function, liver function, blood vessels, skin, and fur growth, says Denckla, there was no deterioration with age. And in every respect they looked and performed like much younger animals. "Our ability to consume oxygen at high rates falls with age," he says. "A seventy-year-old man cannot run as fast as a thirty-year-old. But our [older] animals could run [like much younger ones]. As a matter of fact, our gross overall indices of cardiovascular fitness showed that the animals were like eighteen-year-olds. They look better, their hair grows back, and the quality of their skin is like that of a young adult. Whereas the old animals look like they need a shower and shave."

Most impressive of all were the life spans he achieved. While the mean life span was only slightly increased in the treated rats—26.5 months as against 24 months in the controls—the difference in maximal survival was startling. As of 34 months of age, when Denckla was forced to terminate the experiment for lack of funds, 23 out of the 93 treated animals were still alive, while there were only 2 remaining out of 155 control animals. "I stopped aging," he says. "I stopped it dead in its tracks. There was no Gompertz curve, no death curve. Every animal study has shown an accelerated rate of death toward the end of life, but our animals died at the same rate at two years of age that they did at three."

Although Denckla's findings had yet to be replicated, and neither he nor anyone else had been able to isolate the putative hormone, Schwartz's work on DHEA was a powerful boost to the idea that aging was primarily a hormonal or neuroendocrine phenomenon. In a sense, the basic quarrel about aging—whether it occurred in the cell or outside of it—had been going on since the time of Weismann. On another level, it was the argument between Hayflick and Carrel all over again, between mortality and immortality, between the cell and its media. Either the cell, in Hayflick's words, had a "mean time to failure," or there was something in its habitat, some hormone or peptide, DECO or DHEA or some other yet-to-be-discovered substance, which, if added or subtracted, could slow aging or prolong life perhaps indefinitely. Now, more than one hundred years after Weismann, fifty years after Carrel, and twenty-five years after the discovery of the double helix, these questions were yet to be resolved.

But it was not until the third day of the conference, when Cutler presented his work, that the emotions that had been building up in the first two days started spilling over. He had expected that his work showing a correlation between life span of a dozen mammalian species and an enzyme, superoxide dismutase (SOD), which protected the DNA against damage from superoxide, one of the most toxic molecules formed during the breakdown of oxygen, would be welcome news to his fellow gerontologists. Instead, he met with severe criticism. His methodology was attacked, his failure to distinguish between two kinds of SOD present in the cells was held up as an example of poor biochemistry, and his results were dismissed as a statistical sleight of hand.

It was the last issue that most infuriated his critics. They attacked as specious his idea of relating SOD to the total amount of oxygen consumed by an animal over its lifetime. The fact was, they contended, that SOD levels were the same in both short-lived and long-lived animals unless you divided the amount for each species by its specific metabolic rate. Only after you did this did you get a correlation with longevity. The problem was, they contended, that you could do the same with any factor that was constant among all animals, such as the fact that they have four limbs, and get a correlation between the number of limbs that an animal has and its life span.

To Cutler's consternation, they had missed the point. The amount of SOD an animal required had to be related both to its metabolic rate and to how long it lived. A mouse, which burns up oxygen like a house on fire, lives a very short time while an elephant, which has very low levels of oxygen consumption, lives seventy years. Therefore, the important figure is going to be what its total oxygen needs are over its lifetime. And from that point of view, the elephant had a lot more available SOD than the mouse had.

It was an especially bitter occasion for the already embattled Cutler. "I got nothing but ridicule," he said. "Most of them didn't believe me. One of the scientists even turned during the discussion period and asked, 'Is Bob Butler here? [Butler at that time was the head of the National Institute on Aging.] This is an example of the type of work that we want to get rid of in the field.' "

The attack did not stop at Cutler; instead, it became directed generally against much of the data that had been presented over the past three days. "It was the first time that all the studies had been synthesized and presented with evidence to the audience," says Hart, "not theory, but evidence. You had Larry Loeb on the fidelity aspects, bringing up the idea of gene expression; you had Joan Smith-Sonneborn's findings on repair and life span; you had Schwartz on metabolism; Cutler on scavenging; Roy Walford on the relationship between the immune system and repair; and George Sacher putting everything into an evolutionary framework.

"People were overwhelmed when they saw the whole thing put together with data. There was a tremendous positive acceptance to the whole approach, too much so. Because I think at that point a kind of schism began developing between those who were using the evolutionary-comparative approach, looking across species to get at the mechanism of aging, and those who were using the ontogenic approach, where you study the changes in a given system as a function of age. There was a tremendous defensive posture among those of the ontogenic type. Some of them were, I believe, unduly critical, not of the data, which in most cases were very fine, but of the approach. They would say things like, 'People don't care *why* they grow old. They just don't want to lose their hormonal balance or become senile. Our main job is to find out things like that, why man has more or less of whatever it might be with age, not what the mechanism is.'

"And that is when you started to see the division you have now. But I prefer to think that it came about for humanitarian reasons. Some of the people in the audience who were from the National Institute on Aging, the people who fund the research, were saying that the overwhelming correlation between these systems and longevity was really impressive and might be a basis for a mechanistic approach. And so it dawned on people that their laboratories and their staff might be in jeopardy if funding switched substantially to the comparative-evolutionary approach or anything that was different from what they were doing. There is only so much pie to go around. And if one approach gets a bigger slice, that means another approach will get a smaller piece. And then what happens to your lab and the people who may have worked with you for five or ten years? You suddenly had a lot of competition coming into gerontobiology that you did not necessarily have before."

Some people blamed Hart himself for the divisiveness. "Ron needlessly antagonized many people, because of his insistence on a central role for DNA," said one of the scientists. "It was not just what he said, it was the way he said it. He really let them know that nothing else was important. He stepped on their toes and, quite understandably, some of them had it in for him."

Others criticized him for building a case on very little evidence. "All Ron has is a correlation," says Caleb Finch. "And correlations can be due to anything. Because a horse was stolen and a man left town at the same time, [it] doesn't mean he left town on that horse. Let me give you another example. Radiation causes mutation—no question about it. Radiation also shortens life span. That does not mean that radiation shortens life span by causing mutation. The process of mutation is random. Aging is not random. It is incredibly predictable. So that's the problem."

For his part, Hart is equally critical of Finch: "I don't pretend to understand neuroendocrine effects or hormonal effects any more than he understands molecular biology. But I do know that his hormones have to be templated off a macromolecule, and that macromolecule is DNA. And I do know that if I change that DNA, I can change that hormone."

After the Gordon Conference, the November 1979 Gerontology Society meeting in Washington, D.C., was anticlimactic, with one striking exception—the last session of the last day of the symposium on "DNA Repair and Aging," headed by Ed Schneider. Perhaps there are times in science when an idea is suddenly in the air, like a joke making the rounds or a tune everyone is humming. Whatever the reason, all four session speakers had independently become interested in the same area, which stood at the frontier of knowledge about DNA. This was the area of DNA supercoiling, or DNA superhelicity, as it is also called. These terms refer to nature's ingenious packaging job. If one were to remove all the DNA in a single human cell and stretch it out into one unbroken line, it would measure three feet end to end. How is it possible that all this material occupied a space far smaller than the eye can see? The answer is that in the chromosomes, the DNA is coiled into a double helix and then twisted into even fatter supercoils. The result resembles a coiled telephone wire that has twisted and turned into bunches and kinks and is now compressed into a much smaller space.

Hart ended his talk by describing several recent experiments in his laboratory on DNA supercoiling. It was known that the supercoiling controlled the genetic function in bacterial cells, and now one of his students, Phil Lipetz, had shown that the state of DNA supercoiling in human cells might be related to aging. The next speaker, Jerry Williams, a DNA repair worker at George Washington University, indicated that he, too, thought DNA superhelicity was "an interesting way to go"; and David Kram, a member of Ed Schneider's lab at the Gerontology Research Center in Baltimore, commented that changes in supercoiling might be modulating the chromosome repair system that he and his colleagues were looking at.

Finally it was Smith-Sonneborn's turn to speak. It was now late afternoon. The session had run almost two hours over the schedule, but the small audience sat glued to its seats. Glasses perched above her forehead, an incandescent smile on her face, and almost dancing across the stage as she wrote on the blackboard or pointed to a slide, Smith-Sonneborn did not lecture so much as she shared the material, offering it around like pieces of a treasured collection. After describing her by now famous life-extension experiment using both UV light and photoreactivation, she spoke about her recent attempts to zero in on the phenomenon. In her first experiment, she said, "my goal was to treat the paramecia with a high-enough radiation dose so that I could shorten life span and then try to reverse it with photoreactivation. Now my goal was to look at life-span extension." Her hypothesis was very simple. If she was inducing a repair system, then most likely there was a critical threshold for the level of damage necessary to initiate the process. Too low and there would be no effect; too high and the bad effects of the damage would outweigh the beneficial effects of repair. In that case the life span would be abbreviated rather than extended.

By experimenting with various dosages of ultraviolet light to see which gave the longest life spans, she found, much to her amazement, it was a very low dose; in fact, it amounted to the same dose that the cells in her original experiment had been left with after they had been treated with UV and photoreactivating light. At that point, it looked as if the ultraviolet light, a potent DNA damaging agent, was in and of itself the cause of the greatly extended life span. Photoreactivation only served to bring UV light down to the level where it helped rather than hurt.

"Now what is it [the ultraviolet light] doing?" she asked the hushed audi-

ence, pointing to the diagram she had drawn of the various UV doses used.
"My Lord, I don't know," she said with an infectious giggle. She and her
students had found that the ultraviolet treatment induced a higher level of
one of the DNA repair enzymes, but that effect lasted only six to eight
hours. "It's hard to imagine that the kind of repair you are inducing in six
to eight hours is going to give you a dramatic extension in life span," she
said.

There had to be some other explanation. She said, "Perhaps it could be
something like what I call my 'Slinky' and what Hart is calling supercoiling.
Everyone knows the Slinky toy. The idea is that you start out with your
Slinky exposed and then as you age, the DNA coils more tightly." The
coils have to unwind in order to be accessible to repair enzymes, she explained, and maybe that was what the UV-photoreactivation treatments
were doing in her original experiment—stretching out the Slinky so that the
damage sites were available for repair.

She cited other evidence for her idea, along with a recent experiment in
her lab with DHEA. With just one treatment of the substance over a
twenty-four-hour period, she had achieved a significant lengthening of life
span. Whatever was happening, she decided, it had to be something that
changed the physical structure of the DNA in some way. "As cells age in
culture, they lose function generally," she said, "not only the ability to repair. The ability to transcribe their DNA and their fission rate also goes
down. Many things happen. A Slinky would take care of everything."

She finished her speech to tumultuous applause. Quickly she was surrounded by a small crowd of people, energized by what they had heard.
Even though the hour was late and the conference had ended, they were
reluctant to go home. They went upstairs to the hotel coffee shop and, for
the next hour and a half, talked excitedly about DNA repair, gene expression, and superhelicity. Again, as at the Renegade Repair Conference and at
the last Gordon Conference, there was the feeling that somehow their separate endeavors in the laboratory were beginning to overlap; connections
were being made like tributaries that flow from many different directions
into a single stream. Just as one tends to forget the endless hours of tedium
and frustration that precede a successful experiment, during the times when
ideas are being freely interchanged, one blocks out the long periods of isolation and the occasional feelings of competitiveness, envy, and resentment
toward one's peer. At those times, the scientist can be swept up in a wave
of intimacy, a kind of love for one's fellow practitioners.

Back in their labs, the scientists were continuing their separate projects

but were influenced by the ideas they had woven together during the
Gordon and Gerontology Society conferences. Schwartz was now more
excited than ever by the prospects of developing a drug with DHEA-like
qualities. Walford was exploring other facets of the supergene for aging that
he had identified. Cutler, buoyed by Smith-Sonneborn's talk, was intent on
developing a kind of antiaging vaccine that would trick the cells into upping
their levels of repair and protection. Smith-Sonneborn was anxious to explore her Slinky model, perhaps with the help of Phil Lipetz in Hart's lab.

Only Hart had shelved his ideas for aging research for the moment as he
prepared to embark on new directions. He had been offered a job as director of the National Center for Toxicological Research in Jefferson,
Arkansas. Tucked deep into a forest outside Little Rock, the center, an
FDA research facility, worked on the health problems engendered by modern technology—the synthetic chemicals in food, drugs, and the environment. Directing research science at a national laboratory was something
that challenged him. It also offered him the opportunity to pursue his twin
interests in toxicology and gerontology, since in both cases DNA damage
was a common element.

One of the things that interested him at the moment was research, done
in Israel by Ruth Ben–Ishai, that indicated that the level of excision repair
was very high during embryonic life and then was set at a much lower level
by the time of birth. The work was very preliminary, but if this were the
case, it meant that there may be far higher levels of DNA repair stored in
the genetic material, but how to get the genes to express these was anybody's guess.

When I asked Hart how he might go about doing it, he said, "If I knew a
way to raise excision repair in the cell, don't you think I'd be doing it
now?"

Chapter Eight

Taking It One Step Further

" **I** think I have a way to jack excision repair up and down in the cell."

Joan Smith-Sonneborn stared at the tall, intense, bearded young man, with straight brown hair falling over wire-rimmed glasses, who spoke those incredible words. "Phil, you've *got* to tell me what you're talking about," she implored.

His excitement matched her own. Waving his hands and arms in the air, discharging words like "nicotinamide-adenine dinucleotide" and "poly ADP ribose," Phil Lipetz rushed through his latest findings and ideas like a brush fire through the canyons of southern California. With her vigorous nods and murmurs of "right, right, right," Smith-Sonneborn fueled the fire.

If Hart was right that DNA damage played a role in aging, then manipulating repair levels in either direction might have a direct effect on life span. Smith-Sonneborn had already manipulated repair levels in paramecia by using ultraviolet light, but sitting under a sunlamp was clearly not the way to go for human beings. There had to be a way to get into all the somatic cells of the body, and now this young researcher who had not yet received his doctorate was telling her he had one.

Lipetz is a rarity among researchers, a third-generation scientist. His grandfather started out to be a rabbi in Lithuania, but switched to science after immigrating to this country. While getting his master's degree in botany, he noticed that certain molds had a lethal effect on bacteria. He had, according to Lipetz, accidentally stumbled upon antibiotics years before Fleming found penicillin. Although he documented his results with photographs, his mentor refused to believe him, declaring that there was no mention of such an effect in all the scientific literature. Discouraged, his grandfather left research and became a teacher, suffering the fate of most people who are ahead of their time, says Lipetz.

His father, Leo Lipetz, started out in electrical engineering with a physics background and, after World War II, participated in one of the first biophysics doctoral programs in the country, at Berkeley. A researcher in the electrophysiology of vision, he discovered that radiation on the retina could produce images, a phenomenon that was later to explain the flashes of light "seen" by the astronauts in outer space.

Phil Lipetz, the oldest of three boys, still remembers when his father was in the lab. It was his private playground, where he learned to do dissections and use a microscope as easily as other children learn to ride a bike or put together a model. Born in Oakland, California, he spent a sabbatical year with his father in Paris, and then, at the age of seven, came to Columbus, where his father was and still is a member of Ohio State's faculty. In elementary school, where he wavered between boredom and rebellion, he learned one skill that gave him a competitive edge—speed-reading, not rapid-scanning, which is what most speed-reading is, but the ability to take in every word at a vastly accelerated rate. To this day, he can flip through a technical journal as though it were a deck of cards, lighting on the relevant phrases with the alacrity of a cardshark filling out a full house.

A cradle scientist, he spurned it as a career. It was his father's domain and he wanted nothing to do with it. His mother, however, was an artist, and perhaps it was this side of his upbringing that made him decide, by the time he had finished high school, to become a playwright. At Antioch he majored in creative writing. And it was not until his senior year, after a near-fatal accident, that the prodigal son returned to the fold.

In a supremely foolish act, Lipetz was climbing Cathedral Ledge cliff in the White Mountains of New Hampshire. Rated very difficult under normal conditions, it presented an almost impossible climb on that freezing, rainy November evening. He and his buddy were rappeling down, when Lipetz lost his footing and wound up dangling upside down with his safety rope looped about his neck.

In the four and a half hours that followed, Lipetz experienced the well-defined psychological stages that manifest themselves in the face of death, and then some: panic ("God, help me. I'm going to die"); resentment ("Why me? It's not fair"); bargaining ("Lord, get me out of this one and I'll give up drugs, alcohol, and tobacco"). When it seemed to him that he had been hanging there forever and a large crowd had assembled below while searchlights played about him, he entered the last stage—resignation.

He was going to die; that much was apparent. But while he came to that realization, he began to hallucinate. "I start seeing lights everywhere and the lights are alive," he recalls. "And at the same time, I see everything that is going on, the rocks, the people below waiting to see my body fall, the rope, myself, the air, and there is no difference; there is only unity, it is all a continuum.

"Then the lights start going through stages, and finally they concentrate on a blue light, and it is like I am seeing everything, everywhere in the world through this blue light. And I am being absorbed in that and I am expanding out in the entire world. And the world is me and the world is arising from me. And I am not dying. Do you understand? Because if everything is arising out of me and I am a part of everything, how can I die?"

When he was finally rescued, Lipetz felt as though he were being wrenched away from the most exquisite experience he'd known. It took him months to recover. His back continued to bother him long afterward, and it appeared God was determined to make him keep his side of the bargain. He was no longer able to tolerate alcohol, tobacco, or drugs of any kind. But most serious was the possibility that the lack of oxygen to his brain during those four and a half hours had left him permanently impaired. Everywhere he went, he could still see the blue spot of light before his eyes, which the neurologists ascribed to possible brain damage. "You'll never be able to go back to school," they told him. "And if you do, it will only be part-time and in a field that doesn't demand much intellectual effort."

Thumbing his nose at their gloomy predictions, Lipetz switched his major to science when he returned to college. Starting out in environmental science, he later opted for biology because he wished to translate the visions he had seen that night into scientific reality.

He chose his father's institution, Ohio State, for graduate school because of the presence there of Karl Kornacker, "a man of genius," he says. A mathematician, Kornacker had ventured into the thicket of biophysics, hoping to place the study of life on the molecular level upon the sturdy foundation of mathematical principles. In other words, he was trying to do for biology what had already been accomplished for physics: move it from an observational science into a theoretical science with great predictive power.

From Kornacker, Lipetz learned how to read through the literature, looking for anomalies that did not fit the model but kept unaccountably cropping up, and, from these little grains of truth, how to build a new model from which to predict experimental results. It was an invaluable skill, and one Lipetz still relies upon to jump upon the wave and ride it in before others even see it coming.

Since Kornacker was primarily a theoretical scientist, Lipetz had to look elsewhere for lab experience. With his uncanny ability to spot the wave, he joined Hart's group in 1972, soon after the latter had set up shop at OSU and two years before he would publish anything significant. It was the beginning of a stormy eight-year relationship during which Lipetz would quit three times.

Hart and Lipetz see themselves as opposites. "If you want to see the difference between us," says Hart, "just look at our desks." The older man is meticulous, compulsive, a stickler for details, while the younger is impulsive and works in an atmosphere of creative disorder, literally letting the chips fall where they may. It was not unknown for Lipetz, in the throes of an experiment, to hurl used pipettes to the ground as he worked.

But a researcher who has worked with both of them sees the similarities between the two men as more striking than the differences. "They both have the same need to dominate, to be the center of attention, to be absolutely intolerant of others' shortcomings," he says.

Additionally, there was the same love-hate, father-son type of tug-of-war that Hart experienced with Dick Setlow. "The problem with Ron is that he never stopped treating me like a kid, even after I got my Ph.D.," complains Lipetz, who was only twenty-three when they first met. For his part, Hart demanded the same high standards from his students that had been asked of him in his graduate-school days. "Like Dick, I expect perfection from people. At the same time, I feel no compulsion to compliment people. And it's not because I don't like my students. I'm extremely close to them. It's just . . . [and here he stumbles seeking the right words] part of, you know, the classic American framework, the strong, silent father. You expect people to do a good job not for some oftentimes fake stroking but because they really love science."

To top it all off, Lipetz found religion. Scientists are no more united in their opinion about the existence of a deity than the rest of us. Walford has his mysterious mathematical mysticism, while Smith-Sonneborn, although no longer a churchgoer, remains a true believer. Once when I asked her how the immortal strain of one-celled animals called tetrahymena came into being, she answered as though nothing could be more obvious, "God made them."

Cutler, on the other hand, who had a religious upbringing, is an agnostic who believes that the practices of science and religion are mutually exclusive, the one directly interfering with the pursuit of the other. Perhaps the most vociferous is Trosko, who was branded an "Antichrist" and "the devil incarnate" by enraged fundamentalist students at Michigan State University. During a debate with a creationist, he explained his idea that the mutations in the germ line have an adaptive function, allowing the species to survive, while mutations in the somatic tissues have a devastating effect. "Evolution to me explains why one billion people on the face of the earth will get cancer," he said. "If I have to believe in a God who would deliberately make one billion people get cancer for the price of Adam and Eve eating an apple," he stated firmly to the nine hundred people present, "then I will tell that God to stuff it and go to hell."

Lipetz did not see a contradiction between his mystical and scientific beliefs, but for a long time, he could not figure out how to live in both worlds. After his cliff-hanging experience, he had sought out various teachers, gurus, and psychics, hoping to find someone who could offer an explanation for the images that exploded in his brain that night on Cathedral Ledge. Finally, five years after the accident, he went with a group of friends to meet a Yogi master, Baba Muktananda, who had recently arrived from India.

His initiation into the world of Siddha Yoga was accompanied by visions, images of the purest white: a white cobra, white swans, white peacocks, a white elephant, a snow-covered mountain, snow-covered ground with white flowers growing out of it, and in the midst of all of this, a luminous blue light, the same blue light he had seen that night on the mountain and that had followed him around for months.

Call it hallucinations, autosuggestion, or cosmic consciousness, but Lipetz was hooked. He began going to yogic retreats as often as his schedule would allow and for the next few years, he was torn between working in the lab and living at the ashram. On one side was his fervent desire to be a holy man, which, to him, meant giving up the world and devoting his life entirely to meditation and Siddha Yoga. On the other side was the need to get his degree, something that Muktananda himself had urged.

After passing his general exams, Lipetz decided to enter the ashram in Boston and work on his doctorate at the Harvard University library. Rather than resolve the crisis, he felt more and more depressed. Finally, at a retreat one Thanksgiving, a young American swami put his finger on the problem. Lipetz was unhappy, he said, because he was not following the guru's teaching. "What gave you the idea that in order to be holy, you had to go into an ashram?" he asked. Yoga could be practiced anywhere, in a lab, in an office, in a classroom. Realizing that he was right, Lipetz "surrendered" to the idea of returning to OSU to get his degree.

In 1978, after Lipetz had gotten his degree, a young Indian molecular biologist, Sohan Modak, joined the group. Lipetz credits Modak with turning him from a purely theoretical scientist into a hands-on laboratory worker. "He not only taught me technique and how to run an experiment, he gave me the intensity to feel the molecules," he says.

While Lipetz and Modak were doing research on cancer, Modak observed that a crude protein extract they were working with had an astonishing effect on bacterial DNA. It appeared to change the very structure of the DNA coiling in the cell. Lipetz believed that the extract could be a "nicking-closing enzyme," one of two enzyme systems that controlled DNA supercoiling. In 1973 James C. Wang first reported the existence of such an enzyme in the bacterium *Escherichia coli*. Now Lipetz believed they had found the same enzyme in another bacterium, *Micrococcus luteus*. But before he could prove it, Modak returned to India.

Lipetz wanted that enzyme badly, but while he was trying to purify it, Wang and his group beat him to it, publishing the purification of a "nicking-closing enzyme from *Micrococcus luteus*." For Lipetz, who was just starting out in science, it was not so much a disappointment as a confirmation that he was on the right track. "Hot damn!" he yelled when he saw the report. "We got a live one."

That was his start in DNA supercoiling, and he began to haunt the library to learn everything he could on the subject. The first time I met Lipetz, he performed what I came to think of as the superhelicity dance, writhing and twisting his long body like a serpent under the influence of a snake charmer. "DNA is not the simple little double helix that you see in pictures," he explained while tying himself into impossible knots. "The coils of DNA are organized into huge supercoils of about 140 base pairs long, and then you get about twenty thousand of these supercoils together in a huge loop and you have a *domain*, which behaves almost as though it were a separate piece of DNA."

In 1965 Jerome Vinograd of the University of California introduced the concept of supercoiling, or superhelicity, to describe the circular rings of DNA he had found in a small tumor-causing virus. Over the next decade, the DNA of all organisms was found to be supercoiled, but with an essential difference between *procaryote* cells such as bacteria, which lack a well-defined nucleus, and *eucaryote* cells, which have the nucleus set off by a double-layered membrane. In procaryote cells the supercoils of DNA form a closed circular molecule. In eucaryotes, which include everything from fungi, amoebae, and paramecia to multicellular human beings, the supercoils of DNA are wrapped like thread around a series of protein spools called nucleosomes. Scientists began to speak of levels of DNA, with the first and second level being the nucleic acid bases with their sugar-phosphate backbone, and the third and fourth levels being the supercoils and the domains.

Researchers in the United States and Europe found that DNA supercoiling in bacteria was associated with virtually every physical, chemical, and biological property of the cell, including the regulation of cell division, gene expression, and DNA repair. Nor did the state of supercoiling remain static. Like a yo-yo, the supercoiling contracted and expanded, relaxed and rewound. Two complementary enzyme systems controlled this activity. One was the nicking-closing enzyme, which like its name implies, breaks one of the DNA strands, allowing it to unswivel, and then closes it up again. The result is a relaxation of the DNA supercoiling. The second enzyme, gyrase, winds the DNA back into its original configuration.

In contrast to procaryote cells, the supercoiling of the DNA in eucaryote cells was what scientists call a black box, a container the contents of which cannot be discerned. It was known that the DNA was tightly bound with proteins in a network of fibers called chromatin, but the pattern of its twists and turns was unclear. Nor was it believed to move about as it did in procaryote cells, since no enzymes capable of rewinding the supercoiling had been isolated in higher-order cells. Perhaps, as some scientists claimed, DNA supercoiling in the eucaryote cell was just a good packaging job—a convenient way to fold the far greater amounts of eucaryotic DNA into the chromosomes—and had no further function.

But Lipetz believed, more as an article of faith than anything else, that this could not be the case. For one thing, evolution generally preserves successful mechanisms for survival throughout the species and there was no reason why DNA supercoiling should be an exception. Second, it offered a mechanism to explain how hormones, nutrients, or any other outside signal, could tell genes to turn on and turn off; and finally, DNA superhelicity had the potential of linking up the most important aspects of the cellular function, including replication, gene expression, and DNA repair. It was the scientific equivalent of the vision he saw that night on the mountain, a means of bringing unity to seemingly disparate phenomena. Proving the significance of DNA supercoiling in higher-order cells, he decided, would be his life's work.

He put together a small lab with a technician and high-school summer student, but when he submitted his first experimental results for publication, they were rejected by the reviewers. Soon after that, he was sitting in his office, feeling angry and at loose ends, when Hart came in to ask him where he was heading with his research. Lipetz shrugged. They talked for a while about the limitations of somatic mutation theory and how the field of gerontology could use some good new ideas. If he could find a way to tie in DNA superhelicity with aging, Hart told Lipetz, it would be a big step up in his career.

Lipetz leaped to his feet. "That's like shooting fish in a barrel," he exclaimed, using one of his favorite phrases.

"What do you mean?" asked Hart.

"Well, we know that DNA strand breaks increase with age. And we know that strand breaks decrease the superhelicity. So it follows that the DNA superhelicity goes down with age and, with it, everything that it controls."

"Prove it and I'll present it at the Gerontology Society meeting," Hart promised him.

With only two months to go until the 1979 meeting, Lipetz had to work like a demon. His first problem was how to do the experiment. Up until then, he had been measuring DNA supercoiling in bacteria. Now he would have to do it in human cells. To do this, he would have to learn the mysteries of the gradient.

In order to make the invisible visible, molecular biology, like magic, requires a kind of sleight of hand. The investigator builds upon the work of others, borrowing a trick here, a manipulation there, often adding a stratagem of his own to obtain the desired effect. Progress in the field may depend upon a slight variation in technique—the way the DNA is prepared, the type of "label" used, how long it is centrifuged. At the same time, unlike the conjurer, the scientist has to guard against illusion; whether through craft or cunning, the ends achieved must be real.

The first trick in looking at DNA supercoils was to sustain them. Most experiments in molecular biology call for extracting the DNA from the proteins bound to it. But doing this removes the supercoiling. To avoid this, Peter Cook and I. A. Brazell, two British scientists, devised a technique that stripped off most of the protein but left just enough to retain the supercoiling. The resulting structure is called a "nucleoid."

The second trick was to layer the nucleoid on a solution of gradually increasing density, known as a gradient. The degree of supercoiling is measured by how far the nucleoid travels through the gradient. Tightly coiled nucleoid DNA, like a well-wadded piece of paper, takes up less space and travels faster through the gradient than partially uncoiled DNA, which is bulkier and takes up more space. The third trick was to tag the DNA in some way so that one could tell how far down the gradient the DNA had gone. That part would come later. First Lipetz had to learn the gradient technique, and for that he went to a fellow graduate student, Doug Brash, who was the resident expert.

Brash had come to OSU to do neuroscience, but, under the influence of Ron Hart, had become interested in aging and DNA repair. One of the persistent problems in the field has been the inability to measure DNA damage in the cells of the living animal rather than just the damage in cells in culture. Only by looking at a complete organism would the theory that damage actually accumulates with age be proved. He figured he would spend about a month inventing the assay, measure the damage in both dividing and nondividing cells, and any difference between them, and write it up for his doctoral dissertation. That was three years earlier, and he had just solved problem number one, the assay.

When Brash began his work, the DNA to be examined on the gradient was always "labeled" with a radioactive material. Since only dividing cells can incorporate a radioactive substance, this meant that gradients could be used only for dividing cells, such as the crypt cells of the gut, the basal cells of the skin, or the stem cells of the immune system, but not for cells that were slow-growing, like heart or smooth muscle cells, or cells that never divided, like neurons. Brash compared the use of cell-culture methods to explore what was happening in real life to the joke about the man who was looking for his keys under the lamppost on a dark street. When asked if this was where he had dropped the keys, he answered, "No, but the light is better here." What was needed was a new light source.

After many fits and starts, Brash found his answer, a fluorescent dye, called DABA, which bound to the DNA regardless of the cell type. By placing the test tube in a device that can detect the fluorescence, he could measure how far the DNA had traveled down the gradient. The method, which did not require putting cells into culture, could be used on tissue taken from any part of the living animal.

With the Gerontology Society meeting drawing near, Lipetz began recruiting other people for his crash program to measure the DNA superhelicity in human cells. One was a graduate student, Laurie Joseph, and another was a cell biologist, Ralph Stephens, who had come to OSU a year earlier.

When Lipetz approached him, Ralph Stephens had no idea that his life was about to change—again. The first time, he was about to graduate from the University of Tennessee. He was doing research at the Duke University Marine Labs when he looked through a microscope and saw a sea urchin egg dividing, in textbook fashion, right before his eyes. From that moment on he was hooked. He decided he would devote the rest of his life to understanding how one cell becomes two.

Born, bred, and educated in eastern Tennessee, Stephens still retains the drawl, style, and charm of a hillbilly. Slightly built, with short wavy hair, eyes of the lightest blue, and an elfin smile, he is, like country music, easy to take. Although almost forty when he teamed up with Lipetz, he had yet to achieve tenure or to head up his own laboratory. In his long and checkered career, he had often been a bridesmaid but never a bride, coming within a hairbreadth of several major discoveries. Some of the misses were due to ill luck, but mostly he attributes them to a distaste for conflict. His goal, he says, is not to be rich and famous but, rather, to be left alone to work.

Don Quixote had his Sancho Panza; Robinson Crusoe, his man Friday; and Lipetz, although he didn't know it at the time, had his Stephens. What one lacked, the other had in abundance. Lipetz loves the limelight, addressing crowds, giving interviews, meeting people. Stephens hates it "out front." Lipetz dashes off scientific papers; Stephens, an elegant writer, crawls through them. But when it comes to running the laboratory, Stephens clearly excels. Lipetz, brilliant when working in the full flush of inspiration, when he "can feel the molecules," has little stomach for the endless details that make up most research. Stephens, on the other hand, sees himself as a conductor combining all the musical elements into a harmonious whole.

Lipetz entered the lab building on a fine, crisp morning in late November. His stomach felt tied up in knots. The lab looked like a restaurant kitchen before the morning rush, with the glassware hung gleaming on wooden pegs, the test tubes stacked neatly in their holders, the stainless steel stools tucked under the spotless black counters. In the corner, bent like a stork over a mass of spaghetti-like plastic hoses, Denny Jewett, a tall, graceful technician, was preparing the gradient. While soft-rock music played on the radio, he deftly threaded the ends of each hose extending from the gradient-maker pump into the center of six test tubes. The machine began dripping sucrose of increasing density through the hoses so that it formed a graduated mixture in the test tubes, with the thickest part at the bottom.

The gradient also contained ethidium bromide (EB), a substance that has the remarkable property of being able to slip in between the supercoils of DNA. As increasing concentrations of EB are added, the dye stretches out the DNA, like a child pulling apart a Slinky toy, until the coils flatten out altogether. If more dye is added, the DNA begins to rewind in the opposite direction. This process can be followed on the gradient. The more tightly coiled the DNA, the more EB is needed to twist it about in this fashion.

Working under a sterile hood, Stephens was preparing the cells that would go on the gradient. Invisible sheets of air flowed past him as he added trypsin, an enzyme that unsticks the cells from the glass bottom, to his flask. "Air is your best friend and your worst enemy," he would tell his students. "You have to know where you are and it is at all times." The positive air flow carried the bacteria away from the beaker and himself, but if something blocked the flow, the air itself could become contaminated. He shook the beaker gently to diffuse the trypsin and watched while the solution that had been clear began to turn cloudy as the cells came off the bottom.

"Hi, Phil," said Stephens cheerily as Lipetz came in. Then he took one look at his face and asked, "What's the matter?"

"Goddammit," Lipetz exploded. "Here it is three days before Ron leaves for the gerontology meeting and we've still got nothing." Despite all their work and ideas in the past two months, the two men had been unable to measure the DNA supercoiling in the human cells. And Lipetz had to do that if he were to prove that DNA supercoiling declined with age.

"We're beginning to get a signal," said Ralph.

"But it's not good enough and you know that."

"Still, it means there's something there and it's just a matter of getting it out."

"Yeah, you're right. It's absolutely maddening." He banged his fist down on one of the counters. "The point is, Will we get it in time?"

"Look, Phil, the answer is in those test tubes. If we don't get it now, we'll get it later."

Lipetz could feel the fury rising in him as he began pacing the small room from counter to counter. "The point is, I said we would have it in time for the meeting, and we're gonna have it in time for the meeting if I have to go through every test tube in this building to get it!" He stormed out, leaving Stephens wondering whether all the glassware would go crashing to the floor.

Stephens's immediate problem was that the cells had reached the Hayflick limit and were dying out. These were fibroblasts that had originally been obtained from human foreskin at the time of circumcision soon after birth. Now they were at the very end of their life span, having gone through fifty-one population doublings.

He went out to tell Lipetz the bad news. There were only fifteen thousand cells for each gradient batch—far too few for any definitive results.

"Are you sure?" asked Phil. "Count them again."

"I already did."

"Then we'll just have to go with that."

"That's what I say," said Stephens. "Let's run them. They're all you've got."

They handed the cells over to Jewitt, who layered them on the test tubes containing the gradient. Next he added Triton X, a detergent that gently broke through the cell membrane, exposed the DNA in the nucleus, and stripped away almost all the protein. The result was the "nucleoid"—a nucleus with holes poked through it like a whiffleball. It retained its supercoiling but it was also permeable by other substances.

The next step was to spin the gradient tubes in the ultracentrifuge at great speeds: five thousand revolutions a minute for four hours. The same force that pushes clothes against the walls of a whirling dryer forces the nucleoids through the sucrose solution. The extent of its journey through the tube depends on the degree of DNA supercoiling: Partially uncoiled DNA, stretched out like an extended telephone cord, is bulky and does not travel as fast; tightly coiled DNA offers less resistance and travels faster.

By late afternoon the gradient in the six tubes had been subdivided into thirty test tubes. Each of the tubes contained a fluorescent dye that bound to the DNA and could be picked up by a machine designed for that purpose.

The sun was starting to set when the moment of truth arrived. Lipetz and Stephens carried the trays of test tubes to another building, which housed a prime example of modern wizardry—the spectrofluorimeter. This was the instrument that allowed the rabbit to be pulled out of the hat, the invisible to be made manifest. By detecting the fluorescence emitted by the dye and translating the energy it emits into numbers, the machine made it possible to tell how far down the gradient the DNA went, and from that they could determine the extent of the supercoiling.

Sometimes they had to wait on long lines as people from other labs came with tubes to be read. But tonight the small room was deserted. Stephens turned on the machine; set it to the wavelength of DNA, 360 nanometers; waited for the red numbers on the spectrofluorimeter to reach zero; and began to insert the tubes one by one. But the numbers they were waiting for that would allow them to gauge the state of the supercoiling in the cell never appeared. Just as they had feared, there were too few cells. The fluorescent agent they were using not only reacted to DNA but also lit up non-DNA components, and the only way to distinguish DNA from non-DNA was to use a much larger quantity of cells than they had available.

"They're all the cells we've got," said Stephens. "What are you going to do?"

"I don't know," said Lipetz dejectedly. "But it's taken us months to get this far and I'm not about to give up now. I'm going to get the answer if I have to stay up all night to do it."

Lipetz sat alone in the lab, staring at the rows and rows of gradient tubes. Occasionally, throughout the long night, he heard the sound of footsteps going down the hall as a graduate student went into one of the labs to check on an experiment, but now in the early hours of the morning, it was eerily quiet. He had tried everything he could think of, using up three more batches of gradient solution in the process, and still was unable to get a clear signal of where the DNA was in the gradient. It was infuriating, like looking for a misplaced key you know is somewhere in the room. "The answer is in the tubes. The answer is in the tubes." Over and over, those words ran through his mind like an advertising jingle that wouldn't go away. The answer was in the tubes, but how to get it out?

It was crazy to think that he could come up with an answer in one night. After all, it had taken Brash years to work out his technique. "That's it!" he shouted aloud, bounding off the stool. Taking two steps at a time, he raced up to his office and began tossing the piles of paper from his desk onto the floor, until he uncovered his copy of Doug's dissertation. Tearing through the pages, he reached the section on the fluorescent agents Brash had tried and rejected before finding one that worked in his system. And then his heart nearly stopped. There on the page was a graph depicting the extreme sensitivity of the DNA to a fluorescent agent called DAPI.

Brash had rejected DAPI because he was interested in single-stranded

DNA, and the agent worked best on double-stranded DNA. Furthermore, the alkaline gradient he was using tore up the DNA into little bits. But Lipetz's nucleoids contained the entire DNA in its natural double-stranded state, and his neutral sucrose gradient left the DNA intact. What didn't work for Brash might just be the ticket for him.

The clock on the wall said 3:30 when Lipetz returned to the lab.

Lipetz tried DAPI for the third time. On his trips to the spectrofluorimeter, he was beginning to feel like the sorcerer's apprentice. He placed the tubes in the machine, which "read" the fluorescence bound to the DNA, and began mechanically jotting down the numbers as they appeared. Was this run also going to be a washout? he thought, when he had gone almost halfway through the tubes. Suddenly, a number that was nearly twice as high as he had been getting flashed on the screen. He felt a small surge of hope. Maybe this wasn't just an experimental fluke. He placed the next tube in the machine, and the number was even higher. Now the numbers began popping like champagne corks, until at their peak they were two and a half times over those he had been getting. It was the signal he had been waiting for, the clear indication of where the DNA had migrated to in the gradient.

In his mind, the numbers instantly formed into a graph, and the way the line rose and fell and rose again made the supercoiling of the DNA as visible to him as a range of mountains on the horizon. With DAPI, he had been able to fluorescently label only fifteen thousand cells, about a thumbnail scratch's worth. As far as he knew, he was looking at the most sensitive method for detecting supercoiling at low numbers of cells that had been developed anywhere in the world.

He stepped into the empty hall and roared with all his might. His next reaction was to chant a yogic mantra. "The way I see it," he said later, "something, call it God, call it collective consciousness, wants this knowledge out to the world, and I am just acting as a channel for this force. For me, science is like painting a picture of God; performing an experiment is like meditating; writing a paper is like saying a prayer. I figure that as long as it continues to flow, that means I'm supposed to be a channel for it. And when it stops flowing, that means it is time to do something else."

Now that he had found the technique, he could begin the real work. He had committed everything to a single throw of the dice and he had rescued the information from the tubes. Now he had to get the method down so that it could be duplicated as faithfully as a recipe. It was 5:30 in the morning, and the second wind that had sustained him for the past few hours had suddenly gone, leaving him utterly spent. All he wanted to do was stretch out on a couch somewhere.

At 8:30 in the morning, Stephens walked in and Lipetz handed him the data sheets without saying a word.

Stephens was dumbfounded. "How did you ever do this?"

"I just took a pinch of DAPI, put it in the tubes, and voilà!"

"Well, how in the world will we ever reproduce this?"

"We'll never, never know where that beautiful signal came from," thought Stephens; but in an hour working together they had figured out the optimal dilution of DAPI to use and now they began to play with the system. Lipetz remembered reading that Cook and Brazell had an 80 percent failure rate when they first developed the nucleoid technique. But now he and Stephens were getting more than 80 percent success.

"I got some young cells, only seventeen population doublings," yelled Stephens. "Let's try those on the gradient." They carried out two experiments simultaneously on both young and old cells. In one experiment they asked the question: Do old cells accumulate DNA damage in the form of strand breaks? In the other, they asked: Is there a decrease in DNA supercoiling with age? The two questions went together. If strand breaks, which caused regions of supercoiled DNA to unwind, accumulated in the cell with age, then one would expect the overall DNA supercoiling in old cells to go down.

Previous studies of young and old cells in culture had failed to detect any difference in DNA damage between young and old cells. And yet George Martin, Hart and Setlow, and several other groups had shown that as cells age in culture, there was a growing subpopulation that had stopped dividing. These same cells were also incapable of repair, and thus should be accumulating damage.

But when researchers attempted to measure DNA damage of cells in culture, they were stuck with a Catch-22. The techniques for measuring DNA damage relied on radioactive agents, which were incorporated by the DNA only when the cell was dividing. Therefore, it missed all the cells that were not dividing, and yet these were the cells that were most likely aging in culture. This was the same trap that previous workers in supercoiling had fallen into when they used radioactive compounds for binding to the DNA.

Fluorescent agents, on the other hand, like the ones used by Brash and Lipetz in their respective systems, pick up every single cell in the culture, those that are dividing and those that have stopped. Now their techniques had revealed what radioactive methods had masked: Old cells had significantly more DNA strand breaks than young cells. They were accumulating DNA damage with age.

But for Lipetz, the crowning moment was when they looked at the difference in DNA supercoiling between the young cells and those at the very end of their life span *in vitro*. Just as he had so confidently predicted two months earlier, the young cells were far more tightly coiled than the old cells. DNA supercoiling, at least for cells in culture, declined with age.

Lipetz was ecstatic. "I felt I was on the verge of establishing a new field," he says. "Everyone always said that DNA supercoiling was only interesting in procaryotes [cells without a nucleus, i.e., bacteria]. They knew that the DNA of eucaryotes [cells with a nucleus, i.e., human] was supercoiled, but so what? It didn't do anything. Others had tried and failed to show an association with aging or cancer. This was the first time that anyone had shown that supercoiling did change, that it correlated with an interesting phenomenon—in this case, aging of cells in culture—that it had physiological relevance for the cell. To me, it opened up the possibility of looking at all the things in animal and human cells that had made DNA supercoiling so interesting in bacteria."

If it turned out that supercoiling regulated the same functions in higher-order cells as it did in bacteria, then the implications for aging and cancer were staggering. In bacteria DNA supercoiling controlled *cell division*. Unregulated cell division was the hallmark of cancer, while loss of cell division was a factor in aging. Supercoiling controlled *gene expression*, which genes turned on and off. Altered gene expression was known to occur with both cancer and aging. It controlled *genetic recombination*. In humans the ability of the DNA to combine and recombine in countless permutations made possible the staggering variety of antibodies. Genetic recombination was the key to immune function. Finally, DNA supercoiling governed some forms of *DNA repair*, including excision repair of ultraviolet-light damage.

Here, Lipetz realized, was evidence for a nonmutational theory of aging. The great strength of the somatic mutation theories of aging was that they were testable. And the great weakness of these theories was that they failed most of the tests. For instance, Szilard's idea of somatic mutations in the chromosomes or DNA had foundered on the shoals of probability. The rate of mutation, as far as anyone had been able to measure, was so low, and the number of cells in the body so high, that it would take more than an individual's lifetime before it would cause trouble. The protein-error theories of Leslie Orgel and Roy Medvedev were designed to get around this objection. They suggested a self-generating mechanism for mutation in which errors in the protein synthesis would result in the manufacture of bad proteins, including those involved in the manufacture of new DNA. This would cyclically lead to more and more mistakes in the DNA template until the cell was a virtual bag of bad proteins. But various experiments in a number of different labs had failed to find support for this thesis. For instance, George Martin and his colleagues at the University of Washington in Seattle found that a specific protein they had chosen to follow did not change with the age of a cell. However, two English researchers, Robin Holliday and G. M. Tarrant, did find altered proteins in older cells. "Their cell cultures differed in certain ways from ours," Martin says, "but even they went on to present evidence for some types of enzymes that don't have abnormal forms with age. According to the protein-error hypothesis, all proteins by the end of the life span should be involved. So if you found an exception, that would be an argument against the theory."

Nature itself seemed to rule out a mutational theory of aging. Almost all organisms carry a duplicate set of chromosomes in their somatic cells. But there is a species of wasp that is haploid rather than diploid—it has only one set of chromosomes instead of the normal complement of two. Most mutations are recessive; that is, they must be carried by the same gene on both chromosomes if the trait is to be expressed. In effect, the extra set of chromosomes serves as a protection. Since the haploid has only one set of chromosomes, every mutation is dominant by default. Therefore, one would expect that if somatic mutations played a role in aging, then diploid wasps would live twice as long as the haploid variety, yet their life spans are virtually the same.

Finally, the strongest argument against somatic mutation, according to Hart, was that the cells that were aging in culture could not be accumulating mutation. Mutation, by definition, was an error in the DNA that was passed on when the cell divided. But his own research and that of others had shown that the nondividing cells were the ones that were accumulating the most damage. The problem was that most scientists tended to use the words "mutation" and "damage" interchangeably. But, as he continually pointed out, they were two very different things: Mutations were a change in the DNA base sequence—an adenine in the place of a guanine, for instance—while damage could be many things, such as a thymine dimer, a break in the DNA strand, or a bulky foreign agent stuck onto a base. Cells that were dividing would be accumulating mutations and these would be the cells that were most at risk for cancer, but cells that were no longer dividing would be accumulating damage and these could be the ones most vulnerable to age changes.

The various objections to somatic mutation theory had caused gerontologists in recent years to start casting about for alternate explanations for why cells age. Martin proposed that the reason for the Hayflick limit of cells in culture was that they "differentiated themselves to death." Cells that are continuously made in the body, like those of the blood and skin, start from a pool of mother cells, called stem cells. These generalized cells give rise to descendants that then differentiate into cells with specialized functions. Cells in culture go through a similar transition from stem cells to nondividing differentiated cells. In this way the culture appears to be painting itself into the corner as more and more of the progeny become what Martin calls "end-terminally differentiated." The result, at least with epidermal cell cultures, he found, is that with each successive division, more and more of the daughter cells make keratin; i.e., the culture is literally turning into dandruff.

Instead of an increasing state of differentiation, Cutler became interested in dysdifferentiation, the idea that cells gradually drift away from their specialized state. Hart began to consider what the effects of damage would be on the nondividing cell. While mutations in working genes would cause abnormal proteins to be made, damage might have a more subtle effect—perhaps interfering with the regulatory machinery of the cell, causing the wrong genes to turn on or off. In England, Robin Holliday, known for his work on error theories of aging, proposed that chemical switches on the DNA that controlled gene activities during embryological development and maintained the cell in a differentiated state were lost as the cell aged.

All these ideas had one thing in common: They involved epigenetic, rather than genetic, mechanisms. The term "epigenetic" was first applied to the step-by-step process of development by which a fertilized egg becomes a full-fledged being. It is now applied more generally to processes that turn genes on and off at any point during the life span. The difference between genetic and epigenetic is the difference between written instructions and how those instructions are carried out. While the written instructions are the same in every cell of the body, only a minute amount, an estimated 1 percent to 5 percent of the DNA, is ever executed, that is, translated into protein. Indeed, it is this wholesale repression of genetic information that gives each cell its particular character. Every multicellular organism begins with a single cell containing all the information to make a living being, but after the first few divisions, cells start to differentiate. They become "committed" to carrying out a specialized function and there is no turning back. Skeletal cells make the proteins needed for the body's structure; skin cells make the proteins for the protective envelope; muscle cells make the products needed for mobility; and so on. Only the genes needed to make those products are turned on, or "expressed," in a given cell, while all the other genes, more than 95 percent of the DNA, are turned off, or "repressed." During development, epigenetic changes in gene expression are sweeping and dramatic, allowing an undifferentiated cell to develop into a recognizably human form within 60 days.

It had long been assumed that once the pattern of gene expression had been set in each of the cells, it was maintained for life. But recent research has shown that this is not the case. In cancer cells, for instance, genes that had not been expressed since the time of embryonic life were turned on again. Cutler had found similar events happening in aging cells. And now, Lipetz believed, he was looking at a possible mechanism by which epigenetic changes could occur with age.

It lay in the actual structure of the DNA itself—in this case, the higher levels of organization, which in turn exerted control over the lower levels. What happened to all the DNA that was not being used by the cell in its differentiated state? Like excess grain stored in silos, it was packaged away into the supercoils and domains of DNA chromatin.

Lipetz had now found that strand breaks, which accumulated with age, caused this careful packaging to deteriorate. Other scientists had shown that loss of DNA superhelicity altered control of where the RNA enzymes bound onto the DNA. This meant that the information in the DNA might not be faithfully transcribed and translated into proteins and enzymes. Since much of the DNA superstructure is arranged into huge loops of supercoiling called domains, containing about 100 genes, loss of supercoiling could mean that many genes could be affected at the same time. The fine control of the cell would be lost—unwanted enzymes could turn on or needed enzymes be turned off, with catastrophic consequences to the cell. Along with everything else in the cell, DNA repair would be affected. Lipetz believed he now had an explanation for Hart's DNA repair-life-span correlation, and he couldn't wait to tell him.

According to Lipetz, the next night, a day and a half before Hart was scheduled to leave for the Gerontology Society Conference, he, Stephens, and Hart were sitting in the latter's office shooting the breeze.

"What's new?" asked Hart affably.

"I just won your Nobel Prize for you," said Lipetz. Hart sat back with an amused smile and said, "Really?"

It was a classic moment, the son confronting the father, and Lipetz relished it, walking about with great energy, barely unable to contain the sense of excitement and danger he felt in his moment of triumph. "The problem with your theory all along is that everyone keeps calling it 'somatic mutation,' and you knew that it wasn't somatic mutation but you had no way to show it. Well, I've just figured it out and I proved it. And not only that, Ron, I just figured out what controls your DNA repair correlation and what it arises from. It arises from the DNA superhelicity because that is one of the things that controls UV excision repair."

The next day, Lipetz received a memo from Hart asking him to write up his findings, with two slides for the conference. Although Hart was hesitant about presenting material that was preliminary and had not yet been tested by several different methodologies, he believed the findings were new and significant enough to merit attention. Lipetz and Stephens spent all Saturday putting their results on a graph, rushing it off to a commercial lab that prepared slides overnight. Early Sunday morning, he dropped off the package at Hart's house. It may have taken him somewhat longer to shoot the fish in the barrel than he had reckoned, but Lipetz had made the deadline.

When Joan Smith-Sonneborn called him a few weeks after the gerontology conference, Lipetz could not have been more surprised. He remembered hearing her a few months earlier at OSU on her life-extension experiment in paramecia. Now, of all things, she was asking for a collaboration. As they spoke about her interest in supercoiling and how it might be interesting to test it on her paramecia, Lipetz began to get very interested. Paramecia were eucaryote cells with DNA supercoiling much like that of our own cells and they also had measurable life spans. It might be just the model system he needed. But he was also wary; collaboration was a risky business. Now that he was onto something hot, other researchers were sure to come sniffing around, trying to grab a piece of it for themselves, perhaps even jumping into print before he could act. It had happened to him before and if he were not careful, it could happen again. They spoke together several times after that, and finally Lipetz suggested that they talk further at the FIBER meeting of "Biomarkers in Aging" in April.

FIBER, the Fund for Integrated Biomedical Research, was the brainchild of three very unusual people—a former candidate for governor of Texas,

Don Yarborough; a cancer doctor, Bill Regelson; and a health-minded U.S. senator, Alan Cranston.

Don Yarborough is a quintessential Texan from his Stetson to his out-sized charm. His velvet drawl lures you in and his words keep you there. It's no wonder, you think as he spins his tales with dramatic flourishes worthy of an Olivier, that he won the national collegiate debating championship. The wonder is that he didn't make it all the way to the governor's mansion. But even though he lost the election, he made some powerful, wealthy friends who he believed might support a mission he saw as the most important in today's world.

In his own southern-gentlemanly way, Yarborough is a take-charge type. Upon spotting me at the 1980 Gerontology Society meeting in San Diego, he immediately took my briefcase and escorted me to a chair beside the pool. Then he took away my technological crutch, the tape recorder, insisting that it inhibited the free play of his mind. Finally, he took even my pencil and pad, saying that he would take the notes, that all I needed were a few key words that would jog my mind. For the next half-hour, while he spoke nonstop, he wrote down only the word "culture."

"There are two cultures, the lay culture out there in which people are desperate, literally dying for a solution to the aging problem; and the scientific culture, where the individual is subsumed under the institutional," he said. "The scientific culture is then subdivided into two cultures, the knowledge accumulators and the problem solvers. The knowledge accumulators believe in slowly adding to the sum total of knowledge for knowledge's sake. They act as though they have all the time in the world. For them science is an art. Whether or not they solve the problem in their lifetime doesn't matter. They are content to add their little bit.

"On the other side are the problem solvers, who look at the whole field and say this is where one should go, this is where you can make the hit. They want to solve the problem and only the problem. Theirs is mission-oriented science, like putting a man on the moon. These are the knowledge synthesizers, the ones who can bring everything together and make the breakthroughs.

"In the scientific culture, the institution dominates and the knowledge accumulators dominate the institutions. The granting process, the peer-review system which looks for 'scientific excellence,' rewards those who amass bits of data and penalizes the problem solvers. As a result, the knowledge synthesizers are constantly backsliding, backing away from high-risk research, going into 'safe' fields, doing only 'safe' experiments.

"Now we have reached the point where using molecular technology like genetic recombination and DNA sequencing we can really do something about aging. We are in the Garden of Eden, and can taste of the tree of knowledge of good and evil. But instead, what is happening? Survival curves show that, with every decade, the chances of your dying increases greatly. At fifty everything starts to go down and, every decade, it gets progressively worse.

"Why is this allowed to happen? According to the French philosopher Pascal the reason we are always involved in trivia is because we wish to avoid responsibility. That's why we have committees and institutions and the peer-review process, and large meetings like this one involving thousands of people—to avoid responsibility. It would be better to put four problem solvers into a room and tell them they can't come out until they've solved the problem. That way they would all be responsible.

"We need leadership. We need to support the knowledge synthesizers, the problem solvers. We need mission-oriented scientists—large problems like the Anderson project at Argonne National Laboratory, to get the molecular sequence of every protein in the human body. We need to get a computer into every lab. We need to work out programs in different areas. We need to have telecommunication between labs. And we have to do it now. The time for playing around in the Garden of Eden has ended."

Then there is Bill Regelson. Dark, earthy, expansive, energetic, he has an intellect that darts and pounces on a dozen different topics in medicine, like a cat chasing a moth; and a manic enthusiasm, with a knack for drawing people out, listening to their problems, looking for solutions.

Finally, there is Senator Cranston, a fitness advocate whose interest in life extension is not merely academic, who diets, jogs, and consumes large amounts of vitamins in the hope of living as long as he can. He is a person who has always looked at the big picture, he says, not the small details. By tackling the problem of aging as a whole, he believes, one might discover the means for wiping out its various manifestations, like arteriosclerosis and cancer.

Yarborough had the idea and the access to people with money; Regelson, the scientific expertise; and Cranston, the political know-how and contacts. Over dinner one evening, the three men decided that what was needed was a private-sector alternative to the public-sector scientific establishment. As they saw it, biomedical research on aging was being generated all the time, but there was no mechanism for bringing the pieces of the puzzle together. It could be five, ten years before the fruits of basic research reached the clinical table. This lag time could be greatly reduced by simply putting the right people in touch with one another. Just as an enzyme speeds up the interaction between a protein and its substate, so might such an organization act as a catalyst between one researcher and another, bringing together the separate pieces of the puzzles. Instead of large grants to a few, they would provide "seed money" to the innovators, the knowledge synthesizers. Instead of huge sprawling conferences, they would hold small meetings on a single topic, where the actual people doing the work could rapidly exchange information. The idea for FIBER was born—a "center without walls," an institution that would avoid the pitfalls of institutionalization.

Regelson is sitting in the FIBER office one day amidst an avalanche of books, manuscripts, reprints, and grant proposals. Most of the time, he is on the phone, talking up current research, making arrangements, weaving an informal network of communication. "You ought to get into dipulsed electronics; heals by radiowaves without producing heat," he tells one caller. A researcher from Seattle calls, requesting $25,000 to continue his work on thirty-six-month-old rats. Regelson dials someone else, making his pitch: "This one is crucial. The rats will die out before the study is completed." To yet another person: "You really got to go to Philadelphia and speak to Dr. X and see his lab there. I'll pay your way.

"The National Institute on Aging was set up to fund research in aging and the diseases of aging," he says between phone calls. "But you can't expect the National Institutes of Health to support high-risk, innovative research, because peer review is intrinsically very conservative. It is also very competitive. And so research that is on the fringe in times of tight money is not going to make it. The innovative research is in a classic bind. You can't put anything speculative in a grant unless you have data to support it and you can't get the data unless you have the grant.

"In addition to innovation, what we need is what I call fulcrum research; that is, key research which, if it succeeds, [means] things will tilt in a very specific direction. [Leo] Szilard and others have indicated that it isn't necessary that a tremendous number of experiments be done. What counts are the key experiments that bring about a total change of direction. Unfortunately, under the present grant system, it takes a long time for a lot of key areas to be recognized. That's where FIBER comes in."

"The Biomarkers in Aging" was the first of FIBER's conferences. The idea behind it was simple: If aging treatments were to be developed, there had to be accurate and rapid measures, or biomarkers, of their effectiveness both in experimental-model systems and in the human body. The conference was designed to bring together people who were looking at different aspects of this problem.

The atmosphere of the meeting, held in Washington, D.C., was only slightly more formal than that of the Renegade Repair Conference. Twenty-eight speakers were scheduled to give their spiel in eight hours. It was "rapid-fire gestalt," according to Regelson, the bottom line without the fine details, so that people in different disciplines could cull the entire field of aging in a single day.

Lipetz, who has trouble speaking as fast as he can think, who prides himself on "going for the jugular" in an experiment, and who has the patience of a hungry child just before dinnertime, found the format most congenial for his maiden speech to the gerontology community. Smith-Sonneborn, like some of the others present, had heard some of the material earlier at the Gerontology Society meeting when Lipetz's preliminary data were presented by Hart. But now when he talked about some of his latest experiments, she was convinced. This had to be the way to go.

That evening they talked for hours and proved FIBER's point about the spark that could be ignited just by bringing together two people working in different fields along different lines. He wanted to know how supercoiling controlled life span, DNA synthesis, and repair in eucaryotic cells; she was trying to figure out how supercoiling was responsible for the life span extension of her paramecia. She was expert in cell biology, he in molecular biology. He had chemicals he believed could increase or decrease the superhelicity, while she had the system that could rapidly screen their effectiveness. She was a workaholic with a passion for science that was all-consuming, he was mystical, driven, idea-obsessed. Two lovers could not have been better matched. "Joan is the only person I have ever met," he was to say later, "who could keep up with me, and then bury me."

Smith-Sonneborn felt that the collaboration she had always longed for was about to happen: a meeting of the minds, where the whole is larger than the sum of the parts.

"What does it feel like to carry out research on the forefront of knowledge," I said to her as we sat in her backyard in June of 1980, when their experiments on superhelicity, DNA repair, and life-span manipulation were just getting under way.

"I'll tell you exactly what it feels like," she answered without hesitation: "a roller-coaster ride. As you do the experiments, you're sort of scared;

you're not sure you're right. Then you're on a high and you think you know what it's all about. The next experiment . . . [and] there you are on the bottom again. You thought you knew what it was all about and something comes up and it's not that way at all. You reach the top and down you go again. It's a mixture of highs and lows, anxieties and triumphs.

"I really love roller coasters. My favorite is the Space Mountain in Disneyland. It's a roller coaster in the dark. And it has an enormous lighting effect on the order of *Star Wars*. So you combine the thrill of up and down with the highs of visual stimulation, and your sensation of speed is even more intense because the lights are going in the opposite direction. Then there are all these warning signs as you enter, but I keep on going, just for the reason I keep on going here, because for all the lights and for all the speed and for all the anxiety and for all the thrills, you got to go all the way."

Chapter Nine

Life Extension 1: Supercoils

Just as Smith-Sonneborn had predicted, the experiments were a roller-coaster ride. "Well, we're up to something," Smith-Sonneborn told me, when I visited her in June 1980. "What we hope to do," she confided, her brown eyes glowing intently, "is change the level of excision repair. And since Hart's hypothesis is that aging is determined in part by the relative rates of accumulation of damage and repair, if we could alter the levels of repair, then theoretically we should be able to alter the rates of aging."

The plan was that Lipetz would provide compounds that change DNA supercoiling. She would test their effect on DNA repair in paramecia, while he and Ralph Stephens looked at the same phenomenon in mammalian cells. This would provide a rapid prescreen for compounds that had the potential to increase repair and extend life in human cells. FIBER had given them some seed money so that they would be able to do some traveling back and forth between their labs.

Added to the excitement she always feels, when beginning a series of experiments, was the heady sensation that they might be breaking new ground. Only a handful of laboratories in the world were working with DNA superhelicity, and among those that were looking at the relationship between the higher-order structure of DNA and aging, there might be only Lipetz, Stephens, and herself. For now they were keeping their work a secret from the outside world, a not unusual practice among scientists who want to safeguard their new ideas until they have results to present.

At the lab, things are just getting under way. A young woman with blonde hair that almost reaches her cut-off jeans is starting the coffee. Five young men in various stages of hirsuteness—mustaches, beards, or both—walk in wearing T-shirts, jeans, sneakers, or sandals. Smith-Sonneborn is amused that three of her students have begun smoking pipes. "There must be something about pipe smoking and paramecia," she says. "Tracy Sonneborn always has a pipe in his mouth, like it's part of his face."

Upon observing that supercoiling declined with age in human cells, Lipetz wondered if he was looking at a means of intervention. Changing genetic function, such as increasing the amount of DNA repair in the cells, presents formidable obstacles. The genetic-engineering techniques necessary to do that in multicellular animals is proving to be more difficult than was once thought, and it may be years before it becomes feasible. Lipetz believed that DNA supercoiling could be the door to DNA repair. And substances known to affect DNA supercoiling might be the key to opening that door.

"Right now many people in science are so enamored of the fact that the DNA molecule controls everything that goes on in the cell, they've lost sight of the fact that there has to be a pathway from the outside in," he says. "There has to be a hormone or some other chemical signal. Otherwise, how does the nucleus know what enzymes to make and how much is needed? I don't regard DNA as necessarily the primary causal event in every case in a senescent progression. Rather, it could be an intermediate step in a cascade of events. For example, you could have a change in hormonal levels at the cell membrane that changes substances which modulate the superhelicity, which then affects DNA synthesis and perhaps gene expression."

With this idea in hand, he began casting about for compounds that could change the DNA supercoiling in the cell. The first ones he found were those on the negative side; they decreased DNA supercoiling and lowered DNA repair. One of them was the antibiotic novobiocin, which other researchers had shown relaxed DNA supercoiling in the cells of bacteria and mammals. Novobiocin also interfered with DNA synthesis and inhibited excision repair. Lipetz and Stephens confirmed these findings and then showed that another antibiotic, nalidixic acid, also decreased repair and DNA supercoiling in a mammalian cell. He sent vials of both novobiocin and nalidixic acid to Laramie for Smith-Sonneborn to test on her paramecia. This is the "down" side of the experiment. He also hopes to send her compounds that will go the other way, increasing both DNA supercoiling and DNA repair. But first he has to find out whether his idea of trying to affect changes in DNA repair by altering the supercoiling has any validity at all.

In today's experiment, Smith-Sonneborn will look at the effect of novobiocin on DNA repair in paramecia. To test this, she will expose the cells to ultraviolet light. If novobiocin decreases DNA supercoiling in the paramecia, then it should also decrease the cell's ability to repair the damage induced by the UV.

The first order of the day is the lab meeting. In 1976 she received an award as outstanding teacher of the year at the University of Wyoming. Her student evaluations attest to her fairness, her enthusiasm, her caring, her ability to communicate with students, her availability to them, her obvious desire that they learn. "When I teach," she says with feeling, "it's for life." All these qualities are evident as she talks quietly with her crew.

They discuss the number of groups of cells they will need to look at all the experimental variables, including the doses of novobiocin, the length of time the cells should be irradiated with ultraviolet light, and the age of the cells. The student in charge of the day-to-day operation of the lab disagrees with her on the dosage, and after a bit of dickering, Smith-Sonneborn compromises by agreeing to use both their doses.

"So far we have four groups," says a student who is taking notes. "One with novobiocin only, one control, and two with novobiocin and two different doses of UV."

"Oh, c'mon," she says with a cheerleader's enthusiasm. "Let's get those groups up. We've got a good culture here, so picking up cells will be no sweat."

They add more groups, varying the possibilities, until they end up with sixteen. Smith-Sonneborn gets up from her squatting position, looking quite pleased. "Let's go, okay?" she says. The rock music is turned on and the lab swings into action. She checks the culture in a Petri dish under the microscope and then tells me to take a look. I have seen human cells growing in tissue culture, but this is completely different. At one-hundred-times magnification, it is a living world of miniature animals moving in a miniature sea, each individual maintaining its own space like a swimmer in a pool lane. "They don't bump into one another," I marvel.

"Aren't they pretty?" she asks proprietarily. "There are plenty of cells, but few dividers." Suddenly two cells come into view, locked together like Siamese twins—the dividers she is looking for. There are highly sophisticated methods for "synchronizing" the cells so that they are all at the same stage in their reproductive cycle, but these require chemicals that can affect the cell's biology. Smith-Sonneborn, who prefers "natural" solutions where possible, simply extracts the cells from their media when they are in the process of division, then waits two hours before treating them, when she knows the micronucleus is most resistant to DNA repair.

She isolates a single cell, stains it, and shows it to me in all its glory under the fluorescent microscope at four-hundred-times magnification. For the first time, I can appreciate the *in vitro/in vivo* nature of her model system. All the internal structures of the living animal are revealed—the dominating macronucleus, which contains the genes for the cells' everyday functioning; the much smaller micronucleus, which houses the DNA for reproduction; the many food vacuoles, which look like bright pennies; the contractile vacuoles, which blow out and explode like a nova as they expel their contents. It is as though I could look into a person and see the heart, lungs, liver, kidneys, intestines. On the outside of the cell, the stubby hairlike projections of cilia beat in food like thousands of tiny fingers. She disturbs the cell and points to arrowlike structures that appear on its surface. "Those are trichocysts," she says. "He puts them out when he's mad."

Fascinated, I begin to play with the controls of the microscope, moving the stage up and down. Suddenly there is a bulge in the cell membrane, which continues to blow up like a balloon until it bursts and all the inner structures go sliding out. "Oh, my God, what's happening?" I ask. She takes a look and laughs. "You've squooshed the cell with the stage. It's just gone splat, like a person who's fallen from a twenty-story building."

Although the debacle has left me feeling like a proverbial bull in this china shop of sterile glassware and delicate microscopic creatures, she insists that I "get a feel for laboratory work" by isolating some cells. This means starting out like everyone else by making my own pipettes, the hollow tubes with suction bulbs at the end. Beginning with a long, thin, glass cylinder, I am supposed to rotate it back and forth over the flame of a Bunsen burner until it melts; stretch it out like taffy to about 100 microns in width, about the thickness of a human hair; and then snap it back on itself so that it breaks off in just the right place, leaving an opening large enough to accommodate a single paramecium. In what seems like a single motion, she makes one pipette after another, lining them up like angel's-hair pasta.

It looks incredibly easy, but it takes a handful of broken tubes before I learn to gauge the moment at which to pull the tube out. Wait too long and it melts in half; pull too early and it breaks in two rather than elongates. Finally I make one that fits all the specifications. Then comes the hard part, fishing out the dividers. This calls for keeping the prey in my field of vision, trying to stop the Parkinson-like shaking of my hand, and not disturbing the medium as I move the pipette, which has taken on harpoonlike dimensions under the scope. After twenty minutes of sucking up what I am certain are a dozen paramecia, I squeeze the rubber bulb at the end of the pipette, squirting out my "catch." The yield: two cells.

Smith-Sonneborn sits down, her hand like the Rock of Gibraltar, and after what seems like half a second, announces that she has netted thirty cells. It takes from two days to two weeks to become a proficient cell isolater, she says. And some people never quite get the hang of it. Unlike mathematics, physics, or even chemistry, biology requires the sure hand of a surgeon; and molecular biology, the skill of a microsurgeon.

Sitting at the fluorescent scope, one of her students checks for autogamy, or self-fertilization. Using an automatic pipette that can pick up four samples at a time, he stains them with acridine orange, which colors the body orange and the macronucleus green. When the nucleus has broken up into sausagelike fragments, the process of autogamy is under way.

Later in her office, Smith-Sonneborn describes her mutagenesis assay, which measures how harmful a substance is by looking at the rate of mutation in the paramecia. She will treat the cells with novobiocin, with and without UV, and then let the cells go through autogamy. Any mutations that the cells have incurred will be expressed in the daughter cells either in the form of stillbirths or slow growers. Since the cells are kept in the dark, away from photoreactivating light, the only repair they are able to carry out is dark repair, that is, excision repair. Therefore, the number of survivors in the experimental group versus the number in the controls represents the amount of excision repair that has taken place. If novobiocin is inhibiting excision repair, then it should make the treated cells far more sensitive to the mutating and killing effects of ultraviolet light.

Requiring only five days to carry out, the mutagenesis assay does double duty for Smith-Sonneborn. For the Department of Energy, she uses it as the equivalent of the Ames bacterial assay to identify potentially mutagenic and carcinogenic substances in the environment. For aging and longevity studies, the assay provides a rapid prescreen of chemicals that might alter life span. Once she has identified a compound that has an effect on DNA repair, either increasing it or decreasing it, she will carry out the much more demanding and time-consuming life-span study.

Excision repair not only repairs damage from ultraviolet light, it also patches up damage from certain noxious chemicals. Even if their experiments do not prove the hypothesis that enhancing DNA repair can lengthen life span, just finding substances that could raise repair levels and protect against the mutating and cancer-causing effects of environmental pollutants would be of enormous public-health benefit.

Beyond this there is always the tantalizing possibility that Lipetz might be right about a controlling role for DNA supercoiling in eucaryotic cells. If their experiments can tie together supercoiling, DNA repair, and life span, they could point the way to chemical intervention into the aging process.

Later, as we sit under a tree enjoying the soft summer day, Smith-Sonneborn tells me about her belief that the control of aging lies in the interaction of the cytoplasm and nucleus. Unlike most of her colleagues, she does not rule out the possibility of immortal life for human cells if some way could be found to prevent or reverse the aging process. There are precedents, she says, immortal one-celled creatures, called tetrahymena, that have been cultured for thirty years in the laboratory with no sign of diminished growth. Amoebae are immortal but can be made mortal just by changing their medium. "This says that immortality may be a fairly fragile thing since just slight changes in the environment can flip them into the other mode of life," she says. Lest any argue that protozoa are in a class by themselves and bear no relationship to multicellular animals, she points out that "what is crystal clear in all organisms is the immortality of the germ line. No species of any kind would continue from generation to generation, unless it could form itself anew. So what is going on? What happens to the immortality?"

There are a lot of data, she says, that indicate that when embryological development takes place, the potential for immortality is lost. "But clearly the germ cell had it. And as soon as it differentiates, it seems to lose it. The real question is, Has it lost it?"

She tells me about some experiments she has undertaken, at the instigation of Regelson, that, if anything, are even more revolutionary in their implications than the superhelicity project. They involve the use of electromagnetic radiation fields (EMF), which are generated by coils wrapped around magnets. Other scientists have found that these fields that emit very low currents of electricity have a profound effect on living cells. They believe that the fields induce changes in the cells that closely mimic the environment during embryonic development, allowing long-repressed genes to turn back on. Among the claims made for EMF are that it accelerates bone healing in humans and grows back amputated limbs in lower animals that ordinarily are incapable of doing this.

In her own experiments, she has subjected her paramecia to various EMF frequencies. "The cells picked out two frequencies that are beneficial to humans," she says. Although her experiments are very preliminary, they show a small, but significant, life-extension effect, enough for her to order bigger machines that will allow her to place whole trays of cells within the coils.

"Theoretically, the idea is, you can get the cell to become totipotent, that is, to express its full potential as an embryo," she says.

"You're talking not only about extending life, but going backwards. Rejuvenation. Do you think that's possible?" I ask.

"I think it is," she says with conviction. "I'm arguing that the experiments with limb regeneration using electromagnetic fields say the somatic cell is still capable of embryonic tricks. If the conditions were right, maybe you could get some of that immortality back."

The results of the novobiocin experiments came in time for the Gordon Conference in August 1980. Just as Lipetz said it would, the antibiotic greatly increased the sensitivity of the paramecia to ultraviolet light. It doubled the lethal effect of ultraviolet radiation in vegatively dividing cells—that is, paramecia that have not gone through autogamy. The effect was even more dramatic in the mutagenesis assay. After the paramecia went through autogamy, over 70 percent of the cells in the next generation were stillborn, compared with 2.9 percent of the cells that received UV alone. On their very first try, they had taken a compound known to decrease DNA supercoiling and shown that it had a devastating effect on living cells.

Smith-Sonneborn's first emotion was relief. "When something doesn't work in the lab," she says, "it's really the devil to get in there and find out what's stopping it. Is it your idea or the way you carried it out or something about the organism that is stopping it? That's a real bottleneck which may take years to unravel. But right from the beginning, it looked like we weren't in that situation."

From that point they were on a roll. Although they were on a very tight budget, she decided the results were promising enough to go for the far more complicated life-span experiment. Not wanting to stop the other work in the lab since it paid the bills, she assigned the project to a work-study student. Because it was his first real experiment, she made him repeat it three times. Each time the answer was the same: The antibiotic lopped 15 percent off the expected life span. Again the premise seemed to be holding up: There was a direct association between a decrease in DNA supercoiling, a corresponding fall in DNA repair, and a shortened life span.

But there was still the question of whether or not the abbreviated life expectancy was due to a decrease in DNA repair. To answer this, she turned to the model she had worked out in the earlier experiments on UV light and life span. Once again she treated the cells with novobiocin and ultraviolet irradiation, but this time, instead of keeping them in the dark, she allowed them to repair the UV damage with photoreactivating light. If the novobiocin worked by interfering with excision repair, then the results should be the same for both treated and untreated cells. If the antibiotic had some other adverse effect on the cells, then the results should be significantly different for both sets of cells. To her intense satisfaction, the treated cells reacted just like the untreated cells—no mutagenesis, no increased deaths. The simplest explanation for these results was that novobiocin worked by inhibiting excision repair of UV-induced damage. "The fact that photoreactivation brings the level of mutation back to that of the controls," she says, "implies that the target for novobiocin is excision-repair capacity." In other words, they had taken a substance known to decrease DNA supercoiling and shown that it interfered with DNA repair and shortened life span.

Throughout this period, the telephone wires between Laramie and Columbus were burning up. "I think that Joan had her doubts about supercoiling before that, but when she started getting results, she became a convert," says Lipetz.

"It was a very lovely time," she agrees. "With each additional success, we became more excited. And we were not yet telling anybody what we were doing. We were just reveling in the joy of finding a correlation between what we thought ought to happen and what was happening."

When they had presented their first results at the Gordon Conference, the consensus was that the work was very preliminary. Lipetz and Smith-Sonneborn agreed with that judgment but, in the context of the Gordon Conference, found it particularly galling. "I had been to Gordon Research Conferences in other fields," he says, "but this one was a joke. Some of the data were literally years old." Smith-Sonneborn agrees: "It was bad enough there were so many papers that had been published three or four years ago, but when a session chairman singled out one of them to say, 'There's an example of what ought to be presented,' I thought, 'Whoa! Our stuff is unpublished, preliminary data. If you want a beautiful, complete picture, I can pull out my data from three, four years back, too.' "

But one criticism struck home: They still lacked physical proof that the reason novobiocin decreased repair and shortened life span in the paramecia was that it decreased DNA supercoiling in the cells. Until they showed this, and it could only be done using the gradient technique, they could not rule out the possibility that the novobiocin worked by some other mechanism. In the early fall of 1980, Lipetz went to the University of Wyoming to try the novobiocin experiments again, but this time he would put the paramecia DNA through the gradient.

At this point the roller coaster started downhill. They had expected a smooth ride since Lipetz and Stephens had already done a preliminary experiment at OSU that showed that novobiocin reduced DNA supercoiling in paramecia, but they ended up proving only Murphy's law.

Their problems began from the moment Lipetz arrived. Since Smith-Sonneborn did not have a gradient maker, Lipetz brought one with him on the plane. It arrived with several bulbs broken and its sensitive instrumentation thrown out of whack. Although FIBER footed the bill for his plane ticket, there was not enough money to bring out technicians. They had to rely on her crew to carry out procedures for which they had no experience. And then there was the matter of the ultracentrifuge.

The few machines scattered about the Wyoming campus, which are as essential to molecular biology as a washing machine is to a mother of young children, were in constant demand. Using all her powers of persuasion, Smith-Sonneborn managed to get her friends in the agriculture department, several buildings away, to give up their instrument for a few hours. Their arms laden with test tubes, chemicals, and instruments, she and Lipetz made their way to the "ag" building, spun the tubes, "read" them, only to find that they had made mistakes in preparing the gradient, and had to start from scratch. After a few days of disrupting the other lab's experiments, they were asked to find another centrifuge, which they did in the botany building. But without an experienced technician to make the experiments run like clockwork, they ended up an hour behind schedule and dashed over to the building with all their paraphernalia, only to find themselves locked out without a key.

But the worst part was that the very last step of the experiments was sabotaged by the lack of a spectrofluorimeter to "read" the DAPI fluorescence. They tried several more-primitive fluorescent detectors, again going from building to building, but none of them was sensitive enough to pick up the DAPI signal. They were stymied on the final step of the procedure—locating how far the DNA had traveled in the gradient, which would indicate the degree of supercoiling.

The stress imposed by the working conditions took a toll on both of them, and by the time Lipetz had left, it was apparent the honeymoon was over. Lipetz's rages are legendary in his own lab. But there they are tempered by the fact that everyone is used to them and whatever damage is done is deftly and rapidly repaired by his collaborator. A running joke at his lab is that Lipetz fires everyone in the morning and Stephens hires them back in the afternoon. But to Smith-Sonneborn and her crew, his temper was far from funny.

"We were working fifteen, sixteen hours a day with really lousy equipment," says Lipetz. "And I did get boiling mad in her laboratory. But that was because of idiotic things that ruined the experiment. But she gets the same way. When an idiotic thing is done, she goes into this frosty state and talks supercalmly, and you better go into the mountains for a week or two and be careful not to leave a trail. Then she gets over it, calls a lab meeting, and everyone goes, 'Whew.' Joan and I are absolutely alike that way."

Whatever hopes they still had for the experiment were literally washed out on the plane ride home. Since they were unable to obtain clear-cut results on the fluorescent monitors at the University of Wyoming, they decided to pack the hundreds of DAPI-containing tubes, and label each one of them according to its location in the gradient batch—a painstaking, time-consuming job—and ship them back to Ohio, where they could be read properly. But pressure changes on the airplane caused the tubes to literally flip their tops, leaking their contents and washing off the labels.

Even though they were stalled on the molecular level of their experiment, they had attained half of their stated goal to jack DNA repair up and down in the cell. Granted, it was in a direction that no one wanted to go—lower repair and life shortening. But as Smith-Sonneborn pointed out when others raised this objection: "If you can modulate repair with a chemical, it implies that the flip side should be possible."

In order to continue their investigations, they had to have more than FIBER's start-up money. Separately, they had submitted grant proposals to the National Institute on Aging (NIA), which were still being reviewed and, even if approved, might not be funded. Smith-Sonneborn was also waiting to hear from the National Science Foundation, which had supported her aging work in the past. Her only grants at this point were from the Department of Energy, and this meant mutagenicity and toxicology studies, not life span and aging.

It looked as if FIBER was their only hope. Bill Regelson had interested the MacArthur Foundation in funding an aging project. From two dozen proposals he had submitted, including one from Lipetz on supercoiling and one from Smith-Sonneborn on the paramecia model, the foundation asked him to select three. These were Schwartz on DHEA, Denckla on DECO, and if Lipetz and Smith-Sonneborn could combine their proposals, he told them, they could be the third.

A few months after his earlier fiasco, Lipetz flew back to Laramie. The fall air was still warm and fragrant, and this time, all the fun and excitement that had marked their first meeting returned. "We didn't do experiments, we just wrote," says Smith-Sonneborn, "long hours day after day, getting it down on paper. But it was thinking, and that's what Phil does best. It was a delight."

While she was still recovering from the whirlwind activity of getting out the grant proposal, Yarborough called. The MacArthur Foundation was not going to buy their project unless they could automate the lab techniques for isolating and working with paramecia. She and Lipetz had driven themselves to exhaustion, getting in a grant proposal when they could have been doing experiments, and, after all that work, the foundation was going to turn them down because their techniques weren't automated. She hung up the phone, feeling that she had had it with FIBER. The idea was even too silly to consider.

Lying in bed that night, she flashed on the one person in the world who could automate her system. It was Don Glaser, her postdoctoral mentor at Berkeley. Winner of a Nobel Prize in physics for his bubble chamber, he was the inventor of Cyclops, a computer-driven, one-man-laboratory band that could plate colonies, assess their speed and shape, pick out mutants, measure their growth rate, and so on, in the time it took thirty trained technicians.

"I've got just the man for you," she told Yarborough the next day. "Someone I used to work with: Don Glaser."

"I don't believe you said that," he exclaimed. "Because we've been trying to get support for Glaser and his Cyclops. You check with him, and if he agrees, you get right on the next plane to Berkeley, you hear?"

The next day she was basking in the summery warmth of the tree-lined Berkeley campus, marveling at how it seemed like only a day, rather than twenty years, since she had been a student there. Glaser welcomed her and, within a few minutes, was spinning out ideas, diagramming on the blackboard just how his device could be adapted to work with paramecia. It would pick up cells, isolate them, count them. Instead of having one person per compound, it could do a hundred, recording and storing the data with the objectivity possible only with a computer. The prospect of doing research a hundred times faster thrilled her. She could look not only at superhelical coiling, but at antioxidants, vitamins, hormones, anything her heart desired. There would be no need to pick and choose among compounds or, for that matter, theories. She could test them all. "You're not talking about chicken feed," she told Glaser, "you're talking about the whole ranch."

Glaser shared her enthusiasm. His problems of getting enough money to keep Cyclops alive were well known and had recently been chronicled in *Science*. Although the government had already sunk millions of dollars into its development, the priority rating on his latest grant proposal was just under funding level. Without help from FIBER or some other private group, the marvelous machine was in danger of becoming a white elephant.

Arriving home late that night, she threw herself into bed, exhausted but exhilarated. By seven A.M., the telephone was ringing. It was Yarborough waiting for a debriefing.

"Glaser is fantastic," she told him, suddenly wide awake. "There's no question in my mind that he could automate the system. It's going to cost plenty. But it can be done."

"Get to Washington by five P.M.," he told her, "and you're on." The time zones in flying East worked against her, and the Denver airport was a two-and-a-half-hour drive away. Nevertheless, less than twenty-four hours after leaving California, she found herself pulling up to the entrance to the Capitol building in a black Mercedes, having no idea why she was there. Upon entering Senate Democratic Whip Cranston's office, she learned it was a dinner for the MacArthur Foundation. Over food and wine, they discussed the projects competing for MacArthur's approval. Smith-Sonneborn spoke about her work with Lipetz, where Glaser would fit in, and the dual role of DNA repair in the aging process and environmental mutagenesis.

Senator Cranston was particularly interested and asked that she come to his office in the morning to speak with a venture capitalist about her ideas. The businessman listened intently to her lecture and, when it was over, pronounced it "the most lucid scientific presentation I've ever heard."

Back in her own office the next day, she tried to sort out the hectic events of the past three days. MacArthur, Cranston, and the venture capitalist all seemed interested. They were now talking in terms of an enormous grant, perhaps $2 million to $3 million. But what thrilled her most was the prospect of using Glaser's machine to expand and accelerate her work on a level beyond her wildest imagining.

"I was like a little child," she says. "I said, 'I want. I want to be able to do this.' Instead of moving at a snail's pace, we could go full speed ahead and really do it right. We'd work with the best people, perfect an assay, and find the promising compounds. It's too much to hope for. And it was. Because nothing happened."

While the automation idea was still under consideration, Lipetz threw her another curve. He had heard, in leaks from MacArthur, that they wanted a breakthrough. "We don't have one, Phil," she said. "All the information we have is in our proposal. And it is going to take money and plodding to get there. What they're asking for is an already established breakthrough the world can sit back and recognize. And we're not at that stage." What she didn't know was that Lipetz thought that they were.

When Lipetz first told Smith-Sonneborn about raising DNA repair, he had not yet worked with Alan Galsky. A plant physiologist at Bradley University in Peoria, Illinois, Galsky had come to OSU on a three-month sabbatical that fall. He had brought with him the Ti-plasmid system. A plasmid is a circular piece of DNA in a bacterium that functions as an accessory chromosome. It is the basic tool of genetic engineering, the vehicle by which genetic information is transferred to a cell.

The Ti plasmid is a natural gene machine, recombining with the genetic material of certain plants, causing tumorous growths. Since DNA supercoiling controls genetic recombination, Lipetz reasoned that if they used novobiocin to reduce the supercoiling in the Ti plasmid, it would sharply limit the ability of the bacterium to recombine with the genetic material of the plants, resulting in fewer tumors. They did the experiment, and as Lipetz predicted, there was an enormous decrease, about 80 percent, in the number of tumors that normally occurred. He had prevented the occurrence of tumors by interfering with DNA supercoiling.

Galsky was also interested in aging, but in plants. Did Lipetz know, he asked, that there was a hormone called kinetin that retarded senescence in plants? Lipetz shrugged. "I'm not really interested in plant hormones," he said. "But it's not only a plant hormone," Galsky persisted. "It's also found in fish and other vertebrates." A few days later, one of Lipetz's graduate students walked in with an article from the *Proceedings of the National Academy of Sciences* on a related substance called isopetanyl adenine (IPA), which increased DNA synthesis. As the three of them gathered around to look at the paper, Lipetz, who had been skimming it with his usual speed, skidded to a halt at one of the sentences. "Alan, do you realize what this means?"

All the sentence said was that the action of IPA on DNA synthesis could be prevented by nalidixic acid. But Lipetz felt a triumphant flash of "aha" in his mind. He and Stephens had just shown that nalidixic acid decreased

DNA supercoiling in mammalian cells. Maybe what was happening was that both nalidixic acid and IPA were modifiers of DNA supercoiling. Nalidixic acid went in one direction, decreasing supercoiling and interfering with DNA synthesis, while IPA went in the other direction, increasing supercoiling and promoting DNA synthesis. Now Galsky's earlier comment about kinetin's retarding aging took on the significance it failed to have the first time. Kinetin belonged to a class of hormones called cytokinetins and so did IPA. In other words, it appeared that with IPA and kinetin, he now had not one, but two substances that might stimulate supercoiling, raise repair, and lengthen life span.

Realizing that the compounds might be the ticket to the breakthrough FIBER wanted, he told Joan to gear up for testing them. She would do the same experiments they had done with novobiocin, but this time in reverse. She would do mutagenicity studies to see whether the substances made the paramecia more resistant to the damaging effects of ultraviolet light as well as to the combined effect of novobiocin and UV, and she would also do a life-span study to determine whether the compounds were life-extending.

Lipetz had reason to believe that IPA might be the more potent of the two, but since kinetin was the first to arrive from the chemical company in January 1981, that was the one she tested first. Because a longevity study takes forty to sixty days, she began that experiment before doing the much shorter mutagenesis studies. Within a few weeks, she began getting the strangest results. First thing every morning, she looked at the data sheets on the cells that her students had isolated. Some days the kinetin group was running 20 percent ahead of the untreated group in terms of survivors at a given age, and her hopes would soar. Four days later, as the kinetin group came crashing back to the level of the controls, so would her aspirations. The data went up and down until the survival curves looked like the foothills of the Rockies. There was no way to tell how this would end up. While all this was going on in March 1981, Ralph Stephens came out for two weeks.

Once more they were about to try what she and Lipetz had failed to do: measure the amount of DNA supercoiling in the paramecia on the gradient. They needed to be able to do this in order to prove their contention that novobiocin and kinetin were acting directly on the supercoiling. This time they had a spectrofluorimeter, supplied by multimillionaire science patron Paul Glenn, who had been approached by Yarborough. They also had the benefit of Stephens's temperament, which is like a bridge over troubled waters. But an improbable series of mishaps, similar to those that had plagued Lipetz's visit, continued unabated.

No sooner had Stephens walked into the laboratory than he made two horrifying discoveries. Peering down the fluorescent scope, he realized that when he and Lipetz had done a quickie experiment on the decline of DNA supercoiling with age in paramecia, they had been working essentially blind. Through Smith-Sonneborn's scope, he could see what he could not see with the light microscope at OSU: the sausagelike fragments of paramecia nuclei indicating that some of the cells were going through autogamy. But the funny part was that he and Lipetz had gotten results. "Probably we were looking at a small percentage of the population which still had intact nuclei," says Stephens. "And we got exactly what we had predicted. But it was pure, dumb, stupid luck."

The second discovery came when Stephens tried to turn the dial on the new spectrophotofluorimeter to zero and it wouldn't budge. Some of the parts had been broken in transit. While Smith-Sonneborn called the company in Washington to send a repairman, Stephens, who prides himself on "having a way with machines, cells, and people," began putting it back together as best he could. By the evening they were able to get a preliminary reading.

The next night, their hopes for a result were blown by a shattered bulb in the machine. Finally, the following night after the repairs were made, they ran the gradients, turned on the machine, inserted the tubes, and the fluorescent indicator went wild. Impossibly high numbers were flashing at them. Since these were the first tubes in the gradient and would not be expected to contain any DNA, it made no sense at all. Tube after tube gave the same ridiculous readings. Finally Stephens inserted an empty test tube. There was no difference. "Joan," he said in a tone of utter amazement, "the tubes are autofluorescing. They light up without anything in them."

In anticipation of his visit, Smith-Sonneborn had ordered ten thousand tubes, and now she realized that each one of them had an imperceptible flaw that, in most experiments, would not make a difference but in this instance was crucial. Sitting at the lab bench, her head in her hands, she managed a wan smile. "Ralph, do you think the gods are trying to tell us something?"

"Don't worry. You still have tubes from before this shipment, and I can wash them out so well, we'll still be able to use them."

"Ralph," she said, brightening, "you're a godsend."

Throughout all the snags, Stephens kept his cool, meticulously washing out each tube between runs. Finally they began to get results, but they weren't good enough. The clear signal of where the DNA was in the gradient, which would indicate the degree of supercoiling, still eluded them. Lipetz's technique, which worked so well for human and animal cells, was not working for paramecia. Whatever "dumb luck" Stephens and Lipetz had had in the past was deserting them now.

As soon as Stephens left, she put her students, who had all been making gradients, back to work on the kinetin experiments. This time they did the mutagenesis assay to see whether or not kinetin could reduce the number of mutations in the offspring of cells that received ultraviolet light or UV light plus novobiocin. By the second day of the experiment, she was beside herself with excitement. The kinetin worked. Not only did it cut down on the number of dead and slow-growing progeny of UV-irradiated cells, but it was even more effective in blocking the lethal combination of UV and novobiocin. Here she had taken a drug, novobiocin, that was known to inhibit DNA supercoiling and had shown that a naturally occurring hormone, kinetin, blocked its action. The most likely explanation for kinetin's effect was that it, too, acted on the DNA supercoiling but in the opposite direction from that of novobiocin, with opposite results: Where novobiocin decreased DNA repair and supercoiling, it appeared that kinetin raised DNA repair and restored DNA supercoiling.

She ran to the telephone: "Phil, we've got it. The kinetin is acting on the same mechanism as the novobiocin. It is interfering with novobiocin mutagenesis. We're modulating repair in both directions. I don't know what it is going to do to longevity, but it looks extremely promising. And that's the way we've got to present the data, as promising."

"Will you write it up?"

"You bet I will. I wouldn't write anything up before now, but I sure will today."

The next five days, she and her lab went into a flurry, writing, editing, proofreading, while the typists pounded out the succeeding drafts. All this time, they were continuing to accumulate data on the life-span experiment, but in order to make the deadline, they had to send off the paper before the cells in either the treated group or the controls had died off.

One week later, they had the answer to the life-span race: The kinetin-treated cells beat the controls by a small but significant margin. The 7 percent increase in longevity, she believed, was important enough to merit including it in the report to FIBER. Once again she threw the lab into turmoil, replotting the data and sending off copies of the revision to MacArthur, FIBER, Paul Glenn, and Lipetz.

On the biological level at least, they had accomplished everything they had set out to do a year earlier. They had jacked repair up and down in the cell; they had shortened and lengthened life span; and there was evidence, but by no means conclusive, that they had done these things by acting on the level of superhelical coiling.

It occurred to Smith-Sonneborn that the reason they got the spurts of survival all along the life-span curve might be due to the fact that the supercoiling was unwinding with age and the kinetin was winding it back up. There were several findings that pointed in this direction. First, the earlier study on novobiocin showed that the enhanced mutagenic effect of UV was greatest on young cells and scarcely existed in old cells. The reason for this, she and Lipetz believed, was that the supercoiling was already so decreased in the aged paramecia that there was nothing for the novobiocin to act on. On the other hand, kinetin produced its greatest effect if novobiocin, which also decreased the supercoiling, was given first. It all pointed to the observation she had made in her first life-extension experiment with ultraviolet light: The best way to raise repair levels, and perhaps increase life span, might be to damage the cell first. It was akin to a vaccine containing a harmless dose of a virus, which threw the body's defense system into high gear.

Smith-Sonneborn finds this concept incredibly appealing. "The idea," she says, "is to utilize your natural defenses. And one way to do this might be to stimulate your body's compensatory mechanisms by first inducing damage. And if you do so in just the right amount, you won't harm the cells, but you're left with all the goodies."

But just when the roller coaster was reaching its zenith, FIBER was unable to get any money from the MacArthur Foundation. Indeed, FIBER was having trouble staying alive. Said Regelson in retrospect, "The main idea behind FIBER was informational exchange, to facilitate the movement of basic research from the laboratory into the clinic. We hoped that by providing seed money, we could set up a catalytic group, and make things happen. We estimated that we needed a million dollars a year, which we would raise through private philanthropy. But after the first year, in which I helped Phil Lipetz and Joan Smith-Sonneborn and Art Schwartz and other key people, we never had the money. The most that FIBER ever raised was between $200,000 and $300,000."

Not getting the MacArthur grant was the least of Lipetz's problems. In the spring of 1981, the NIA had rejected his proposal for looking at the relationship between aging and changes in DNA supercoiling. With no research money to support him, he was in a vulnerable position. There was a state budget crunch and the university was among the state institutions affected. Adhering to the last-hired, first-fired rule, the head of the department informed him he was out of a job as of June.

Moreover, two recent papers had just been published that forced him to reconsider both his experimental methods and his interpretation of the results. One of the papers, by David Pettijohn of Colorado State University, had the effect of shooting down his first aging experiment. Lipetz had assumed that since DNA strand breaks increased with age and strand breaks caused a relaxation in the supercoiling, the first caused the second, which is why there is a decrease in supercoiling with age. Now Pettijohn's experiments indicated that this could not be the case. In a higher-order cell, such as our own, strand breaks would not cause the supercoiled DNA to unswivel like a cut telephone cord—which is what happens in a bacterial cell—because the proteins attached to the DNA would act as a restraining force. The nucleoid technique, used by Lipetz and most researchers in the field of supercoiling, called for stripping off almost all the proteins from the DNA. Under laboratory conditions using the nucleoid technique, strand breaks *would* cause the DNA to uncoil, but in life, Pettijohn was saying, this would never happen. In other words, Lipetz's observations of an increase in strand breaks and a decrease in DNA supercoiling, on which he based his entire supercoiling theory of aging, may have been an experimental artifact.

In the second paper, one of the leading figures in the field of DNA supercoiling, Abraham Worcel of Princeton University, proposed a model, for how the DNA was packed into the chromosomes of eukaryotic cells, that differed substantially from Lipetz's own view. Lipetz envisioned a gyrase enzyme, similar to the one found in bacterial cells, that would introduce DNA supercoiling. But Worcel's model eliminated the need for such an enzyme. If Worcel were right, Lipetz's idea that novobiocin and kinetin were acting on the gyrase enzyme—in the first case by interfering with it and in the second by promoting its activity—had to be wrong. In effect, he was back to square one.

Sitting on the floor of his living room with his infant daughter on his lap, Lipetz was planning his comeback. "Now you can see why NIA turned down the grant," he said. "The irony is that I requested Worcel as a reviewer, and then two weeks later, his paper, which was probably used as the basis for turning down my grant, appears in the *Proceedings of the National Academy of Sciences*. Now I'm trying to regroup and to do this, I have to pass my brash-kid stage, accept what Pettijohn and Worcel say as the current dogma, and sell my ideas in the narrowest, most orthodox manner."

To do this requires putting the laboratory seal of approval on Lipetz's ideas. "We are the chutzpah kids," he says. On a shoestring budget, Stephens and his ragtag crew of work-study undergraduates, half-time technicians, Ph.D. candidates donating their time, and people who "just came out of the woodwork," are simultaneously carrying out half a dozen basic experiments to lay the foundation for the role of DNA superhelicity in higher-order cells, from paramecia to man.

"I still believe I was right, but I may have been right for the wrong reasons," says Lipetz. He cites other work indicating that supercoiling declines with age but he believes that the "strongest evidence," albeit indirect, comes from Smith-Sonneborn's studies. "You put in novobiocin, which decreases the supercoiling, and it affects young cells, which are tightly coiled, and not old cells, where the supercoiling has come apart. You put in kinetin, which increases the superhelicity, and it has its greatest effect on the old cells, which is what you would expect. This adds up to a pretty powerful picture that there is a decrease in supercoiling in the paramecium system with age. And the fact is that when we do things that increase the supercoiling, we get an increase in life span, and when we do things that decrease the supercoiling, we get a decrease in life span."

If he is to get the roller coaster moving again, Lipetz has his work cut out for him. He has to prove that the changes he sees in DNA supercoiling are real rather than an artifact, that supercoiling regulates gene function in the cells of higher animals and not just in bacteria, and that it plays a significant role in aging and age-related diseases. And, most pressing of all, he must find some means of supporting his research.

In the last week of August 1982, I returned to Columbus, Ohio, to try to catch science in the making. Smith-Sonneborn was spending a month working at OSU, taking one last crack at getting the nucleoid technique to work in the paramecia. This time they had everything going for them—a fluorescent microscope, the latest-model Amico Bowman spectrofluorimeter, in the lab rather than in another building; a back-up crew that knew all the techniques; and the three collaborators—herself, Lipetz, and Stephens—all working together.

Since my 1981 visit, Lipetz's fortunes had shifted dramatically. He scored several scientific coups in the laboratory, the most recent reports in the field of DNA supercoiling started to go his way, and he found what he hoped was a new route to financial solvency. Although he and Smith-Sonneborn had so far failed in their attempt to use the nucleoid technique for detecting DNA supercoiling in paramecia, they had one incredible moment of excitement in which they hit upon what they believed was nature's own "antiaging pathway."

Wearing a prairie-style dress with ruffled hem, and with gold earrings dangling from double-pierced lobes, Smith-Sonneborn prepares a sample of the paramecia for the day's run. After staining the sample with acridine orange, she checks it under the scope. A number of the cells display the green-frankfurter bits of the nucleus during autogamy.

"It's a lousy culture," she declares. "Some cells are in autogamy, some haven't even started, and some are already through. If we superimpose all this variability on our test, we're done before we start."

Most of the morning is spent discussing ways of overcoming their major problem: the breakup of the nucleus in its passage through the gradient. With the pride of a parent, Stephens shows me their new acquisition, the spectrofluorimeter. No longer is it necessary for someone to insert the gradient tubes and note the numbers that flash on the screen, indicating where the fluorescently bound DNA is in the gradient. Now the machine does it all, moving the tubes along on an assembly line and graphing the results with a moving pen like an electrocardiograph. "You see how that kinda looks like a jump rope with a lot of slack on the bottom?" he says, pointing to the spectrofluorimeter printout from the previous day. "Well, we'd like to get a nice, high peak in that rope that'd show us where the DNA went."

Lipetz comes in shortly before lunch, carrying an attaché case, and wearing a vest, suit, and tie instead of his usual T-shirt and dungarees. He has been at business meetings all day.

The first time I heard Lipetz talk about forming his own company was at the 1980 Gerontology Society meeting in San Diego. And he was not the only one. Everywhere I went at that meeting, it seemed that the search for riches was vying with the search for truth. Discussions about setting up a business, foundation, or connecting up with a corporation, dominated the informal gatherings between sessions. Walford and his associate, Kathleen Hall, had set up a foundation to receive funds from private individuals and companies that wished to support their research. Schwartz, hoping to take out a patent on an analogue of DHEA, was talking to a pharmaceutical firm. Others spoke to me about negotiations with venture capitalists who would support the research and development of their ideas in return for a share of the profits.

Since World War II, the government had been the huge trough at which the scientific research establishment fed. The National Institutes of Health alone gave two-thirds of all funds for basic university science and funded 40 percent of all biomedical research. It was, as one young frustrated scientist put it, like "having only one bank in town."

Attempts to change this system were fraught with difficulties. In one highly publicized case, Leonard Hayflick was excoriated for selling his WI38 cells, the human cell culture system that had transformed gerontology and was used around the world. In 1976 he had been offered the position of head of the NIA. But an NIH investigation of his handling of the WI38 strain ended with charges that since the cells had been developed under NIH grants, they belonged to the government and were not his to sell. Hayflick, who resigned from his post at Stanford University, sued the government for title to the cells and the profits from their sale. Although it took six years, a settlement was reached in which he received all the back profits with interest, a total of about $900,000, as well as title to some of the original cells. According to a letter in *Science* (January 19, 1982) signed by ninety-five scientists and scholars, the settlement was an "exoneration" of all the charges against him. For Hayflick, it was not only a personal victory but an affirmation of the right of researchers to profit from their own work.

"The government's contention was wholly wrong," he says. "What about the thousands of products that are developed under government grants that are given to industry or the universities? Why should the universities get fat at the expense of the taxpayer? If the university can benefit, why shouldn't the scientist? By winning the suit, I established a principle that has now changed many of the rules in respect to the ownership of intellectual property rights by scientists. Today the biologists are discovering what the electronic engineers and the chemists learned twenty years ago. They have finally agreed to surrender their virginity."

In the fall of 1980, two other events took place that were to change profoundly the relationship between academia, the government, and research biologists. Genentech, founded by the University of California scientists who held the patent on the *E. coli* plasmid—a discovery for genetic engineering that was equivalent to the invention of the wheel—went public. Within hours, they made Wall Street history when their opening stock offer of $35 vaulted to $88 a share. One month later, Ronald Reagan was elected president, and his election was immediately perceived as a swing of the pendulum away from public support and toward the private sector.

For Lipetz this shift could not come too soon. On a personal level, he had had it with the hassles of trying to break into what he saw as a "closed club, the old-boy network of established scientists who referee each other's journal articles, and review each other's grants." With the threat of unemployment looming near, no grants (either public or private) in sight, a baby to support, and a monthly mortgage to meet, the formation of his own company seemed the only solution—and he had the means.

"The company was set up for profit as well as to do breakthrough research," he says. "It became obvious to me that the governmental system of peer review is not set up for breakthroughs but to ensure that the next small step is taken. Big advances in knowledge are accomplished either on their own or by a company. And since we are a capitalistic society, it makes sense that they would be realized by capitalistic means, that is, through private enterprise rather than government."

His achievements in the boardroom have been paralleled by those in the lab. He and Stephens have now answered one of the objections of their critics: that the decrease in DNA supercoiling that they observe with age is not real, but, rather, an experimental artifact. They have refined the gradient technique so that they can clearly distinguish when a decrease in DNA supercoiling is due to a change in the actual structure of the DNA, and when it has been brought about by strand breaks that are introduced as part of the experiment. Once they had proved that the changes in DNA supercoiling they saw were real, they had to confront the second charge: that the changes had no "physiological relevance"; that is, that they played no role in health or disease.

Here they were aided not only by their own research, but that of others. Two Cambridge University researchers, F. H. Yew and R. T. Johnson, had shown that at least for one disease state, chronic lymphocytic leukemia, the superhelicity was abnormally increased. At first glance, Lipetz admits, this sounds like a paradox, since cancer goes up with age and supercoiling goes down with age. But he believes his most recent experiments suggest why this may be so.

Jim Trosko of Michigan State, whom Lipetz had known from the days when he had collaborated with Hart, had recently shown that a class of chemicals called tumor promoters were like double agents, working both sides of the street. In cells that had been mutated for any reason, such as chemicals, X-rays, or ultraviolet light, they stimulated division, moving the cell in the direction of becoming a cancer. In cells that were already cancerous, they blocked cell division, pushing it in the direction of normalcy.

Lipetz was struck by this observation as well as by another one: When the tumor promoter, TPA, was applied to the cancerous cells of leukemia patients, it caused the cells to function more normally. In other words, the TPA had restored some of the differentiated state the cells had lost when they became malignant. It seemed to Lipetz that if TPA were changing the state of differentiation, making cancerous cells more normal and normal cells more like cancer, and if DNA supercoiling had anything to do with the state of differentiation, then changes induced by TPA should be reflected in alterations of the DNA supercoiling.

And this is just what they found. TPA had opposing effects on the cell, depending upon its prior state. It increased the DNA supercoiling of normal cells, making them more like that of malignant ones, and relaxed the increased supercoiling in leukemic cells, making them more like normal ones. It was a major victory in Lipetz's battle to prove that the DNA supercoiling was "physiologically relevant" in eucaryotic cells.

"In our experiments," he says, "we took an agent known to change the state of differentiation in a cell and showed that it changed the supercoiling in the expected direction. This is the first hard evidence *in vivo* that DNA supercoiling may be related to the state of differentiation." Now the idea that DNA supercoiling increases with cancer and decreases with age, he believes, makes sense. "There appears to be a normal operating range for the DNA supercoiling," he says. "If you get too far out of it in either direction, it is going to affect gene expression, either in the direction of further cell division, which is cancer, or in the direction of further differentiation, which is aging."

Over lunch, Smith-Sonneborn and Lipetz let me in on their big discovery of the past month. Even now the excitement is apparent in their eyes as they recall the moment. They had been talking in the lab one day about mevalonic acid, one of a class of compounds called isoprenes that interested Lipetz because they were involved in regulating DNA replication and might work, he believed, by acting on the superhelicity.

Smith-Sonneborn had had a brainstorm. Mevalonic acid was a precursor of cholesterol. Perhaps the reason why eating too much cholesterol was bad, in addition to building arterial plaques, was that it shut down the body's own cholesterol-synthesizing machinery. If this happened, you would no longer be making the intermediate products, like mevalonic acid, that regulate the manufacture of new DNA.

"Great idea," said Lipetz. "Let's look at the chart and see what other compounds are on the pathway leading to cholesterol synthesis." They hurried into the small office just outside the lab. There on the wall was the intricate road map of the body's chemistry, the innumerable highways in which compounds that sustain life were broken down or synthesized. Way down on the bottom, one or two compounds behind cholesterol, they found mevalonic acid. But that was not all they found.

Feeding into the cholesterol-synthesis pathway were all the isoprenes, including all the steroids. Moving back up the chart along the pathway, they got to a number of antioxidant compounds, including vitamin A, coenzyme Q, vitamin E, and the retinoids, near relatives of vitamin A that had known anticancer activity.

"Joan," said Lipetz, "I don't know whether your idea about the regulation of DNA synthesis is correct or not, but do you realize that you can come with almost every antiaging substance in the world and put it on a pathway to these substances? What we have here is the pathway that unifies all of molecular gerontology."

Lipetz's big push now is to get all the chemicals on that "antiaging" pathway, run it through Joan's paramecia system, and put the paramecia nucleoid problem on the back burner. As far as he is concerned, his lab has already wasted too much time on it over the past two years. "The aggravating thing about it," he says, "is that we can get nice, sharp, nucleoids on almost any human cell. I mean we spent years developing this technique and then we get this mishmash."

But while he and Smith-Sonneborn have found compounds that interfere with nalidixic acid and novobiocin, known inhibitors of DNA synthesis and supercoiling, and have shown that they reduce mutagenesis and extend life, they have yet to prove these effects are due to modulating DNA supercoiling. And the only way to determine the extent of supercoiling is to get the paramecia nucleoid to stay in that whiffleball state, with most of the proteins removed but all the supercoils intact, as it moves through the gradient. This is the goal that still eludes them. Without this, she says, "we're not talking hard science."

Lipetz leans back in his chair and smiles knowingly: "What you see here is a difference in philosophy. She wants to do careful, careful science and I want to go for the jugular, make some intelligent guesses, get the breakthroughs, and skip the intermediate stuff."

She smiles back. "It's great if you can do it," she says, "but often in the process you fall down the gully."

"All I'm saying is that there is a ton of molecular stuff to be done. Let's go for the pathway and let's not get hung up in this mopping-up operation."

Back at the lab, she announces that she has discovered the best culture of the day. That morning she had refrigerated some in the centrifuge in order to slow their metabolism and prevent autogamy, and had forgotten all about them. She glances at the clock: 5:30. Too late to run them.

"If you got cells, Joan, I've got gradients," says technician Denny Jewett. "Holy Toledo," she cries. "I'm gonna move." Suddenly, the lab snaps into action. "Come on, come on, baby," she mumbles to the cells as she shakes the flask. Denny checks the spectrofluorimeter as she gets the paramecia nuclei ready.

It is now five minutes to six. "All right," she yells. "I got some good-looking ones." Denny puts them on the gradient. Suddenly, Smith-Sonneborn is spent, leaning against the black Formica counter with a Mona Lisa smile on her face. "I'm in another place," she says happily.

First thing next morning, we check the gradient printout. There is a small blip in the rope but still too much slack. "We've got to get that peak a lot higher," Smith-Sonneborn says. Throughout the morning, she and Paula, another technician, work quickly to make an eleven o'clock gradient run. She asks Ralph to look into the microscope. "Know what I did? I added acetic acid to stabilize the nuclei."

"They look good."

In the coffee room, they pore over the printouts from last night's run as though they were navigational charts. "The nucleoids are swimming to the top of the gradient," says Ralph. Once more they discuss ways to keep the nucleus intact—different kinds of stabilizers, varying the speed or the length of time of centrifugation.

As usual, Lipetz is impatient. "You got these nuclei that, under high salt conditions, chomp up the macronucleus. The damned 'mac' is designed to fall apart when the cell divides, so we are trying to beat that."

"Yeah," says Joan, "but something is holding it together for most of its life span."

Late that afternoon, they watch the moving pen of the spectrofluorimeter as it records the gradient tubes with the acetic acid.

"Phil, look at that," says Smith-Sonneborn, pointing at a small glitch in the rope as it slides to the floor.

Lipetz: "I'm not impressed."

Stephens: "That looks promising."

Smith-Sonneborn: "Promises, promises."

The last two days of Smith-Sonneborn's stay are spent working on the four papers they plan to get out. Although they are now getting a consistent bump on the gradient, it is still not where it should be. "It looks like it's giving us the finger," she remarks ruefully.

Each morning, when we went to look at the printouts of the previous day's runs, I would feel a surge of anticipation. But while so much of their collaboration had been a success, the attempt to get Lipetz's technique to work on the nucleus of the paramecia has so far been futile.

Trying to do something no one has ever done before is fraught with pitfalls. There are no guidelines, only seat-of-the-pants instinct. Basically it's trial and error and inspired guesswork. Then it's sit and wait, and try again. "Doing research is like scaling Mount Everest every single day," says Stephens.

Chapter Ten

Life Extension 2: Supergenes

Unbeknownst to Lipetz and Smith-Sonneborn, while they were carrying out their collaboration on manipulating life span, Cutler was trying to do the same thing. And like them, he was not saying anything to his fellow scientists until the results were in. I first heard about it at the 1979 Gerontology Conference in Washington, D.C. It was late afternoon, and the session had ended when a small group, including two graduate students, a gerontologist, and me, sat down to talk with Cutler.

Over the next hour and a half, he regaled, intrigued, and provoked us with his contention that although the aging process was probably very complex, intervention might be comparatively simple. "At least in regard to the hypothesis and data, we are in about the same state as they were when the polio vaccine was developed," he said. "And yet there are many hard-nosed people in aging who say you can't really do anything about aging until you know a lot more. Well, if scientists had taken the attitude that we first have to know about nerve conduction, the mechanisms of paralysis, the function of the immune system, and how polio virus interacts with cells, before we can do anything, we'd still have polio epidemics."

This kind of buoyantly sweeping statement continually gets him into trouble with his colleagues. Even now, one of the students, Angelo Turturro, fairly exploded. "The difference between what Jenner was doing in the eighteenth century when he was using cowpox to protect against smallpox, and what Koch and Pasteur were doing in the nineteenth century, was that they started the *science* of vaccination," he said. "They evolved a number of theories and tried to use vaccinations to probe what was going on, and this work actually led to the modern lock-and-key hypothesis. This is a big difference. If something works, you try to find out *why* it works and how to modify it so it works better. You don't say, 'Ha, ha, ha, let's keep plugging things into people until we find a vaccine against aging.' "

"No, no, no, no," protested Cutler. "My point is that you're able to develop vaccines and prevent very complicated diseases without understanding too much about it, like with polio."

"But we first had to find out that polio is a disease caused by something, rather than being genetic."

"That's right!" shouted Cutler, thumping the table. "That's exactly where we are in regard to aging. I could state that the life span of man and other mammals evolved on the basis of different levels of common sets of repair/protection processes. There it is. It's being tested right now. This carries with it the implication that there could be comparatively simple methods for enhancing these processes to high levels. In other words, if a mouse carries within its cells—and I suggest it does—enzymes to protect against free radicals, DNA repair, the whole works that the human does, it should be theoretically possible to produce a mouse that lives ten, fifteen, or twenty years rather than two. You don't have to invent anything new, you don't need surgery, genetic engineering, a new chemical. You just have to find ways to bring these processes up naturally, the way longevity evolved."

By October 1980, Cutler's situation at the Gerontology Research Center (GRC) in Baltimore had worsened considerably. After the debacle at the 1979 Gordon Conference in which his finding of a correlation between life span of various species and the antioxidant enzyme superoxide dismutase (SOD) was attacked and ridiculed, his financial support had been substantially reduced.

On his desk, books, magazines, reprints, and manuscripts rise like barricades. A few feet away at another desk, where the literature barrier is only slightly lower, Cutler's wife, Edith, taps away at a typewriter. Except for pictures of their three children, the walls are bare. Convinced that he could not get a fair review for his SOD paper in a gerontology journal, he had gone another route—the *Proceedings of the National Academy of Sciences*. Unlike other journals that handle submissions through an editorial board and anonymous reviewers, *PNAS* first sends articles under consideration to a member of the academy, who assumes sole responsibility for its contents. He or she also gives the manuscript to external reviewers but may override their objections.

Some scientists put down publication in *PNAS* as being more a matter of whom you know than what you know, but Cutler vehemently disagrees.

"Every paper in the journal is published with the words 'communicated by,' followed by the academy member's name. In other words, he puts his reputation on the line." With that in mind, he sent his paper to the late Philip Handler, then president of the academy. Handler sent the paper for review to Irwin Fridovich at Duke University, who codiscovered the anti-oxidant enzyme. "Here I was," says Cutler triumphantly, "with all the criticism, and the same damn data is published in *PNAS*, communicated by the president of the National Academy of Sciences and approved by the codiscoverer of SOD."

But the victory is nominal. With no funds for graduate students, technicians, or secretarial help, he and his wife not only do all the experiments, but all the chores generally performed by a full range of personnel. The only thing keeping him going, he says, is a small grant from millionaire philanthropist Paul Glenn.

With all of this, the last few months have been among the most exciting of Cutler's life. Not only have his experiments been going extremely well; his early ideas on aging have been confirmed and extended into a new "integrative hypothesis." Theory and practice are now interlocking in ways that he had not foreseen and his hopes for life-span extension are higher than ever.

Considering his precarious status at the GRC, Cutler is skating on the thinnest of ice with his latest experiments. They are the kind of high-risk, possibly no-win, ventures that make review committees tremble. Both NIA head Robert Butler and GRC Director Richard Greulich are on record as saying that life extension is definitely last on their list of priorities. In an interview with me, Greulich had said that if a "silver bullet" were to be found against aging, he, personally, would be against it. Yet here Cutler is trying to find that bullet.

Code-named "project enhancement," Cutler's brainchild has a kind of swashbuckling, derring-do about it. When it first occurred to him that a few "longevity-determinant" genes might control aging, he immediately began casting about for a way to test this hypothesis. The logical straightforward method would be to try and identify each of the genes and look for correlations with life span. He could spend the rest of his life in such a pursuit, so the only way to do it was to proceed as though the knowledge were already there. He would prove his case not by the preponderance of evidence but by the result. He would produce the first six-year-old mouse, the equivalent of a two-hundred-year-old man.

The idea was simple, audacious, and ingenious—to trick the cell into turning on repair and protection processes by making it "think" it was under attack. Smith-Sonneborn was moving along the same track when she used small doses of ultraviolet-light damage to induce large rates of repair in her paramecia. But, as she recognized, if people were put under sun lamps, the UV would harm the skin cells while leaving the internal tissue completely untouched. To get around this, Cutler came up with an idea that was stupefyingly obvious. He would use the damage product itself—the thymine dimer.

In the lab, he and his wife made gram amounts of dimers by placing strings of thymines together in a frozen solution and UV-irradiating them. Injected into the mice, the dimers found their way readily into the cells, but because they were not incorporated into the DNA, they posed no actual threat. "During the process of repair, the thymine dimers are excised and not metabolized," says Cutler. "It could be that the level of these excised dimers governs the level of repair enzymes, perhaps by interacting with a regulatory protein. Our hope is that the cell will see the injected dimers and react as though it were the real thing, and that it will turn on not only UV repair but SOD and other protective processes as well."

Since it would take two to three years before they would know whether they were affecting the animal's life span, he conducted a short-term assay to verify that they were headed in the right direction. The simplest one, he decided, would be to measure the ability of the animals to resist X-ray irradiation. He bombarded the mice with high levels of X-irradiation, using control animals that had been injected either with saline solution or thymine in its natural form. At the end of two weeks, all the controls were dead, but the thymine-dimer-treated animals lived another two weeks.

"It was unbelievable," he says. "We got a two-fold increase in survival. We know that when you inject SOD into animals, they become more radiation resistant. And it's reasonable to assume that higher levels of DNA repair may increase the level of resistance. So the increased survival in the treated animals may be due to enhanced levels of DNA repair and protection."

The thymine dimers were not the only "antigens of aging" he was testing. The Cutlers irradiated chromatin, causing cross-links to form between the DNA and its associated proteins. They removed purine bases from the DNA, simulating a form of damage that occurs naturally. They exposed the genetic material to various mutagens, carcinogens, and free-radical-like elements, such as hydrogen peroxide. These damage products were then injected directly into the mouse's bloodstream, or sometimes packaged into lipid protein envelopes, called liposomes, to facilitate entrance into the cell.

But while he was in the midst of "project enhancement," a startling series of revelations unexpectedly supported his "few-genes" hypothesis—that a relatively small number of genes may control life span—and at the same time lent credence to his tricking-the-cells experiments. Walford's supergene theory of aging was suddenly in the ascendancy, and it looked as if Cutler's star could rise along with it.

Kathleen Hall, a vivacious young woman with a rollicking sense of humor, runs the DNA repair lab in Roy Walford's complex at UCLA. At Ohio State, Hall worked with cells and DNA repair in Hart's lab. Now at Walford's lab she turned her attention to nailing down his preliminary observations on a correlation between DNA repair, life span, and the immune function. To do this, she used classic Mendelian genetics.

Using Walford's inbred mice strains that differed from one another only at the major histocompatibility complex (MHC), the supergene cluster regulating the immune function, she bred a short-lived strain with a life span of three hundred days to a long-lived strain with a life span of nine hundred days. The offspring of these matings known as F1 (first filial) was a genetic mixture of both parental genotypes. She then crossed the offspring with each other. According to the laws of Mendelian segregation, the F2 generation would be 25 percent long-lived, 25 percent short-lived, and the rest, hybrids with intermediate life spans. Next she tissue-typed cells from each mouse to determine which genes they had inherited and, finally, she measured the ability of the animals' cells to repair UV-induced damage.

The cells used in the study were lymphocytes, the white blood cells of the immune system. Most studies of DNA repair, including the ones done by Hart, used fibroblasts, for many years the only cells that could be reliably grown in the test tube. The problem with fibroblasts is that they are early, undifferentiated stem cells and are not typical of the highly specialized cells of the body. Walford and other researchers had succeeded in culturing lymphocytes. These white blood cells, which are the cornerstone of the immune reaction, are differentiated cells and carry markers for the MHC genes on their surface.

"The results were just beautiful," she says. Mice that had inherited the short-lived genes had low repair, while the genetically endowed long-lived ones had high repair, and those who carried genes of both types had repair levels in between the other two. This study not only reinforced the correlation between DNA repair and life span, but appeared to show that genes in the major histocompatibility complex, the supergene which controlled the immune function, might, in part, regulate DNA repair.

When Walford's preliminary experiments on congenic mice in 1979 first showed that mutations in the major histocompatibility complex were related to life span, the California scientist called Cutler. Could the MHC, he asked, possibly be the "few genes" that, Cutler had predicted, regulated longevity?

"No, I don't think so," Cutler told him. "I believe these are regulatory genes, and the MHC hasn't been shown to control levels of protection and repair of the DNA." But when Walford and Hall later demonstrated that mutations in the MHC did indeed correlate with DNA repair, Cutler thought to himself, "Roy just may have something there."

Still, it wasn't until a paper appeared in *Science* in January 1980 that Cutler realized that he and Walford were headed down the same track. In the article, by a group of Hungarian researchers, it appeared that the MHC, Walford's supergene complex, might regulate the levels of SOD, an enzyme directly involved in the protection of the DNA.

"Boy, that set a fire under me," says Cutler. "I'd just finished establishing that levels of SOD were important in governing life span, and here were Roy and Kathy's work on MHC and DNA repair, and this report on SOD showing that the changes in MHC regulated both. He [Roy] was right. The MHC might be the longevity-determinant genes I had been looking for."

How many repair/protective processes are related to the MHC? Cutler wondered. Reading up on the supergene complex, he found that the gene for catalase—like SOD, a naturally occurring DNA-protective, antioxidant enzyme—was part of the MHC. In addition, work was in progress indicating that the mixed-function oxidase system, the body's primary mechanism for detoxifying environmental chemicals, was on the same chromosome that housed the MHC. This was particularly interesting in light of Art Schwartz's study showing a correlation between this metabolic system and life span. Furthermore, mutations in the MHC had also been found to be associated with a number of age-related diseases such as diabetes, systemic lupus erythematosus, and rheumatoid arthritis.

He also learned that the MHC controlled the levels of two very important cell-function regulators. These are the cyclic nucleotides and they are found in the cells of all forms of life from bacteria to man. Cyclic nucleotides come in two forms, GMP and AMP, and they have a seesaw relationship—when one goes up, the other goes down. The comparative levels of these substances in a given cell determine such important gene functions as cell division and differentiation.

Walford also was interested in cyclic nucleotides and their connection to the MHC supergene. In earlier research he and other immunological gerontologists demonstrated that the strength of the immune response declines with age to about 10 percent to 15 percent of its peak youthful capacity. What, he wondered, happens to the levels of cyclic nucleotides in the immune cells as we grow old? He assigned the problem to a postdoctoral fellow, Chick Tam, who found that the levels of both cyclic AMP and cyclic GMP change dramatically with age. Cyclic AMP, which is high in youth, is five times lower in old cells, while the level of cyclic GMP goes up sevenfold, making the ratio between the two substances fifty times lower in old age. Most significant, perhaps, he found that the lymphocytes of people with Down's syndrome, the disease which shows more features of accelerated aging than any other, were markedly abnormal. Cells from thirty-year-old people with the disease had the cyclic AMP levels of cells of an eighty-year-old.

Like Cutler and Sacher, Walford had long been interested in the idea that mutations in a small number of genes could determine life span and aging. In 1974 he first announced his "limited-gene theory," and his belief that the MHC might fill the bill as a supergene for aging. Now in 1980, as the evidence mounted for his idea, he wrote, "The main histocompatibility complex may be one among this finite set of genes controlling aging. It is of interest to note that genes regulating superoxide dismutase (SOD), mixed function oxidases, and the level of cyclic nucleotides are on the same chromosome and genetically linked to the MHC. Because SOD and the mixed function oxidases protect against the damage by free radicals that may contribute to aging, and cyclic nucleotides are involved in proliferation and differentiation, genetic linkage of all these factors suggests that chromosomes #6 in man and #17 in the mouse, which carry the MHCs for these species, contain identifiable families of life-maintenance-process genes."

Looking at the same evidence, Cutler also saw in it a vindication of ideas he had been expressing since 1972. At the same time, he was bringing these ideas to a new level of integration. Like a conductor assembling the scores for instrumental parts so that he can view the whole, Cutler laid out in front of him the Hungarian paper on SOD, Walford and Hall's work on DNA repair, and Tam's study on the cyclic nucleotides. All the experiments involved the same strains of congenic mice, whose only difference from one another were on the genes of the MHC. Together, the papers made beautiful music. The strains that had the longest life span had the highest levels of SOD, the highest levels of cyclic AMP, and the highest levels of DNA repair.

"Okay," he thought, "let's add it up. For years we've known that there are specific functions in the body that do nothing but protect and repair the cells. There's the immune system, the mixed-functional oxidase system, DNA repair, antioxidant enzymes like SOD and catalase. All these have one thing in common: Their regulation is controlled by the major histo-compatibility complex."

As a student of Howard Curtis, Cutler had started out as a strong believer in somatic mutation theory. But more and more, it seemed to him that the idea of his mentor, and that of Szilard, Orgel, and others, that aging was an accumulation of mutations in the DNA could not be right. "It was like the old-fashioned wear-and-tear concept—cells and tissues wear out like an automobile. But the problem is that you can take a cell from an aging kidney or a liver or any organ, and it is functioning nowhere as well as it did when the organ was young, and yet when you look at its DNA and its protein, there's nothing wrong. So the accumulation of somatic mutations can't be the answer, or at least all of it."

While still working in Curtis's lab, he began to consider the idea that changes in gene expression—which genes are turned on and which off—might be playing a key role in aging. He found support for this idea in his first aging study in 1972, when he showed that the patterns of gene expression, in terms of which DNA was transcribed into RNA, were not fixed at sexual maturity but continued to change throughout life. In the late 1970s, other gerontologists flirted with the idea that alterations in gene expression played a dominant role in aging, but they lacked evidence. Support for this idea was already accumulating in cancer, where, for example, in transformed cells, previously repressed embryonic genes suddenly became active again. Then in 1978 Cutler showed a similiar phenomenon in aging cells. It was, to use Regelson's term, a "fulcrum" experiment, the kind that can tilt an entire field.

It had long been believed that once a cell was "committed" to a specialized function during development, it stayed that way forever. A liver cell was always a liver cell; a neuron, a neuron; and so on. Cutler, who takes nothing for granted and delights in playing devil's advocate, decided to take on this obvious truth. He asked, What if with age a kind of dysdevelopment takes place? What if the alterations in transcription activity he saw meant that the genetic program was unraveling, that the liver cell, the neuron, and all the other specialized cells of the body were becoming less differentiated? What if growing old was just a special case of the general tendency in the universe toward entropy?

Although others had suggested this might be the case, Cutler decided to see if he could actually demonstrate it. The question he asked was, Do cells "drift away from their proper state of differentiation with age?" For example, if he could show that neurons, in addition to transmitting the electric and chemical impulses of the brain, "lost their way" as they got older and began synthesizing hemoglobin, something only red blood cells were designed to do, he would have the perfect test for his dysdifferentiation idea.

Using a DNA probe for hemoglobin that could bound to its complementary RNA hemoglobin partner, he and his coworker, Tetsuya Ono, were able to detect the capacity of neuron cells in mice to synthesize globin, a protein constituent of hemoglobin. "It was a really sensitive assay," says Cutler, "where we could measure one or two RNA molecules in the cell. The changes we were looking at were not on the order of, say, going from 30 percent to 50 percent, but from zero percent to the presence of something." What they found confirmed Cutler's view that aging was not only genetic, but epigenetic; not only a mutation in the genes, but a change in which of the genes were expressed.

"All the nerve cells we looked at were turning on hemoglobin genes," says Cutler. And the phenomenon was age-related—the older the cell, the more globin molecules they detected. They repeated the study in liver cells, with the same results: Genes essential to the manufacture of hemoglobin, which had been repressed since embryonic life in the cells of the nerve and liver, had turned on again.

In another experiment, carried out at the same time, they found further evidence of gene repression with age. In this case they looked at mice that carry leukemia viruses in every cell of their body. These viruses are inherited by the animal, but they remain repressed for life and the mouse usually dies of other causes. When Cutler and Ono looked at aging cells from the brain and liver, they found that the mice were losing the ability to repress these viruses.

"I tend to look at unorthodox ideas," says Cutler. The idea suggested by these two experiments, which now had him in thrall, was that aging was not a continuation of development, as some gerontologists had hypothesized, but just the opposite—development in reverse. He called his new idea the "dysdifferentiation hypothesis" of aging.

"Look what happens with aging in human beings," he says. "First there is the conception of the individual, then growth, development, and finally, the fully matured person. All this is the result of many, many different cells doing different things. This is maintained by the protective/repair processes for a certain period of time. For humans that may be a total of twenty-five to thirty-five years, because throughout most of our evolution, few individuals ever lived beyond that point. There was no selection process to maintain these processes any longer than that.

"Now we have artificially lowered our environmental hazards and people are living far longer. And now we can see that aging is really dysdifferentiation, the falling apart, in a random, haphazard manner, of the very processes that created the organism. Eventually all our cells drift away from their differentiated state. Genes that have been repressed are derepressed. The pinnacle of tightness and control which characterizes the young cells is lost. Energy is required to maintain the differentiated state against the forces of entropy, but it is only maintained for a certain time and then it is just relaxed. So you don't have to invoke aging genes or anything else. Senescence is basic to the very processes that created us."

Now he saw that the latest revelations on the MHC as a "supergene" of aging fit into his idea of dysdifferentiation like a plug into a socket, shedding light on both concepts. The genes of the major histocompatibility complex made it possible for genes to "know" themselves. They conferred on the surface of the cells of every individual a mix of antigens as unique as a fingerprint. They determined whether our cells and tissues "tolerate" substances as "self" or rejected them as "nonself."

Simple laws govern complex events. It is Cutler's guiding philosophy, his faith, his hope, that biological systems, like planetary systems, are subject to this rule. To him, the fact that the same gene cluster that controls self-recognition of cells also regulates the processes for DNA repair and protection has the intrinsic beauty and simplicity of a physical law.

"Might it not be," says Cutler, "that the basic, fundamental concept behind preservation of health is really the preservation of self? What does the immune system do but recognize the difference between self and nonself? It removes and protects the organism against nonself, things like bacteria and foreign antigens and proteins. It also removes mutated cells—that is, cells which have lost their differentiated state. DNA repair also works by recognizing a mutation in the cell, which is a deviation from self. SOD and the mixed-function oxidases are involved in preventing an alteration in the membrane. And proper membrane integrity is fundamental to maintenance of the proper differentiated state of cells.

"A theory of aging must answer all the phenomena that we see associated with growing older. The coarseness and graying of hair, the changed texture of skin could be explained by the cells, losing their proper state of differentiation. Alzheimer's disease, which some people see as due to slow viruses, could result from the derepression of these viruses with age. Autoimmune disease could represent a derepression of genes that code for embryonic proteins. Our immune system only develops to its full potential when we are a few years old. And so we become tolerant and consider as 'self' only those proteins that represent the state of differentiation at that time. If at a later age, the genes coding for embryonic proteins are derepressed, the cell would now look like nonself and would be rejected by the body. In other words, you would have an autoimmune reaction. Even the *in vitro* aging in culture, the Hayflick limit, can be explained in this way, because the cells don't die; they just change their state of differentiation from dividing to nondividing. All these phenomena of aging can be explained by alterations in the state of differentiation, the inability of the cell to maintain its proper self."

In a few hectic months, Cutler saw his ideas from the past and the latest findings fitting together. But even as he incorporated the new knowledge on MHC, Cutler began to worry that he might experience with Walford a replay of his priority fight with Sacher. To forestall this, he suggested to Walford that they write a joint paper on the link between Cutler's longevity-determinant-gene hypothesis and Walford's supergene ideas.

Walford, according to Kathleen Hall, could not care less about who gets the credit for what. "I have never seen anyone less involved with the usual competitiveness and backbiting that goes on among scientists," she says. "All he cares about is that someone discovers the cure for aging. Of course, he'd like to be the one who does it, but if someone else does, that's just fine with him." Nevertheless, it was Walford who said drily, "Now Dick is talking about the idea of the supergene all over the place. Well, don't forget that I first broached the idea in my book *The Immunologic Theory of Aging* in 1969."

While Cutler rapidly assembled these ideas for presentation at the next gerontology conference, he learned of work from other labs that not only supported the supergene hypothesis but indicated that with his "project enhancement" scheme to increase life span by raising the levels of several protective enzymes simultaneously, he may have stumbled onto one of the ways that evolution did it.

In Madison, Wisconsin, Ken Munkrees, a biochemical geneticist, was working with a microscopic mold called *Neurospora*. Starting with the wild type, which lived about twenty-two days, he bred for short- and long-lived mutants, ending up with a full range of life spans from one he called the "mayfly," which lived for a day, to a Methuselah strain that lived eighty-eight days.

Remarkably, he found that the levels of five antioxidant enzymes, including SOD, correlated with the life span of the molds. Short-lived mutants had lower levels of all five, while the longest-lived mutants expressed the higher levels. Genetic studies revealed that all five genes "mapped" at one operon—a cluster of genes that act as a functional unit. He dubbed this supergene the "age complex." Changes in one regulatory gene, he found, affect all five genes at once, either repressing them so that the levels of antioxidant activity are lower, or derepressing them so that they can express higher levels.

"Presumably, all these genes have been kept together throughout evolution, so that they can act in concert," says Munkrees, who believes his work supports Walford's and Cutler's. Without these enzymes, he points out, free-radical activity would exert its destructive force on the cells far more rapidly, aging would be accelerated, and life span shortened considerably.

Indeed, it appears as though the concerted regulation of these enzymes made life on earth possible as the oxygen content in the atmosphere gradually increased from zero to its present levels. In studies done by Hosni Hassan and Irwin Fridovich, codiscoverer of SOD, at Duke University, *E. coli* bacteria mutants that were unable to make three major antioxidants, SOD, catalase, and peroxidase, had lost the ability to live in the presence of oxygen. "This would support Munkrees's idea that they are a gene cluster," says Fridovich. "How could one mutation knock out all three enzymes if they weren't all on one operon?"

The work of Munkrees and Fridovich also helps explain how longevity could evolve so rapidly, Cutler points out. "If you had to change the SOD itself, or one of these other protective enzymes, then it might take a hundred mutations before life span evolved. But if the level of all these enzymes were under the control of a master gene, then all it would take is one mutation." In this light it is particularly interesting that both Munkrees's age complex and the MHC have much higher mutation rates than other genes.

From Cutler's point of view, the most thrilling aspect of a supergene, which had now been shown in microorganisms, mice, and men, was that it indicated that coordinated enhancement of repair and protection mechanisms was in the cards. And Cutler believed he knew what the master regulator was—cyclic GMP, one of the two cyclic nucleotides that had so interested him and Walford.

Cutler's interest in cyclic GMP was first piqued by a serendipitous finding by one of his colleagues. Tetsuya Ono, who had collaborated with Cutler on several projects including the SOD-life-span correlation, had a friend at another laboratory who was measuring guanylate cyclase, the enzyme that generates cyclic GMP. Since he still had the tissue extracts from the various primates used in the SOD study, Ono was curious to see whether the levels of guanylate cyclase might also differ with life span. The tissues from the different species did indeed have different levels, but Ono, who was involved in other projects, turned the data over to Cutler. "I plotted it out and, my God, he was right," says Cutler. "There was a correlation. Only it was in inverse proportion to the life span, exactly opposite to what we had found with SOD."

What could possibly account for this species difference in guanylate cyclase? he wondered. Unlike cyclic AMP, which was known to act as a "second messenger" relaying the messages of certain hormones to the cell's chemical-manufacturing machinery, almost nothing was known about the role of cyclic GMP. Searching the literature, he came across two recent papers that set his mind racing. It appeared that guanylate cyclase was activated by carcinogens, mutagens, and free radicals, things like cigarette smoke, estrogen and progesterone, and the hydroxyl free radical. Could this be the damage detector that he had been looking for in his tricking-the-cell experiments, the spigot that turned on the flow of life-maintenance processes?

He injected cyclic GMP into his mice, and it worked beyond his expectations, greatly increasing the animals' resistance to radiation. The only problem was that cyclic AMP also worked, but not as well. Since the two nucleotides are presumed to have opposite effects, the results were difficult to explain. But the experiments gave him the germ of an idea that he would later develop into a model for tricking the cell.

He came across two other papers in 1980 that provided a way to unite both the somatic mutation and epigenetic theories of aging. Using a classic test of mutation, the change in eye color in fruit flies, a husband-and-wife team of British researchers, M.J. and O.H. Fahmy, had demonstrated that very low levels of carcinogens and free radicals were highly mutagenic. They exerted their effect by interacting with highly unstable portions of the DNA. Known variously as migratory DNA, transposons, or, as their discoverer, Nobel Laureate Barbara McClintock, called them, "jumping genes," these transposable genetic elements do not appear to play by the rules. Rather than stay in their place on the gene, they leapfrog about the genetic material, bringing together completely unrelated segments of DNA.

According to the Fahmys, the carcinogenic agents stepped up this migratory process, which plays a controlling role in differentiation and gene expression. In other words, the mechanism by which the agents acted to change eye color in the fruit flies was not mutational but epigenetic, not a change in the genetic code, but in how that code was expressed.

The work of the Fahmys, Cutler realized, offered a clue to the mechanism by which cells were nudged away from their state of differentiation. He had long postulated that there were two kinds of "biosenescent processes," the "continuously acting" and the "developmentally linked." The former were the insults of daily life, the toxic by-products of oxygen metabolism, foods, industrial pollutants, ultraviolet light, while the latter were the hormones, steroids, growth factors, all the other substances tied to growth and development. As oxygen both nourished and poisoned the cells, the agents of development had similar multiple—or pleiotropic—action. For instance, estrogen, a vital element in the female reproductive cycle, after menopause became a potential carcinogen. So deeply embedded are these dual-purpose processes in growth, maturation, and reproduction that the only way that evolution has been able to deal with them is by stretching out the period of development. The longer-lived the animal, the longer the period of infancy and childhood, the longer the organism is protected from the hormones' double-edged effect.

What both types of aging processes had in common was they produced damage. This damage could act directly as a mutation, or, in the new idea, as an epigenetic mechanism. The free radicals, the carcinogens, the mutagens, the thymine dimers, the hormones could perturb the cell by interacting with DNA "migratory elements," or perhaps by affecting the DNA chromatin, or supercoiling. The take-home lesson was that mutation was not the only way a cell could be done in. The damaging elements could enter the cell, do their dirty work, be repaired, and when one went to look for them, there was nothing there. They had disappeared like footprints in the falling snow.

After two years of the enhancement project, Cutler felt it was time to come in out of the cold. Although the project looked "very interesting," he explains, "it was not good enough to be published. I could see another two years' work ahead before I'd have anything. And I did not want to be unproductive in terms of publication."

He decided to take another tack in looking at life span, one that would give him answers regardless of how the experiment turned out. In this way, he would not only have the material for scientific papers but any "yes" answers he obtained could be the basis for a human longevity-enhancement program.

Chapter Eleven

"The Cell Controls
Its Own Destiny"

Somatic mutation, DNA damage and repair, free radicals—all have gone in and out of fashion as explanations for aging. By the end of 1982, the idea that intrinsic changes in the genetic material of somatic cells played a causative role in the overall deterioration of the body, which had been put forth so powerfully only four years earlier at the 1979 Gordon Conference, was on a downhill slide.

Kicking off the 1982 Gerontology Society meeting, for example, was a symposium entitled "An End of Errors! The Disproof of an Attractive Hypothesis." It was an attempt to bury not only Leslie Orgel's theory that a buildup of errors in the protein could reach catastrophic levels in the cell, but any role in aging for somatic mutations. One of the speakers was David Gershon, an Israeli molecular biologist whose early experiments had supported Orgel's theory, but whose subsequent work now ruled out a role for the genes in senescence. Any changes he saw in proteins, he believed, occurred after the protein was made. These changes could be due to free-radical-like components acting on the cell membrane, proteins, and cellular components, but not on the DNA itself. "We have absolutely no evidence," he told me emphatically, "that the DNA is damaged to such an extent that it would have an effect on the life span of the cell."

From an entirely different direction, David Harrison, an expert on the hemopoietic, or blood-forming, system of the body, had come to a similar conclusion. In a number of different tests, he failed to find an accumulation of mutations, autoantibodies, or any other genetic factor in the stem cells of older animals. "It could be," he said, "that there are some intrinsic factors that are related to the loss of physiological function, which we define as aging, but we don't see them, at least not with the simple linear correlations that we look for. We hope we can find some underlying relationships, but

219

more and more I am driven to the opinion that we don't have anything that is consistently correlated with anything else in the aging process."

On the eve of a 1982 FIBER conference on "Intervention in the Aging Process," rumor had it that a Washington, D.C., molecular biologist, Jerry Williams, was about to reveal an important finding that would breathe new life into the DNA damage theory of aging.

Short, with a bushy mustache, Williams has a gentle, cushiony quality, accented by the residue of a southern drawl. If anyone illustrates Kathy Hall's dictum that a gerontologist is someone who loves life, it is Williams. In fact, it was what drew him to biology in the first place. He remembers the day. In 1967 he was sitting at his desk at the General Dynamics Corporation, when he asked himself what in the world he was doing there working as a physicist. "My job," he thought, "is to design a shield for tanks against atomic weapons. Not to save a person's life, but so the machine can function five or six hours longer. This is morbid stuff and not what I went to school all those years for."

Perhaps it was the spirit of the late 1960s that made Williams do the unthinkable—quit a promising career in a well-paying job and enter graduate school once again, this time to learn molecular biology. A true son of Texas, coming from a long line of cotton farmers and "yellow-dog Democrats—they'd vote for a yellow dog if it ran as a Democrat"— Williams had been the first in his family to finish college. When he got his doctorate from Harvard, he flew his parents to Cambridge for the commencement and then took them by boat—"the first one they had been on"—to Nova Scotia. "It was the realization of the 'American dream,' " he says. "I'm not a particularly emotional person, but that was a real watershed in my life."

From the start of his studies in aging, soon after graduation, he made up his mind to look for a single, intrinsic cause. "Aging is such a universal property of all organisms and seems to be tied so carefully to other evolutionary factors," he says, "that it's hard to believe it's a random process. I don't agree with people who say that because of the multifaceted expression of aging deterioration, there are multiple causes. In science you seek the simplest answer if there is one. And if you say aging is multigenic, then I think you're almost abdicating rigor."

In 1974, when he began, he saw two observations that pointed to a single mechanism of aging. One was the work of Hayflick showing that cells in culture had a limited life span; and the other one, which had just been published, was the Hart-Setlow correlation between UV repair and the life span of various species. To test the Hayflick phenomenon, he chose not human cells, which take almost a year to stop dividing, but hamster cells, which are easy to work with and age rapidly.

His problems started when he found that although he could get the cells to senesce, he and his coworkers also got them to grow forever. Whether or not the cells aged, they found, depended upon their density in the laboratory dish. If they kept them from becoming overcrowded, the reproductive rate of the cells declined in three to four weeks. On the other hand, if they let the population increase without moving some of the colony into another dish, the cells kept right on growing.

Williams decided that Hayflick must be wrong, that *"in vitro* aging" was, as his detractors believed, an artifact of the culture condition. According to Hayflick, the only cells that did not stop reproducing in culture were transformed, or malignant, cells. But Williams's cells never changed in any way, and yet these, too, were immortal. He dashed off a paper to a scientific journal. The journal sent the paper to a reviewer, who gave it a "nasty review." "I said that the cells didn't do any of the things I would consider as transformation," notes Williams. "They don't look transformed, they are diploid [have two sets of chromosomes], and they don't pile up on top of each other in the dish. And the reviewer said, 'If they grow past their transformation time, they're transformed.' " He decided to withdraw the article even though the editor of the journal was willing to push it through "because he wanted to believe the data."

In 1978 Williams left Harvard for George Washington University. A science advisor to the U.S. Environmental Protection Agency as well, he was interested in research in environmental pollutants and cancer. Since the animal model most frequently used for the study of carcinogens was the rat, that became his model system.

"The rat gave us more problems than I ever expected," he says, "but it turned out to be the key to our recent observations." First, no matter how they tried to prevent it, all the cells transformed. Finally, after months of hard work, they were able to get just the right culture conditions that would cause most, but not all, of the cells to age. If he maintained the culture for six weeks, he found that a minute percentage of the cells became immortal, and, just as with the hamster cells, the rat cells were diploid and did not appear to be transformed.

Things went from bad to impossible when he began doing DNA repair experiments. About halfway through the life span of the senescing cells, the

DNA repair of UV-light damage would drop off as expected, but then after a short time, it picked up again. The observation made no sense to him. How could DNA repair first decline with age and then get better? To make matters more confusing, after a few more weeks in culture, the level of DNA repair in the cells fell once more. It was almost as if the cells were getting old, then young, then old. Looking at the wandering peaks of DNA activity on the charts, he felt as though the floor on which he was standing had given way. "My system isn't stable," he thought. "The changes I'm seeing don't mean anything." Williams had committed what he says is "a fatal error" for a scientist. "Instead of saying 'Aha, something very interesting is going on,' I said, 'Aha, something is wrong with the system because we're not getting the data I wanted to see.'"

Greatly discouraged, he shelved the DNA repair experiments and did not look at the data for an entire year. Then David Kram, from Ed Schneider's lab at the Gerontology Research Center, came to work with Williams. He brought with him a technique for measuring chromosome activity that Schneider had helped pioneer. When cells divide, the two identical strands of the chromosomes, called chromatids, can exchange places like partners in a square dance, a process known as sister chromatid exchange (SCE). Although no one knows exactly what the significance of such exchanges are, they increase dramatically in cells that are exposed to DNA damaging agents. The technique for measuring SCE allows the investigator to look at each cell in the culture individually. "It is," says Schneider, "probably one of the most sensitive measures of DNA damage that exists."

"Different people interpret the interchange of DNA in sister chromatid exchanges in different ways," says Williams. "I think of it as a measure of genetic activity that involves both damage and repair." He decided to measure the amount of SCE in his rat-cell cultures and the results flabbergasted him. The cells that were dying off in culture had very high levels of SCE, a finding he could only explain as due to an accumulation of DNA damage with age. But when he looked at the seemingly normal cells in the culture that were continuing to divide long after they should have stopped, in accordance with the Hayflick limit, he was in for another surprise. Instead of having high levels of SCE, like the senescent cells, they had very low levels of SCE. The only other cells of which this was true were transformed cells. In this respect, if no other, they were just like transformed cells.

This last observation converted Williams from a skeptic to a believer in the Hayflick limit. The immortal rat cells *were* transformed. What was needed was the right marker. And it looked as if he had one with SCE: "People always say that the ploidy [the number of sets of chromosomes] is the measure of normalcy in a cell. And we have shown that that's not true. Transformed cells, especially those of the rat, are very happy being diploid [having the normal complement of two sets]."

Using SCE, he and Kram began to focus on the fine details of what was happening inside the rat cells. Every time the cells filled the dish, they would transfer some of them into a new dish, to see how many would continue to grow. Some cells would divide vigorously for three or four passages, and then slow down, while another group went eight to ten passages before entering into senescence. What he originally thought was one population of cells all aging at the same rate was actually two distinct groups, both aging but at different rates. There were two waves of senescence.

Although he was at a loss to explain why cells in the same culture should age at two different rates, he found other reports of this in the literature. Suddenly all the inexplicable findings of the year before made sense. He said to his staff, "Get out all the work on DNA repair in the human cells, in the rat cells, in the cat. Let's take a look at everything."

They dug out the data on DNA repair. There were the wandering peaks of DNA repair with age that had so confused them. Now at last the mystery was solved. When they looked at DNA repair, they were looking at all the cells in the culture as a whole, but with SCE they were able to focus in on each cell individually. In the DNA repair experiments, he had seen two separate precipitous declines at two different times in the life span. With SCE, he had uncovered the fact that there were two distinct populations in the culture, each aging at a different rate. Putting all the data together, he found that the two declines in DNA repair matched the two waves of senescence like the halves of a broken ring.

DNA repair did decline with age and Williams's faith in his system was renewed. "I could have tied all this down a year ago," he says, "if I had done what I tell my students. The first step in the scientific method is to reject authority. Don't believe what people have told you. Look at the data."

And that is what he did in the next few weeks of the summer of 1982, whipping himself and his group into a frenzy of activity. He reviewed the data, was seized by an idea, assigned one student to do a quickie experiment, sent another one to the library to research the literature, and then saw where the new pieces of data fit in. He was doing the thing he loves best in science, looking for patterns, making connections, pulling together fragments of information like an archaeologist assembling an ancient amphora from scattered shards.

"We had everybody in the laboratory plotting data and writing," he says. "It was just an exciting time. Amazing, really. I don't think ever in my knowledge has anything, . . . has so much work for me . . . come together in such a short amount of time. It was a heady experience."

During this time he made several observations that added up to a most astounding conclusion. Not all the DNA damage to the cell came from the outside. As strange as it seemed, the cell was putting damage into its DNA and it appeared to do so not haphazardly, but purposely.

Williams returned to an idea that had been explored by R. J. Wilkins and Ron Hart at Oak Ridge National Laboratory in 1974. The question they had asked was, Why wasn't all the DNA that was damaged by ultraviolet light repaired? Others had shown that only 50 percent to 75 percent of UV-induced dimers were repaired, while the rest of the dimers persisted in the cell for at least twenty-four to forty-eight hours later. In mammalian cells, part of the DNA is wrapped around proteins called histones, while part of the DNA is free of proteins; the combination of the bound and unbound DNA is called chromatin. When Wilkins and Hart stripped the proteins from the DNA in the chromatin, they literally unmasked what was going on. Most of the repair of the UV damage occurred in the free regions of DNA that were readily accessible to repair enzymes. The DNA that was not repaired was hidden by a mask of protein that prevented the enzymes from acting on them. The persistence of these lesions in the DNA chromatin, they suggested, might lead to trouble years later if the damaged genes in the masked DNA became expressed. (Although the DNA is supercoiled around the proteins, they were not looking at this because by removing the proteins, they were also removing the coils.)

Williams decided to do a similar study, but this time comparing cells from rodents with those of humans. In the first two hours of repair, the cells of both species rapidly removed the damage so that the difference in repair between them was not very large. But after that time, the story changed dramatically. Rodent cells stopped removing the damage altogether, while human cells continued but at a reduced rate. Most of the unrepaired damage was hidden away in the hard-to-reach areas of the chromatin, where the DNA was shielded by protein.

In another study, he looked at cells that were taken from young and old animals. These were fresh-dividing cells that had been in culture only forty-eight hours and had not been exposed to any outside DNA-damaging agents. To do this, they used enzymes called endonucleases, which recognize UV-induced damage and break the DNA at what is called endosensitive sites. By seeing how fast the DNA moves through a gradient, they could then measure the extent of UV damage. DNA that contains breaks moves more rapidly than intact DNA. Now they found that there was no difference between the young and old cells if they just looked at the DNA as a whole. But if they stripped the proteins off the DNA using high salts, as Wilkins and Hart had done in the earlier experiment, they found that the old cells had far more damage than the young ones. Again all the damage had been hidden away in the inaccessible regions of the chromatin and would never have been seen if they had not removed the proteins.

The experiment posed a most intriguing puzzle. These were fresh-dividing cells that had been in culture only forty-eight hours and had not been exposed to any outside DNA-damaging agents. Furthermore, they had been grown in the dark, so that UV dimers could not have been induced. Where had the damage come from?

As mind-boggling as it seemed, there could be only one explanation. The only way the damage could have gotten there was if the cell put it in. The kind of damage produced by the cells appeared to be a dimer, since they were attacked by the same enzymes that attack dimers produced by ultraviolet light. The more Williams looked, the more it seemed this unlikely event was taking place.

In another experiment, he hit the cells with a large dose of ultraviolet light and then put the DNA into 100 percent formic acid at 180 degrees Fahrenheit—a sledgehammer process that takes everything apart in the cell, *except* for the dimers. In the first hour of repair, he found, the cell had 10 percent more of the dimerlike lesions than he had put in with the UV light. Again it looked as if some of the damage was originated by the cell.

Dimers produced by ultraviolet light occur with the randomness of lightning striking the ground. So Williams next asked the question, Were the dimerlike lesions he found in the cells random or nonrandom? They put the results of their gradient studies into the computer and found there were two different kinds of lesions. One was random, as might be expected with DNA damage, but the other was not. The nonrandom ones were regularly spaced throughout the DNA as though something were placing them there.

Was there a difference between the amounts of random lesions versus nonrandom lesions according to the age of the animal? There was, and it was the kind of difference that resonated with his physicist's view of natural phenomena. In the cells from the older animals, the number of random lesions far outnumbered the regularly spaced ones, "almost as though entropy were taking over," says Williams.

Finally, he asked, Was there a difference in the number of lesions between species with different life spans? In the year they had worked on DNA repair, they had looked at cells from a human, cat, and rat. Now he laid out all the results from these experiments. If these lesions played a determining role in life span, then the number of damage sites should be highest in the rat, lower in the cat, and lowest in humans. That is exactly what he found.

All this happened in two glorious weeks in the summer of 1982. "I was on cloud nine," says Williams. "It was one of those rare times in a scientist's life, when you think you have a glimpse of the truth with a capital T."

In the same way that his doubts about the Hayflick limit were overcome by his own experiments, so were his initially negative views about Hart and Setlow's original observation. The first time I heard Williams speak was at the 1979 Gerontology Society Conference in Washington. He had just followed Hart's enthusiastic presentation linking together his own work with Lipetz's on superhelicity. "The question," Williams said at that time, "is whether the fidelity of DNA is important in aging as cause or as an effect. I suppose that I have come up with a more pessimistic view than Ron has expressed in the state of our knowledge and the ability to say where we are in terms of this hypothesis."

I reminded him of his words and he agreed that he was "quite negative on Hart's data at that time. Hart comes on so strongly that I tend to draw back. But everywhere I go—the technique we use, the DNA repair correlation—he's been there."

As Hart and Setlow pointed out at the time of their study, UV-induced dimers from the sun, which were literally skin-deep, could not be the cause of aging. But excision repair, which patches up UV damage, also repairs other forms of damage, such as that caused by chemical pollutants in the air we breathe, which, unlike the sun, reaches the internal organs. Conceivably, those animals that could better handle insults from various DNA-damaging agents would live longer.

Williams had long had his own questions about the DNA repair/life-span correlation. If one just considered ultraviolet-light damage, why should the process for repairing it be present in fur-covered rats, or, for that matter, in human placental tissue? Most baffling of all, why was there not only excision repair, but at least five other repair systems capable of removing ultraviolet-light-induced dimers from the DNA? He asks, "Why in the world should somatic cells maintain all these systems to repair damage they have not seen for billions of years of evolution?" Now, he believed, he might have an answer.

"Macfarlane Burnet, who wrote the book *Intrinsic Mutagenesis,* is a very brilliant fellow," says Williams. "I heard him speak at Harvard and I remember him saying that it was his observation, after years and years of biological thinking, that everything that's important to the cell is controlled within the cell. So if aging were important to the cell, which he thought it was, the process by which the cell aged itself would be intrinsic. That's why he was always looking for the 'intrinsic mutator.' His ideas influenced my thinking and as soon as I saw these damages which we think are repaired by the UV repair system, I thought here we have a mechanism by which aging can take place."

From an evolutionary standpoint, it all makes sense, he says. Like a carpenter who needs no more than a hammer, nails, and a saw to repair a shelf or build a house, the cell adapts its tools for many purposes. From the beginning of life on earth, the cell has had to deal with damage from ultraviolet light and background radiation. To take out a dimer induced by UV, it must break the DNA strand. The chemical nature of that break is the same as the one caused by ionizing radiation. Removing the damaged bases, synthesizing new ones, putting the repaired strand back together are processes the cell has honed through time. When the cell has to break the DNA in order to replicate or express new genes, it is logical that it borrows the instruments of UV repair that it knows so well.

"When did aging begin in evolution?" asks Williams rhetorically. "It began with eucaryotes. This was the first time that the DNA was organized into chromatin." Over the next hundreds of millions of years of evolution, as the eucaryotes were developing into multicellular creatures, the atmosphere of the earth was changing. The ozone layer formed, acting as a shield against the ultraviolet light, and allowing the first creatures to leave the sea. Suddenly the ability to repair UV damage became far less important, he says. But now the cell was equipped with all the processes it needed to handle the DNA chromatin.

At any given time, the differentiated cells of a multicellular organism use only a minute percentage of the available DNA. The rest is packaged away into the supercoils and domains of the chromatin. But when the cell goes to do its "housecleaning," it must move the furniture and get under the rug. "In order to express itself, in order to replicate itself, in order to repair itself, it must break the DNA and unpackage all or part of it," says Williams.

In other words, the ability of the cell to put in damage is intimately tied to all the functions a cell must carry out to survive.

"If this process is essential to manipulation of chromatin, then clearly it allows differentiation to occur. In fact, if a fetus were defective in this built-in mechanism, it would not be viable," he points out. "The cells could never differentiate into an individual and they would be reabsorbed *in utero.*"

But the price paid for the ability to differentiate, indeed for multicellular organisms to evolve, may be the loss of immortality. The "intrinsic mutator," he suggests, may have two purposes: evolution of the species and aging of the individual.

With age it appears that the cells's capacity to either put in the lesions or take them out again—he doesn't know which—diminishes. When Williams gives a small dose of radiation to young and old cells, both are capable of opening up the DNA and repairing the lesions that have accumulated. But very shortly thereafter, he finds, the random lesions have started to accumulate in the aged cells. At this point, when I visit him in 1983, he tells me, he doesn't know whether the barrier to repair is physical—that is, some kind of deterioration of the chromatin prevents the repair enzymes from reaching the lesion—or chemical, the enzymes themselves go bad. He suspects the former is true.

"I tend to think that there may be a deterioration of chromatin with age, for whatever reason," he says. "And that this restricts the amount of repair. It is a dynamic situation. The sum of the forces that puts the damage in and takes it out is always going to be less in the rat than in man."

When Williams arrived at the FIBER meeting in November 1982, having just completed the experiments on the intrinsic-mutating mechanism, he had still not made up his mind about how much he would reveal. He hesitated to present work that had not yet been published or even submitted for review, but at the same time, he felt pushed by Lipetz. Although Williams was not looking directly at supercoiling, both men were concerned with how the overall packaging of the DNA in the chromosome affected aging and cancer, and each wondered what the other had to report.

Like Williams, Lipetz was also sitting on top of a new finding, which created a fundamental shift in his view of what happened with the DNA supercoiling with age: As people aged, their cells took longer and longer to regulate the supercoiling after DNA damage. This discovery popped out of data he had collected for a routine experiment. Earlier that year, in an effort to find commercial applications of his work for his genetic-engineering company, he thought of using his nucleoid supercoiling technique to gauge the extent of genetic damage in people who had been exposed to radiation, either in the workplace or accidentally, as with the Three Mile Island incident.

To do this, he had to establish a baseline for the ability of normal cells to handle genetic damage. In the experiment, he and Stephens exposed human lymphocytes to a low dose of X-ray, which causes strand breaks and decreases the DNA supercoiling. With most people, they found, it took about two hours for their DNA to recover from the damage state. But to their great surprise, two people whom they tested had very slow or virtually nonexistent recovery even after five hours. Yet neither one of them had any overt sign of disease.

How many people in the general population showed this response? Lipetz wondered. They decided to expand their original group of twenty, using people from the lab as well as blood samples from Red Cross donors. By the time of the FIBER conference, they had amassed results on ninety-five individuals from age eighteen to sixty. Of this group, they found that 80 percent exhibited "normal" or complete recovery, 15 percent moderate, and 5 percent an extremely slow rate of recovery. Since radiation causes "hits" on the DNA in random fashion, Lipetz believes that the slow responders must have an altered organization of their DNA/chromatin that makes them particularly vulnerable.

Next, he wondered, what role does age play in the ability to recover from X-ray damage? Lipetz and Stephens regraphed the data according to the age of the individual and found that although there was enough variation to make it impossible to predict a person's age from his recovery response, there was a statistically significant decline in the response with age—about two-thirds of 1 percent per year. Unconcerned about the amount of scatter in his correlation, Lipetz says: "If anyone came up with a correlation between chronological age and any biochemical parameter which fell perfectly on the line, I would say that they are faking the data. We all know people who are thirty and look sixty and people who are thirty and look sixteen. So we know that there has to be discrepancy in biological age versus chronological age."

The most important outcome of this finding, he believes, was its effect on his thinking. He had shown a decrease in DNA supercoiling in aged human cells *in vitro,* and recently this finding had been confirmed by Russian researchers who found a supercoiling decrease with age in hamster cells.

But then he and other laboratories had shown an increase in DNA supercoiling in cancer cells. Since cancer was an age-related disease, how could supercoiling decrease with age and increase with cancer? The paradox seemed unresolvable.

But now, with his latest work, he saw a way out. His test had shown a small but significant age-related decline in the cell's ability to restore the supercoiling after it was hit by genetic damage. If this were the case, then it meant that over time, the cell was losing *its ability to regulate the DNA supercoiling*. And if this happened, then the cell could flip in either direction, toward increased supercoiling and the development of cancer or toward decreased supercoiling and aging. Each cell of the body might respond slightly differently to a genetic insult.

"Cells vary according to what they encounter in their environment," says Lipetz. "For instance, they are affected by what hormones bind on. Each cell has a predisposition to go off in one direction or the other. It can be differentiation or it can be a tumor. But the point is that as you get older, the ability of the cell to put the DNA supercoiling back into its proper differentiated state, whatever it is for that particular tissue, declines. The important thing is not that the DNA supercoiling goes up with cancer and down with age in a kind of preprogrammed lifetime progression, but, rather, that as we grow older, our cells are losing their ability to regulate their DNA supercoiling."

The next day of the FIBER conference, Lipetz presented first. After a spirited discussion, Regelson, in keeping with the organization's philosophy of forging links between various pieces of research, asked Jerry Williams, who was standing at the back of the room, if he would care to comment. In one movement, every head in the room turned to see how he would handle it. Williams decided to sidestep. "I have enough trouble interpreting my own data," he said, ducking under the cover of laughter.

Lipetz's speech did push Williams into presenting at the FIBER conference his findings that the cell put in its own DNA damage. But it was not until one year later, when he had entered the territory charted by Lipetz, that he began to understand just what those intrinsic damages might mean. Although as far back as the 1979 Gerontology Society meeting, he had indicated that "supercoiling might be an interesting way to go," he finally "kind of fell into it" in 1983.

The impetus was one of the most successful experiments Williams had ever done. He and a graduate student, Joe Frank, had discovered a molecular mechanism that helped explain a rather dismaying side effect of a beneficial treatment. The disease was psoriasis, in which the dry, scaly patches of skin can in severe cases be disfiguring and debilitating. The treatment was PUVA, an acronym for a chemical, psoralen, plus ultraviolet light of the A wavelength. Although the therapy had proved extremely effective in otherwise refractory cases, the down side of PUVA was that the patients showed accelerated aging of the skin and a cancer rate vastly increased over that of the normal population. Other researchers had found that the patients most at risk of developing skin cancer were those who had been previously treated with X-rays alone. In some unknown way, the cells seemed to "remember" their earlier exposure to X-rays, a DNA-damaging agent, when they were hit with psoralen plus ultraviolet light, another DNA-damaging agent, at a later date.

In their study, Williams and Frank X-rayed cells in culture, allowed the cells to go through many divisions, and then hit them with PUVA. Small doses of PUVA that would scarcely cause a ripple in a normal cell induced a high frequency of mutations in the progeny of cells that had been X-irradiated. In other words, it appeared that cells hundreds of generations down the line inherited a memory of their previous injury that made them hypermutable. In another, related experiment, dual biopsies from PUVA-treated patients, one from an area that had been exposed to the therapy, and another from an unexposed area under the arm, were put into culture. "Invariably the cells from the exposed area senesced first," says Williams. "So the cells we were studying had a memory of their *in vivo* exposure."

But when they tried other mutagenic agents on the progeny of cells that had been X-irradiated, there was no effect. Only PUVA had this unique ability to reactivate the cellular memory of earlier damage. What was it about PUVA, Williams wondered, that could account for the hypermutability of these cells?

In experiments with the agent, Williams found that the most likely answer lay in the ability of PUVA to affect the supercoiling. But more importantly, from his point of view, the agent offered an unprecedented opportunity for looking at superhelical coiling. Like ethidium bromide, used by Lipetz and other supercoiling researchers, psoralen is an intercalating agent—its molecules can insert themselves between the base pairs of the DNA, and, if enough is added, completely relax the supercoiling. But where ethidium bromide slips in and out of the DNA, psoralen can be fixed in place simply by shining ultraviolet light on it. As in Joan Smith-Sonneborn's Slinky model, the amount of intercalating agent that enters the DNA is going to depend upon the tightness of the coils.

By first chilling the cell and then putting in PUVA, Williams was able to measure the state of DNA supercoiling at a given instant. Chilling the cell shuts down its enzymes, inhibiting its response. When he warmed up the cell, the enzymes were able to go back to work and get rid of the PUVA, which is toxic to the cell. The enzymes involved, he believes, are the topoisomerases that control the winding and unwinding of the supercoils.

Performing the same experiment on rodent cells, Williams found that, as the rodent cells went from cold to warm, they revealed a remarkable ability to change their supercoiling and "kick out" the PUVA. The human cells could not do this. The results dumbfounded him. "We are accustomed to looking at a very narrow range of response in cells' ability to deal with DNA-damaging agents. But our technique allowed us to look at the supercoiling much more precisely than other people have been able to. And we saw differences of one hundred- to one thousandfold in the cell's ability to manipulate the DNA," he says.

He immediately started to explore all the differences that, he says, must be considered in any theory of the mechanism of aging—the difference between the cells of short-lived and long-lived species; between young and old cells of the same species; and between cells that live forever, such as transformed cells, and those that are mortal. In every case the differences were striking and revealing.

They found that the cells from short-lived rodents, transformed cells, and the cells of older humans all had something in common—they had far less of the "torsional restraint," the tightly wound Slinky that characterizes the young human cell. The transformed cell had almost none at all, and could whip the supercoiling around with amazing alacrity. "Cells that are transformed, that live forever, have great control," he observes. "They can change their superhelicity dynamically within a few minutes and package everything away." With age, the normal cell behaves more and more like a transformed cell. Part of its supercoiling remains in the tightly wound state, while part of it now moves around autonomously. The cell is losing control over its supercoiling.

"I was sort of skeptical of some of Lipetz's work [on the decline in chromatin recovery response with age] because there was so much scatter in it. It was awfully hard to make patterns. But now I agree that changes in the superhelicity of the DNA may be involved in aging," he says.

Although his investigation is in a preliminary stage and his ideas are still evolving, he has come up with a picture of how changes in supercoiling might affect aging, cancer, and gene expression. What characterizes a young, differentiated cell is that 99 percent of its DNA is packaged away into tight, supercoiled loops of DNA called domains. There are about fifty thousand of these loops in a human cell. Like coiled paper streamers tacked onto the ceiling of a high-school gym, these regions are physically restrained from twisting about. Only the 1 percent of the DNA needed for gene expression can be freely manipulated as the cell goes about its functions. With age, the restraints start disappearing. Areas that should be hidden away are now available to be unwound and rewound by the topoisomerase enzymes that manipulate the DNA. "So now," says Williams, "when the cell starts changing the superhelicity in the regions it normally expresses, it also starts changing the other regions as well, and genes are expressed which shouldn't be."

Williams pictures the domains of supercoiled DNA as being like pieces of a garden hose. If the pieces are very short, you can put only a few twists in them before the hose begins to stiffen. But if the pieces are long, which is what would be happening if the domains were being unhooked in some way, one could put far more coils in before the strand became too difficult to twist.

The same difference between restricted and unrestricted domains holds true between the short-lived rodent cell and the long-lived human one. What Williams and his colleagues find is that the human cells are under much tighter control than the rat cells. "This seems to indicate that human cells have more of these domains and therefore it takes a much longer time for them to lose control over an appreciable portion of their genome. With rodent cells, this happens much more easily," he says. He also believes that the divergence in repair between rodent and human cells has to do with this difference in DNA packaging. The cells of both species, he found, repair equally well in the first two hours, but only human cells continue to remove and repair the damage after that time. The result, Williams believes, is that in both cases the genes needed for cellular function are repaired, but only the human cells take care of the genes that are hidden away in the chromatin and not being used.

Williams does not think of supercoiling in terms of "a decrease" in it with age or an "increase" with cancer. "To ask whether it is more or less supercoiling doesn't mean very much," he contends. "By playing with the stimulus in different ways and inhibiting the enzymes or not, we can have it express much more supercoiling or much less. I think the way to view it is as a dynamic process in which the cell can change its supercoiling very rapidly when it suits its purpose.

"Our hypothesis is that as cells age something happens—whether it is programmed, or random, or free radicals, we don't know—that starts freeing up certain regions of the genome. Incrementally, the cell is losing control of different domains. It begins to act like a cancer cell, in that it can now supercoil that area more freely. It's no longer restrained mechanically from doing this."

The metaphor that comes to my mind is a vast, complicated filing system. In the young cell, the DNA is neatly organized into many different files. Most of the information is stored away in inactive files, while the current data in active files are constantly being gone through. After years of use, the orderly system breaks down. When the clerks go to get out a certain piece of paper, they reach into the drawers that should have been locked. Things that shouldn't be available are now read and transcribed. Papers are not returned to their proper place. There is a certain leakage between the compartments, which interferes with the well-oiled, precise functioning that the young cell enjoyed.

What could such a mix-up in the filing system do? For one, it might lead to the development of cancer. In the summer of 1983, while Williams was in the midst of his supercoiling studies, one of the biggest mysteries in cancer research was cleared up. It had been known for some time that certain genes, called oncogenes, had the power to transform a normal cell into a malignant one. A number of scientists had shown that genetic changes, such as somatic mutations, rearrangements of DNA, or migration of a piece of DNA from one chromosome to another, could activate the normal gene to its oncogenic state. The mystery gene product turned out to be a growth factor associated with normal wound healing. The oncogene made the growth factor, which in turn generated tumor cells. It was like turning on a tap that couldn't be shut off.

"This is the model," Stuart A. Aaronson, a National Cancer Institute researcher who was on one of two successful teams that identified the product, told a news conference. "In normal wound healing this important cellular gene releases this substance called platelet-derived growth factor. This causes limited proliferation of cells, which helps in wound healing. But if through a trigger mechanism—either a genetic alteration in the normal gene in the cell or the addition of the virus that has this gene—we now have the potential for unlimited growth—a continued cycle of proliferation that can lead along with other changes to a real cancer."

In other words, the gene in its normal location performs a useful function for the cell. But if it is moved in some way, such as being shifted to another chromosome and freed from the constraints of its old location, it begins to make the growth-factor product in an unregulated fashion. With a loss of control of the supercoiling, this is far more likely to happen.

"Cancer has turned out to be an extremely fundamental disease," says Williams. "So far about twenty different oncogenes have been identified [along with some of the products], and what happens when we get cancer is, these genes are mutated, or they are moved to another part of the genome, where they can be expressed, or they are amplified in some way. All of these are events that might occur in old people because they are losing their control of their chromatin structure. That, I think, is the basis of the correlation between aging and cancer."

The other consequence of the DNA supercoiling slipping out of control would be the expression of unwanted genes. Indeed, Williams's vision of the cell could be the actual, physical basis for Cutler's theory of dysdifferentiation—the restricted domains characterizing the differentiated cell, and the loss of these restraints corresponding to the cell's slow drift away from the specialized functions for which it was designed. "That certainly is the model we are pursuing," he says. "The cells would continue to do their differentiated state, because these states are turned on, but at the same time, they would start expressing other genes."

Now Williams believes he has a handle on the "intrinsic lesions" he found in his earlier studies. "The amount of the genome [all the genes taken together] that the cell can supercoil seems to deteriorate with age," he says. And it is in these unsupercoiled regions that the lesions accumulate. Also, in keeping with his dynamic view of the DNA, he no longer sees the lesions as "random" versus "nonrandom," but, rather, as a progression from precision to imprecision, from organization to anarchy.

The young cell uses these lesions for its own purpose, unwrapping the DNA, repairing it, and putting it back together in a highly efficient and precise manner—only the right amount of lesions, in the right places, for the proper function. But as the cell ages, it begins to act inappropriately, putting the lesions into regions that it can't handle. "It seems to have lost its purpose. It doesn't put them in to unwind the DNA, but rather places them randomly throughout the cell. And because of the changes in supercoiling, these lesions become hidden away. So you see, it becomes a self-generating process, in which the more lesions it has, probably the more trouble it has controlling the processes needed for repair. It's not that the cell can't repair. When we give them a little damage, they open up the DNA, go through the genome and repair everything. But if our rationale holds, now when it opens up the cell, there is a lot more damage stored away, and it is much more likely to make mistakes when it does repair."

Williams, who has moved from George Washington to a tenured professorship at Johns Hopkins, plans to investigate the idea that loops of supercoiled DNA are becoming unhooked from the "nuclear matrix"—the structural network of protein fibers supporting the DNA. He would also like to answer such questions as, What is the state of the supercoiling in a gene that is being expressed, compared with one that is not? And, ultimately, what controls the changes in supercoiling with age and transformation? But what truly excites Williams is the thought that he is onto a basic mechanism, and that, in pursuing this, he has his life's work cut out for him.

"What I like most of all about this theory," he says, "is that it stays with the intuitively pleasing hypothesis that deterioration of the DNA structure and function is at the heart of aging. You don't need so many of the things that other people have brought in, such as free radicals or cross-linking agents, etc. These may be involved, but it is basically that the cell controls its own destiny; that it is not exogenous, but an intrinsic, genetic process."

The most recent research indicates that the process of disorganization and dysdifferentiation that Williams sees in the chromatin DNA—the most fundamental level of organization in the body—is occurring at every level of organization in the body. Not only is the structure of the DNA falling apart with age, but according to a hypothesis advanced by Robin Holliday of the National Institute for Medical Research in London, the genetic code is going through its own deregulation.

In 1975 Holliday, a brilliant theoretician, became one of the first researchers in aging to propose an epigenetic theory. His interest at the time was to explain one of the central mysteries of development. Starting with one cell, how do you end up with many different cells that have different gene activities? The other side of the coin is that once cells have attained the desired state of differentiation, how do they maintain this state, so that a liver cell, for example, remains a liver cell and doesn't become something else?

The answer to both questions, Holliday and his student, John Pew, proposed, lies in what happens to the genetic code. Ordinarily, one thinks of the DNA as having four nucleic acid bases—adenine, cytosine, guanine, and thymine. But, strictly speaking, this is not true. A very small percentage of certain bases have added onto them a chemical group called methyl, which consists of one atom of carbon bonded to three hydrogen atoms. If a cytosine base in a certain region contains a methyl group, Holliday and others found, the activity of that particular gene will be halted and the enzyme or protein that it codes for will not be made. If the methyl group is removed, i.e., demethylated, the gene will once more be expressed. In other words, methylation or demethylation of the DNA can act as chemical off/on switches for gene expression.

During embryonic development, Holliday believes, the gene switches for each cell are set in a pattern of methylation. This pattern is then maintained by an enzyme he calls maintenance methylase. Any mistakes or changes in this pattern, he predicted, would lead to abnormal gene expression. When he and his colleagues experimentally produced a loss of methylation in the DNA, they were able to show that this was the case; certain genes that had been repressed were reactivated.

It now appears this may be happening in our own cells as we age. When cells from three species—mouse, hamster, and human—were put into culture, they all showed a steady loss of DNA methylation during successive cell divisions. And the rate of loss correlated with the maximum life span of the species.

Whether this is an aging program set in the cells at birth, or comes about as the result of DNA damage, has yet to be determined. But the important thing, Holliday points out, is that once the pattern of methylation is fixed in the genes, "it is like a ratchet, where you can go in one direction, not the other. You can only lose methyl groups, you can't get them back again. You're going downhill all the time. Then when you get to a certain level, you can't maintain the integrity of the cell."

At this point no one knows whether or not there is any relationship between the loss of methylation and the breakdown in the chromatin structure hypothesized by Williams, but the net result is the same: a loss of control over gene expression, a deregulation, a dysdevelopment.

As the DNA goes, so go the proteins, the hormones, and the enzymes. This is the level that Cutler looked at with his dysdifferentiation experiments showing that old brain cells make hemoglobin, a job that should be reserved for blood cells, thus destabilizing the cell.

But even if there is an increase in aberrant behavior of the cell with age, does this have any real meaning in terms of its function? This was the question put to Cutler when he reviewed the evidence for his dysdifferentiation hypothesis at a symposium of the American Aging Association conference in October 1984. Cutler, who was one of the organizers of the symposium, indicated that Phil Hartman might provide some answers.

Hartman, a professor of biology at Johns Hopkins University, has been looking at metaplasia, spots of adult tissue that start behaving as though they belonged to a different organ. For example, in intestinal metaplasia, a group of cells in the stomach acts as though it were part of the intestines. Instead of releasing enzymes that aid in digestion, the cells release enzymes that aid in absorption. They produce less acid than gastric cells should, thus opening the stomach to bacterial invasion. Since intestinal cells are replaced every two days while stomach cells are replaced every four days, the intestinal metaplasias grow at twice the speed of their normal neighbors. It is in these areas of abnormal activity that cancers are most likely to arise. Indeed, the connection between cancer of the stomach and intestinal metaplasia is striking. In Japan, a country with one of the highest rates of stomach cancer in the world, 70 percent of the population, by age thirty, has some intestinal metaplasia, while in the United States, where the stomach-cancer incidence is extremely low, only 35 percent of the population ever develops intestinal metaplasia.

Where do these metaplasias come from? At least part of the answer, Hartman believes, lies in somatic mutations. Experimentally, metaplasias can be induced in laboratory animals, by giving them various mutagens and carcinogens. With age, there is an ever-increasing accumulation of metaplasias of all kinds. Not only do we acquire new ones as we go through life, but the old ones multiply and expand. The abnormal activity of the existing metaplasias actually makes them more vulnerable to mutagens, which in turn leads to more metaplasias and increases the possibility of cancer. These bits of wrong-way tissue may never appear on a death certificate as the cause of death, but as Hartman points out, they are precursors to the kind of functional breakdown in one or another organ that does kill us in the end. As he puts it, "Individually they are benign, but collectively they have a physiological impact."

Still other evidence of a breakdown in the hierarchy of biological function comes from Jim Trosko of Michigan State. In his most recent work, he has been looking at the collapse of normal communication between cells. Although cells are walled off from one another by membranes that keep needed molecules in and harmful molecules out, under certain conditions they form gap-junctions, tunnels between themselves and their neighbors, through which molecules can pass. Cell-cell communication is vital to keeping cells of a particular tissue functioning as part of that tissue, in other words, maintaining the differentiated state. And it is the disruption of these lines of communication over time that Trosko believes is instrumental in causing aging and age-related diseases.

"Somatic mutation is a necessary but insufficient step for aging," he says. "In multicellular organisms like human beings with trillions of cells, how can the mutation of a few cells make a difference? Any deficient cells that are present will be masked by all the normal ones. The only way that aging can occur in my opinion is if you *amplify* the number of mutant cells that result from lack of, or insufficient, DNA repair. And the only way you amplify these single dysfunctional cells in the liver, the eye, the brain, or wherever aging occurs, is by blocking cell-cell communication. This allows the dysfunctional cells to grow into huge clones of dysfunctional tissue. Normal cells have normal gap-junctions and cancer cells do not. But this is not just true of cancer. It may also be true of atherosclerosis, Alzheimer's, and diabetes. All these diseases are due to the organ containing huge masses of mutant cells."

If the Old Testament were to be written today, it might say, "Entropy, all is entropy." It is the original sin, the fruit of the tree of knowledge, the serpent in the Garden of Eden. Living organisms exist for a while as in a state of grace, seemingly immune to the increases in disorder and decreases in energy that inhere in all of nature, but then they, we, all succumb. Aging even looks like entropy. The sharp, delineated features of youth are gradually obliterated by the random collection of lines, wrinkles, odd bits of hair, nodules, bumps, depressions. On every level, it now appears the same thing is going on. The intricate folding of the chromatin is falling apart; parts of the DNA that should be sectioned off, one from the other, are now willy-nilly coming into contact. The cell continues to carry out its functions but it is stumbling, carrying out activities it was never designed to do. The tight organization of the tissues is crumbling. Autoimmune activity increases as cells and tissues literally lose their sense of self and attack their own substance as though it were foreign. Bits of tissue are robbed not only of their identity, but of their identification with the organ of which they are a part. Bit by bit, the tight hierarchical structure and organization of the body are collapsing, with death the inevitable result.

But there is one process that, through billions of years, has worked against the general tendency toward disorder in the universe. And that is evolution. If aging can be viewed as a kind of entropy, then evolution has resulted in the increasing ability of organisms to hold the line against disorganization for the longest period possible. As Ron Hart noted about DNA repair, it is one of the mechanisms "by which living systems hold themselves above the general decline, the increase in entropy, that we see in the universe as a whole."

It is here that we can find a message of hope, here where we can begin to look forward to a healthy, vigorous, extended life rather than a steadily declining old age.

Chapter Twelve

Life Extension—The Long and the Short of It

EAT—DIE, EAT—DIE, EAT—DIE. Like warning signs along a high-way, the three-letter words set inside circles within diamonds blazed across the cover of *Science* on September 23, 1984. The editors of the journal were drawing attention to the lead article, which linked cancer and the diseases of aging with common food substances. Like the signs, the article's message brought the scientific reader up short.

The clear and present danger to human beings, it said, lay not in toxic wastes, or air pollution, or insecticides, or occupational carcinogens, but, rather, in the food we eat. Nature, not man, was the true enemy. Not only were we bombarded by nasty bits of naturally occurring chemicals in such homey vegetables as mushrooms, parsley, and parsnips, but our own bodies were traitors. The very act of breaking down food substances, particularly fat, could generate free radicals, mutagens, and carcinogens. In other words, eating was dangerous to your health.

It was not the first time that someone was making this point. But it created a sensation within the scientific community because the article was a comprehensive roundup of worldwide studies on dietary carcinogens, because it made such a strong case for the role of free radicals and DNA damage in aging and cancer, and mostly because of who wrote it.

The author was Bruce Ames, whose test bearing his name is used in thousands of laboratories around the world for detecting carcinogenic substances. It was the Ames test that first alerted people to the fact that minute amounts of man-made chemicals could cause mutations and that most substances that were carcinogenic were also mutagenic. But now to the chagrin of many people who looked to Ames as a leader in the fight against corporate polluters, he was swinging in another direction. In a subsequent letters column in *Science*, entirely devoted to the Ames article, some hailed him for his view that "cancer is essentially a natural aging process" while others blasted him for failing to give due consideration to the adverse health effect of environmental toxins in cancer. In his reply, Ames wrote: "The most authoritative and thorough study of causes of cancer in America suggests that diet and life-style are major contributors to cancer and that the contribution of occupation and pollution are only a very small percentage of the cause of the major human cancers."

A short, bone-thin man whose bushy gray eyebrows seem the only part of him that has any weight, Ames has a lively, low-key charm that immediately puts others at their ease. He attracts controversy and crowds like a lightning rod. When he addressed the 1984 conference of the American Aging Association in New York, he was treated like a visiting dignitary. He had come to talk about a new assay his team at Berkeley had developed that promised to do for aging what the Ames test had done for cancer. For the gerontology community, which has a dearth of the kind of big-name researchers who have glamorized cancer research, the entrance of Bruce Ames into their ranks was welcome indeed. In the afternoon, as the meeting was breaking up, he held small audiences with a number of scientists. One scientist who had been feeling insufficiently appreciated for his latest contributions was particularly gratified by Ames's attention. "He immediately tuned into what I was saying and saw the wider implications," he said. A young graduate student waiting to bring him regards from her advisor sounded like a star-struck groupie when she said, "I grew up in the 60s and 70s, and Ames's name was like magic to me."

Now age fifty-six—"or something like that, I've stopped counting"—Ames has a new focus on aging, due partly to self-interest and partly to the logical culmination of his scientific career. He grew up in the Washington Heights section of Manhattan, and science has been part of life for as long as he can remember. His father was a high-school chemistry teacher and later supervisor of science for the New York City school system. Ames majored in chemistry and biochemistry at Cornell and got his doctorate at Cal Tech in biochemistry and genetics.

By the early 1960s, he was already concerned with the possible dangers of man-made chemicals leaking into the food supply. At the time, he was working with bacteria, creating mutants by various means. It occurred to him that if he brought these two interests together by using bacteria to detect the presence of mutagens in industrial compounds it might provide a rapid assay for potentially hazardous chemicals. After all, he reasoned, the DNA of a bacterium and a human cell were basically the same and whatever caused errors in the former should do the same in the latter. He began to play around with the notion "sort of as a hobby," and it was not until he realized its wider implications that it became a major part of his research.

The test combines extracts of human or rat liver with a strain of mutant "tester" bacteria. If the compound being tested is mutagenic, either directly or after being metabolized by the enzymes in the liver extract, it will cause a tiny fraction of the tester bacteria to undergo a back mutation, that is, to acquire the capacity for making an enzyme that the strain had lost. Since this enzyme is necessary for life, culturing the bacteria in media lacking the enzyme allows only the reverted bacteria to survive. The mutagenicity of a chemical is clearly visible in a few days in the tiny bacterial colonies that cover the bottom of the laboratory dish like sprinkles on a scoop of ice cream.

For research scientists, industrial chemists, and government regulators, the Ames test was a revelation. Instead of feeding liberal quantities of carcinogens to large colonies of rats and waiting two years for a result, it could be carried out on laboratory dishes by a single technician using minute amounts of chemicals and provide an answer in two days. Although it did not supplant animal testing, it made possible short-term screening of a very large number of chemicals with mutagenic and carcinogenic potential.

But for Ames, the true revelation was what the results showed. Over the next few years, as chemicals that had been shown to be carcinogenic in animal tests were tested with his system, it became clear that the vast majority of compounds that were carcinogenic were also mutagenic, while chemicals that did not cause cancer were almost always nonmutagenic. Here, he believed, was the most compelling evidence for the somatic mutation theory of cancer. Damage to DNA appeared to be a crucial step in the development of a tumor.

What other factors besides chemical carcinogens, he wondered, could be damaging DNA and acting as carcinogens? The quest for answers took him on several paths, which have now all led to the same place. First there was the small but growing concern by a few scientists that certain food substances were inherently carcinogenic. Most of these substances were chemical defenses that plants have evolved to ward off bacteria, insects, and other pests. According to Ames, the "human dietary intake of 'nature's pesticides' is likely to be several grams per day—probably at least 10,000 times higher than the dietary intake of man-made pesticides." Ironically, at the same time that the Ames test was alerting the public to the danger of synthetic chemicals found in a few parts per billion, Ames was becoming convinced that nature posed the greater threat to human health. "The mutagenicity people were finding all sorts of mutagens in your cup of coffee, your celery and mushrooms, your peanut butter sandwich, in your cooking and browning of food," he says. "Every meal is absolutely chock full of mutagens and carcinogens that will give cancer to rats and mice at high levels."

Second, there was the damage created by free radicals. So impressed was Denham Harman, of the University of Nebraska, by the runaway, irreversible, unpredictable reactions generated by these bits of molecules, that, over thirty years ago, he proposed the "free-radical theory of aging." The first free radicals to concern biologists were those produced by radiation. Indeed, a particularly nasty specimen called a hydroxyl radical is the main DNA-damaging component of radiation. But in the 1970s scientists worked out the free-radical-producing pathway of a substance much closer to home—the oxygen in every breath we take.

Electrons prefer to be coupled. The two electrons in each atom of oxygen are unpaired and thus are always seeking mates. Since oxygen is in a position to take on electrons, it is known as an electron acceptor and in fact it is the transfer of electrons to oxygen that generates energy in the cells of our body. When four electrons are added to oxygen, it makes water. The problem is that even though nature is fairly efficient at adding the four electrons all at once, it occasionally takes the easy way out, adding the electrons one at a time. Therein lies the rub. One electron added to an atom of oxygen makes superoxide. Two electrons produce hydrogen peroxide. Three electrons form the hydroxyl radical. All three of these "oxygen species" are mutagens and carcinogens, and behave in the same unregulated way as free radicals. The last one, the hydroxyl radical, is identical to the one that occurs with radiation. In other words, says Ames, "the same thing that does all the damage to DNA from radiation is coming out of your normal metabolism. So living is just like getting irradiated all the time." In addition, there is singlet oxygen. This energetic form of oxygen occurs when the energy of light is absorbed by a dye, such as the pigment of our skin or eyes, and is then passed on to the oxygen.

Food acts as a catalyst to the destructive process of oxygen metabolism. When fat goes rancid, it produces oxygen radicals and other mutagenic substances. Oxygen radicals can start the process of fat rancidity, which in turn creates more free radicals. In this way, fats and lipids act as tinder to the oxygen fire. Not only are radiation, diet, and oxygen metabolism generating varieties of radical species, but research into cancer promoters—the substances that cause mutated cells to start propagating—shows that they, too, may be working through oxygen radicals.

Third, there is the intriguing link between cancer, aging, and evolution. The incidence of cancer rises dramatically with age in both mice and man. At the end of its two-year life span, about 30 percent of the mouse population has tumors. By the end of our life span, we get cancer at the same rate as the mouse. The difference is that we have managed to stretch out the time at which this happens to an average of seventy-five years.

Why is it, Ames asks, that in the sixty million years it took us to evolve from our early primatelike ancestors, the life span increased enormously while the rate of age-adjusted cancer dropped sharply? One reason could be the long-recognized connection between a low metabolic rate and a long life span. The higher the metabolic rate, the faster the organism is churning out free radicals, damaging its DNA, and setting the stage for cancer.

Finally, what tied all these lines of research together was the emerging evidence on the main weapons against oxygen. These are the antioxidants—the naturally occurring vitamins, nutrients, enzymes, and other substances that neutralize the enemy. Vitamin E, for example, is the main free-radical trap in the membranes. Superoxide dismutase mops up the extra electron in the superoxide radical. Selenium, found in many foods, is a component of an enzyme that destroys hydrogen peroxide and fat peroxides. Beta carotene, which gives carrots their characteristic color, is a primary defense against singlet oxygen and is also a radical trap in membranes.

All the antioxidants, says Ames, are turning out to be antimutagens and anticarcinogens. For instance, four different studies by scientists in various parts of the world have found that cigarette smokers who eat green and yellow vegetables, which contain large amounts of the antioxidant beta carotene and related compounds called carotenoids, are far less likely to get lung cancer than their nonvegetable-eating counterparts. And as Denham Harman and others have shown in study after study, antioxidants have antiaging activity, decreasing the incidence of age-associated diseases and significantly extending the average life expectancy of animals.

Like Cutler and others, Ames now believes that "a major factor in lengthening life span and decreasing age-specific cancer rates may have been the evolution of effective protective mechanisms against oxygen radicals." In a surprising paper, which marked his first foray into the field of aging, he revealed that one of the most humble of biological products, uric acid, may actually be one of the most effective natural antioxidants.

His discovery was a spinoff of another, much grander, project. About five years ago, when "all the signs were pointing to oxygen radicals" as a cause of cancer and age-related diseases, he began to think about ways in which he could measure the extent of this damage in human beings. He knew that humans carry a total of 500 grams (about a pound) of DNA in the body, and that every day, some part of that DNA is being damaged. He also knew that enzymes along the DNA strand clip out the damage and repair it. Where did the damaged bases go? Scientists seek the simplest explanation for phenomena, and it seemed to him that the most reasonable assumption was that the damaged bases were excreted along with everything else. He therefore proposed an experiment to examine human urine as a means of determining DNA damage from oxygen radicals.

To find out just what oxidation would do to the genetic material, they took the bases that compose the DNA and began battering them with hydroxyl radicals and other oxidizing agents. In the course of this work, Ames came across a table in a twenty-year-old paper that showed that uric acid, a product of urine, was easily oxidized by the agents they were working with. In chemical terms, uric acid was a powerful "reducing agent," giving up electrons where oxygen accepted them—in other words, an antioxidant.

"When I saw that table it rang a bell in my head," says Ames, "because I knew that at the beginning of primate evolution, we lost the enzyme that destroys uric acid, so we have a very high level of uric acid in our blood, while mice and rats don't. And this occurred just as we began to extend our life span.

"It had been in the literature for years that uric acid was a strong antioxidant but nobody put everything together. You see, it's a waste product of metabolism; we just pee it out in our urine. Nobody ever thought there was a reason for it. But the minute I read about this, I thought maybe the high level of uric acid in our blood does have a function. Maybe there's a reason why our kidneys take 95 percent of the uric acid and pump it back into the blood, so that the level of uric acid in human blood is practically at the saturation point."

Looking further, he found that just at the point in evolution when primates gained the ability to accumulate uric acid, they lost the ability to synthesize vitamin C, another antioxidant. Ames believes that one reason for the switch may be that vitamin C is a two-edged sword. In high amounts it can actually act as a pro-oxidant, generating oxygen radicals rather than getting rid of them, whereas uric acid has all the desirable qualities of an antioxidant without the added complications of vitamin C.

In his paper, Ames referred to the provocative studies linking high levels of uric acid to intelligence and achievement. Gout, which is caused by excess uric acid, has long been considered an "elitist disease," whose sufferers are generally rich, brainy, and successful. These last considerations led Dick Cutler, who collaborated briefly with Ames, to theorize that uric acid may have played a dual role in primate evolution—enhancing both antioxidant protection and intellectual potential.

If antioxidants are the body's main defense against the ravages of free-radical reactions, and if they have played a starring role in the increase in life span and the decrease in cancer that occurred during primate evolution, then perhaps increasing the level in our tissues, either through diet or supplementation, may be the way to go for even greater gains in human health. This is far from a new idea. Self-help books and magazine articles recommend one or another antioxidant regimen, and millions of people flood the health-food stores in search of SOD pills (which are unlikely to be useful since the enzyme is destroyed during digestion), selenium tablets, and high-potency vitamin E. The problem is that unlike the RDAs (recommended daily allowances) that were worked out long ago for vitamins on the basis of what was needed to prevent *deficiency*, nobody knows how much antioxidant is needed to optimize human health, to take up where nature left off.

In this area, Ames and his colleagues may have achieved a dramatic breakthrough. For the first time, it may be possible to take the guesswork out of supplementation and place it securely on a scientific foundation. It took three years, far longer than Ames anticipated when he began, but his fishing expedition for the damaged products of oxidation in the urine was successful.

On the way to creating the assay, he and his colleagues at Berkeley discovered two new repair enzymes for oxidative damage that are called glycosylases. Most repair enzymes are like garbage collectors, roaming the DNA looking for rubbish in the form of "bulky adducts," which are stuck onto a nucleic acid base like a piece of gum on a shoe. These enzymes break the DNA chain and remove the bulky group, whether it is aflatoxin from peanut butter or benzopyrene, a primary carcinogen in all burnt material, such as cigarette smoke, or some other unwanted substance. Glycosylases, on the other hand, are very picky, each one searching for a specific base; and when it finds one, it plucks it out without breaking the DNA chain. Working with a colleague at Berkeley, Stuart Linn, known for his studies in DNA repair and aging, and who had discovered one of the glycosylases in bacteria, Ames found two glycosylases in animal cells. Eight glycosylases in all have now been identified and each one acts on a specific damage product.

"Nature has designed these enzymes to look for only one damage product," says Ames. "And the products [that] the glycosylases we found are looking for are all oxidized bases, which suggests that some of the important damage the cell is trying to avoid is that caused by oxidation. So this again reinforces my idea that oxygen radicals may be important in destructive processes like aging and cancer."

But the big news is that he and his associates, Richard Cathcart, Elizabeth Schweirs, and Robert Saul, have now succeeded in creating an assay that makes it possible to see how much pounding our cells take from oxidative DNA damage every day. Requiring nothing more from an individual than a urine sample, the test employs state-of-the-art technology—high-pressure liquid chromatography consisting of sophisticated pumps that propel liquids, at very high pressure, through extremely dense solutions to detect microscopically small particles.

The importance of this work cannot be underestimated. As Bill Regelson and others have pointed out, for intervention in aging to be successful, there must be biomarkers—physical signposts that allow the researcher to know, in the case of each individual, just how well a particular regimen is working. And if oxidative damage to the DNA is a major culprit in disease and senescence, then Ames's new assay could rival his earlier one as a standard laboratory tool. At the very least, it may finally provide a verdict in the case made by Denham Harman three decades ago for free radicals in aging.

Although the first version of the technique is cumbersome and time-consuming, with a highly trained postdoc taking two weeks to do fifteen samples, Ames is already using it to get very interesting answers. Just looking at two oxidized products of DNA damage, the thymine glycol and hydroxymethyluracil, he found an average of one thousand of these oxidized thymines per human cell per day. The damage rate may actually be many times higher than that since these two products are only a small fraction of the known DNA-damage products caused by oxidative mutagens. "We are measuring the damage that comes through in a day," he says. "But you are getting the equivalent of a body dose of irradiation every day of your life, and not all the damage is being repaired, so you are accumulating damage over your lifetime."

As high as the rate of damage is to human cells, it is slight compared to that of a rodent. When his lab tested rat urine, Ames found the strongest support yet for his belief that oxidative damage was tied to longevity. The rat had fifteen times more thymine glycol damage per gram of tissue than did humans.

"The interesting thing about this is that a rat breathes in oxygen much more rapidly than a human," he points out. "It also has a very high metabolic rate and a very short life span. Our controls support the idea that we are in fact measuring oxidative DNA damage coming out of metabolism, and because the metabolic rate in the rat is so rapid, compared to [the] human, it is churning out much more damage from its metabolism than we are out of ours. And that might be one reason why a rat lives only two years and we live seventy to eighty years."

The first clinical use to which he put the assay was suggested inadvertently by the test itself. Ames used himself and members of his labs when he needed urine samples for the assay. While his own levels of thymine glycol were on the low side and hardly varied from day to day, one of his students had far higher levels, which fluctuated wildly from one day to the next. Since the student, an athlete, was a prodigious eater and expender of energy, Ames wondered whether the variation he was seeing was due to his food intake. In his project, therefore, he will try to answer the question, Does cutting down on calories reduce the level of oxidative DNA damage?

As a researcher in cancer and aging, he has long been impressed with the experiments, going back fifty years, showing that diet-restricted animals get far fewer tumors and live about twice as long as animals that get all the food they want. But while nobody disputes the data, there is an ongoing controversy about their applicability to human beings. One of the more amusing aspects of this continuing debate is that the group in favor of undernutrition for humans tends to be lean while the anti group tends to be, well, substantial. In one corner you have the very trim Roy Walford, who has been fasting two days a week for the past several years. Walford first became interested in restricting his own intake when he successfully achieved a dramatic extension of life in rats who began the regime in young adulthood or even middle age. In the other corner you have Reubin Andres, deputy director of the Gerontology Research Center, who sports a healthy paunch and says that "diet restriction is great, if you're a rat." Andres, who has reviewed all the studies done on the correlation between body weight and longevity, found that older people do better if they are overweight, even by as much as 20 percent. Indeed, the Metropolitan Life Insurance Company has now revised its ideal height/weight chart upward to reflect the fact that fatter people live longer, while the GRC's own weight tables recommend starting out skinny and then putting on about a pound a year after age thirty. Walford argues that the heavier weights at the time of death are partly the result of a statistical artifact, since thinner people who die younger may be gaunt as a result of illness, rather than life-style or genetic makeup. In addition, people who gain weight easily may be starting off with an evolutionary advantage, since their ability to convert food into fat had survival value during times of famine. Based on studies with obese mice, fat people will do even better than naturally lean individuals if they restrict their intake, says Walford, who has now written two popular books on the subject. Cutler, who is neither fat nor thin, thinks that everyone may be looking at the data backwards. Animals that forage for their food in the wild are naturally calorie-restricted, he points out. But when we bring the animals into the laboratory, we turn everything upside down. We look at the underfed mice and rats and say they are living longer, when what we are actually doing is overfeeding the controls and causing them to die earlier.

Ames seems to side with Cutler. "If you restrict the diet of mice even a small amount, the difference in tumors is just phenomenal," he says. "It could be that food itself is going to be the most important carcinogen. That is, if you just take in maintenance calories, you're all right. But the minute you gorge yourself, you have to burn up all the extra calories, perhaps in a more deleterious way, and you get increased DNA damage."

To test this idea, he will look at whether diet restriction in rats causes the level of thymine glycol in their urine to go down. He will also look at the other side of the question, applying the assay to gluttonous human subjects as well as force-feeding himself, and see if his normally low levels rise.

"We would like to use this test to look at individual variations in thymine glycol levels," says Ames, "to look at what is important in the diet, to look at anticarcinogens like selenium and vitamin E, and to get a handle on diseases like progeria and Down's, where people have very high cancer rates and accelerated aging."

For Cutler, Ames's new assay points the way to the future. He is now working along the same lines, trying to develop noninvasive, *in vivo* tests that can be used to assess the effectiveness of various antiaging approaches. "The current strategies of nutrition and exercise leave much to be desired," he says. "There is no information that I know of that one could act on, not one thing."

His recent studies have found that megadoses of vitamins, nutrients, and antioxidants might be counterproductive. Exercise, if started around middle age or later, might actually shorten life, according to data on lab animals found by Israeli researcher David Gershon and others. "Marathon runners and other people who exercise vigorously throughout their lives have better muscle tone and reflexes, but they don't live any longer," he says. Finally, before adapting fasting or near-starvation as a way of life, he believes we should consider the conflicting data showing that rats and mice do well on underfeeding while the longest-lived humans are on the borderline of obesity.

"The bottom line to all this," he says, "is that there is a lot we don't know yet. And by rushing into something, you might screw yourself up. I still think the best rule of thumb—and it's sad to say—is, just doing everything in moderation." (The Golden Mean, as an antiaging regime, has much to recommend it until the kinds of intervention discussed in this chapter come along. In a continuing study of longevity and life-style among some seven thousand people in California's Alameda County, Lester Breslow and Nedra Bellow found that observing seven ridiculously simple rules of good health increased life span eleven years on the average for men and seven years for women. They are: no smoking; moderate weight, not exceeding 20 percent over that recommended for one's age and height; moderate drinking—two to three belts a day were better than abstinence or abuse; moderate physical activity, about three times a week; eating breakfast; regular meals; and sleeping seven or eight hours a night.)

Still, Cutler, who went into aging research seeking solutions, is not about to settle for something resembling a wise grandmother's advice. After putting his "project enhancement" on the back burner three years ago when he realized that tricking the cells was going to be far more complicated than he had bargained for, he has been spending his time on a far more simple task—one designed to require only a yes-or-no answer for every question asked. In doing so, he has gone back to his original query: How do long-lived animals differ from short-lived ones? In other words, how did nature do it? What were the longevity determinants selected over the course of evolution that determined the rate of aging and the length of life span?

For the time being, he has limited his research to antioxidants, because they are easy to look for. He need only select a substance, measure its levels in the tissues of various animals, and see whether it correlates with life span of mammalian species from rodents to humans. So far, he has found four antioxidants that fill the bill and that, he believes, could be the foundation for the first antiaging program to incorporate nature's own design—the protective-repair processes by which the increase in life span evolved.

The first antioxidant/life-span correlation he found was back in 1978, when he did the work on SOD, the enzyme that destroys the first oxygen radical formed during the breakdown of oxygen. The next antioxidant, vitamin E, was scarcely surprising, since vitamin E is indeed a powerful antioxidant. But the other two antioxidants had a long history of being thought of as metabolic defects in humans rather than assets. One of these was beta carotene, the substance that gives carrots, oranges, and melon their color. It is found throughout the brain and body of human beings in such large quantities that our blood serum and fat are yellow-tinged. But its ubiquitous presence seemed inexplicable. The only function it appeared to have was as a precursor to vitamin A, yet humans, compared with other species, had low levels of the enzyme necessary for conversion. Accordingly, most nutritionists held that vitamin A, rather than beta carotene, was the important nutrient.

But when Cutler measured the levels of both vitamin A and beta carotene in various species, he was led to the opposite conclusion: Vitamin A was completely unrelated to longevity, while the levels of beta carotene had an extraordinary one-to-one ratio, all the way from mouse to man, "with no exceptions," he says. Scanning the scientific literature, he found a clue to what may be going on. Beta carotene is important as a precursor to vitamin A, but it is also an excellent antioxidant in its own right and, unlike vitamin A, it is not toxic at high doses. And in a nice tie-in with his dysdifferentiation hypothesis, the carotenoids are closely related to retinoids—compounds that help stabilize the differentiated state of cells and are now being tested clinically for their anticancer properties. So compelling is the circumstantial evidence that Harvard Medical School is now conducting a five-year study on 22,000 physicians to see if beta carotene supplements cut down on the incidence of cancer.

The other surprise was uric acid. Until Ames rediscovered the antioxidant activity of uric acid, the major constituent of urine, most scientists considered it solely an end point in metabolism, an unwanted waste product. As Ames pointed out, the accumulation of high levels of uric acid in the body may have come about in evolution just at the time when the ability to synthesize vitamin C was lost. In Cutler's test, it was uric acid that correlated with life span, with humans having strikingly high levels in the body and brain, while the levels of vitamin C were no higher in a man than a mouse.

While all this research may seem to indicate that just adding beta carotene or vitamin E to the diet is the answer to longer life, it just doesn't seem to be that simple. It is true that Denham Harman as well as many other researchers were able to increase the average life expectancy by adding synthetic antioxidants to the diet of certain animals, but they did not extend the life span beyond the limit for that species. If these compounds are important in determining longevity, one would expect to see a jump in maximum survival as well.

Still, why shouldn't more be better? After all, this is the idea behind megadoses of vitamins and nutrients: not just nutrition, but supernutrition. If free-radical chain reactions are chewing up the cells and mutating the DNA, why not mop up, scavenge, and neutralize the enemy with all the antioxidant weapons at hand? (It should also be pointed out that one would not like to eliminate all free-radical reactions since they play a helpful role in the immune response, destroying viruses and bacteria.) But in another of his recent experiments, Cutler has shown that more may not necessarily be better; in fact, it may even be less.

When he fed animals high doses of vitamin E, their levels of SOD, glutathione peroxidase, and other antioxidants plummeted. Conversely, animals on a vitamin E-deficient diet had dramatic rises in these enzymes. "It is a compensatory process," he says, the antioxidant enzymes rushing in to fill a perceived gap. "So it looks like what people should have been doing all these years is checking to see whether or not there is any increase in *net* antioxidant protection."

Doing just that, he found that the ability of tissue from various species to withstand destruction by oxygen-free radicals was directly related to life span—high in man and low in mouse, even though both species consumed the same nutrients. From his point of view, it makes sense that anything as important as antioxidant protection would not be left solely to the vagaries of diet and life-style but would be under tight homeostatic control. It is the net antioxidant level that is important, he argues, and that is set in our genes the same way that the temperature is set in a thermostat.

This finding now argues for a radically different approach, he believes. Instead of blitzing the body with vitamins and nutrients, which might jack up the level of some antioxidants while depressing the levels of others, what is needed is a longevity prescription tailored for each individual.

Cutler calls his plan "project peak-out." He has partially accomplished step one, identifying antioxidants associated with the evolution of life span. Step two is now under way—developing a series of *in vivo* tests, a kind of DNA-damage-detection kit, that would allow dosages of antioxidants to be adjusted accordingly. He, too, is working on a test for detecting DNA oxidative damage in the urine, but says that "technically, Ames is about a year ahead of us." He is also developing simple tests to measure the lipid peroxides in the blood serum and products of this peroxidation, called pentenes, which are found in the breath. "Our strategy," he says, "is to get a battery of tests for the urine, blood, and breath that would provide an overall picture of the oxidative stress your whole body is exposed to."

Step three is to bring the lab to the clinic, to set up a protocol for each person, based on life-style, diet, and biochemistry. By measuring the amount of antioxidants in an individual's blood and tissues, he could see which antioxidants need bringing up. "We could go right down the line," he says, "monitoring what happens by doing urine analysis of the DNA excision products. We wouldn't have to wait months and years to measure all those various biomarkers. We could get the answers right away. The idea would be to bring your mutation load down to normal."

To begin with, he would correct for any antioxidant deficiencies that might exist. There is an indication that some individuals may be lacking in natural antioxidant protection. For instance, he measured the levels of lipid peroxides produced by free radicals interacting with the normal fat in his own body and in others in the laboratory. He then compared these levels with those of patients at the Baltimore City Hospital. While he found a great deal of variation in peroxide levels among all the people tested, the people who were sick had significantly higher levels of lipid peroxides in their blood.

Once he had brought a person's level of antioxidants up to normal, as determined by his tests, Cutler would "push the system. We would try to make people supernormal by reducing their mutational load as much as possible, to see how far we could go with compensation before we began to depress the net antioxidant levels," he says. "Maybe some people can go farther than others. We will attempt to 'peak you out,' to get the best mileage out of your genetic endowment. To me, this is the first practical, scientific approach to doing something about aging that I know of."

Exciting as this concept is, it is only a "stopgap measure," says Cutler, "until we can directly intervene in the processes that control the longevity determinants." In the thermostat analogy, this would mean, instead of maintaining the heat flow more efficiently, actually changing the set point, raising the entire spectrum of repair/protective processes to superhuman levels—in other words, his original idea of tricking the cells.

Toward this end, he has now published the first model proposing how the cell might detect levels of free radicals and turn antioxidants on and off in response. But learning how to manipulate this system will require money and manpower. Although his position at the GRC is improving, he is thinking of setting up a human-longevity research laboratory in the Baltimore area to explore the possibility of commercializing his dietary-supplementation program and using the profits to develop "the more fundamental, far-reaching approaches."

With regard to all the problems he has had in getting support for his ideas, he says with a shake of his head, "I don't know why my research program hasn't been supported more. It just puzzles the hell out of me. Professional jealousy plays a part but it can't explain everything. Anyway, I'm optimistic that I will succeed if I live long enough and don't get too discouraged."

Now in his late forties, he yearns for graduate students for the same reason some men long for sons—that he might pass on his accumulated knowledge. Ironically, at professional meetings he is surrounded by young people avid to discuss his ideas. "[At] every meeting I go to," he says, "there are people with talent who want to get into aging research and ask for my help. One man who still comes around first approached me seventeen years ago. But I have no fellowships to offer them. It's very sad. You go every day into an empty lab and, at the same time, people are always writing you, hoping to come in. Who's going to carry on my work? Who's going to trick the cells?"

For Arthur Schwartz, like Cutler, it has also been a long haul. Since 1979, the year in which he presented his work on DHEA—the wonder steroid that is anticancer, antiobesity, and antiaging—he has talked about getting out a patentable drug. Now he has discovered that DHEA causes several problems in laboratory animals, the most serious being pituitary tumors.

Far from being dismayed, however, Schwartz is delighted. "It's the best thing that happened to us in years," he exults. Why is he so happy? Because he has filed for a patent on a chemical analogue, which, he says, gets around the problems of the original drug. It does not convert to a sex hormone and it is the estrogenic effect that, he believes, produces the pituitary tumors. So far he has seen no adverse effect with his new synthetic steroid. Not only does it retain the cancer-preventing, disease-fighting, and youth-preserving potential of DHEA, he claims, but it is three times as effective.

In the years since he first started working with DHEA, he and other scientists have found a panoply of benefits that make the compound sound, in the words of California gerontologist J. Edwin Seegmiller, like "a combination of Ponce de León's fountain and snake oil." Among other things, it massively inhibited the induction of colon cancer; it had a therapeutic effect on diabetes, lowering blood sugar within a week; it reduced obese rats to normal size; and it reduced stress, actually interfering with the production of stress-release hormones. Although extensive life extension has yet to be demonstrated, treated animals definitely look younger.

But bringing a drug from the laboratory to the marketplace is a long and complicated process, costing as much as $94 million in 1985. First Schwartz must do three to six months of animal-toxicity tests for determining the lethal dose and any possible adverse side effects. If it passes these tests, he can apply for an IND (investigative new drug) status, which will allow him to go to phase one, short-term clinical trials on volunteers to determine safety. Here Schwartz would like to try the drug in several areas—as a treatment for diabetes and obesity, and as an antitumor drug in colon and breast cancer. Since the compound would be used to *prevent* cancer, he would start by testing it in people who, because of their family history, are at very high risk. The incidence rate for individuals whose family members have the disease can run as high as 50 percent in breast cancer and 80 percent in colon cancer.

Before he can proceed to extended clinical trials—the final hurdle required for FDA approval—he must do additional long-term toxicity studies on animals. Since the drugs might eventually be taken by an individual over his lifetime for a disease he may never get, "there is an even greater burden to prove safety," says Schwartz. Still, if the analogue, or DHEA, which other people are continuing to investigate as a clinical drug, can do for humans what it does for the mouse and rat, it will not only offer hope for three of the most problematic and refractory conditions, cancer, diabetes, and obesity, but will be a portent of things to come: the treatment of medical ills through the body's own chemicals, when nature has started to turn off the tap.

Schwartz is not the only one to try and cash in on a drug with DHEA's amazing potential. In a twist of fate, one of his competitors is someone who has supported his research for years. As scientific director of FIBER, Bill

Regelson made DHEA one of his pet projects—giving Schwartz grants when money was available and trying to put together aid packages for him when it was not. Now FIBER is dead, a victim of lack of funds.

"I had a delightful four years," says Regelson, irrepressible as ever. "I created conferences, went to a lot of meetings, met a lot of scientists. It was a tremendous experience. I put my faith in FIBER, was supported by FIBER, and then when FIBER ran out of money, I wasn't being paid. I let my [medical] practice go down, which is my main source of income, and spent most of my time in D.C. to make it work."

As a cancer doctor and researcher, Regelson was turned on from the moment he first heard Schwartz speak about DHEA. The latest studies, including his own, have convinced him that the compound's unique properties are unprecedented in the history of medicine. "I believe that the discovery of DHEA," he says, "will be as clinically significant as the discovery of the corticosteroids."

Regelson is now collaborating in a study at the Animal Medical Center in New York City, in which cats and dogs brought into the clinic with various kinds of cancer are treated with the DHEA analogue. In seven dogs and cats with mastosarcoma—a form of cancer that is rare in man but common in animals—six animals had regression of their tumor. "One dog literally came back from the dead," says Regelson. "There is no question about it: DHEA is working against a malignant tumor, a cancer that is spontaneous, not one that has been experimentally transplanted."

In 1984 he began his first clinical trial of DHEA on patients with advanced cancer of different types. So far, he has given it to two people and expects to add another twenty to thirty. Even though they are now receiving the highest dose ever given of DHEA, they are tolerating it very well, he says.

When first placed on DHEA, a patient receives no other treatment for two weeks. If the patient remains stable, he continues on this regimen. Should the condition decline, Regelson restores the previous form of treatment, whether it was chemotherapy or radiation, but continues the steroid. The reason for this, he explains, is that the compound may sometimes not work on its own but will "synergize with other forms of chemotherapy." Although it is too soon to evaluate the effect of DHEA, he says, "it seems to stimulate patients' well-being. Their energy level is remarkably improved. But that could be a placebo effect."

DHEA, uric acid, and beta carotene stand as vivid reminders of how much we have yet to learn. For a long time, all three were overlooked or dismissed as having any useful function. Now it appears that they may be part of the body's built-in protective system—beta carotene and uric acid as antioxidants defending the DNA and the cell against free-radical damage; and DHEA as an antidote to stress, via a mechanism that is just now beginning to be understood.

In experiments in Italy, Israel, and the United States, when rats were subjected to a variety of intense stresses, such as total physical restraint or rotation on a turntable, the effect was devastating. The thymus gland, a primary factory of immune white cells, shrank; large numbers of T-cells, which are in the front line of immune-system defense against disease, were destroyed; and the animals developed stress-related illnesses such as ulcers, suffered increased rates of cancer, and died. DHEA blocked the shrinking of the thymus gland, protected the T-cells, and the animals survived. The steroid was even effective against heat stress.

"DHEA is the first example of a buffer action for hormones that I know of," says Regelson. "It is a broad-acting hormone that only demonstrates itself under a specific set of circumstances. In that way it is like a buffer against sudden changes in acidity or alkalinity. That is why when you get older, you're much more vulnerable to the effects of stress. As DHEA declines with age, you are losing the buffer against the stress-related hormones. It is the buffer action that prevents us from aging."

The effect of stress may go even deeper, to the DNA itself, according to a study by Phil Lipetz and Ralph Stephens. In their experiment, they took thirty-five people who were under stress, as determined by a battery of psychological tests, but who were not taking any drugs, and compared them with a control group of thirty-five people who were not under stress. They found that the highly tense individuals had a decreased rate of recovery of their supercoiling after DNA damage, while this was not true of the controls. Since they had already shown an age-related decline in the supercoiling recovery response, this meant that the people under stress were responding to DNA damage as though they were many years older.

Like Jerry Williams, Lipetz sees a tie-in between his work on DNA and the immune and hormonal systems, which have acknowledged roles in the aging process. First, there is the immunological theory; that the ability of the body to ward off disease goes down with age, while the self-destructive autoimmune activity rises. In their studies, Lipetz and Stephens used leukocytes, white blood cells that are the front line of the immune defense system. If these cells, either through stress or age or disease, were losing their ability to repackage the DNA, including the supercoiling, it had profound implications for the immune-system function. Loss of control over DNA supercoiling would mean a loss of control over genetic recombination—the ability of pieces of DNA to recombine into new sequences. This genetic reshuffling is the basis of the immune system's remarkable ability to fashion an antibody that, like Cinderella's glass slipper, is designed to fit only the owner—in this case, the one out of more than a million different antigens. If the ability to repackage the DNA is being wiped out by age, the power to mount an adequate immune response is lost. In cancer this is a double whammy: The cell is increasingly unable to handle the DNA-damaging agents that cause cancer, and the capacity of the body to seek out and destroy transformed cells is progressively compromised. The role of the immune system in protecting against cancer can scarcely be underestimated. In the rare individual born without such a system, the risk of cancer is increased ten thousandfold.

Second, there is the theory that hormonal and endocrine factors regulate the rate at which cells age. Here Lipetz's evidence is as provocative as it was preliminary. One of the individuals who had first alerted them to the existence of a group of people with slow supercoiling recovery rates had developed symptoms of a possible autoimmune disease. When the person was put on the steroid hormone prednisone, Lipetz again tested the cells and found that the recovery rate had returned to normal. After the prednisone therapy ended several months later, they retested and found that the supercoiling response had once more dropped far below normal. It appears that at least in this one case, hormones might play a direct role in maintaining the supercoiled state.

Working with Smith-Sonneborn, he has also identified several other naturally occurring substances that appear to stabilize supercoiling. These include the plant hormone kinetin and a related compound called IPA, both of which increase life span in paramecia. The ultimate goal would be to gain control of the central operating mechanism, to play with the supercoiling of the DNA as though it were a yo-yo, winding and unwinding it at will, decreasing it with cancer, increasing it with age, maintaining it in the full flush of fitness and youth for as long a period as possible.

As it took Hart many years, during which he was establishing his career, to appreciate fully his own mentor, Dick Setlow, so Lipetz, after years of struggling to gain recognition for his work, has gone through a similar process with Hart. "When I look back on my student days, the arguments I had with Ron upset me because I was trying to establish my own independent line," he says, "but I realize that the scientific and management techniques I use are all things I learned from him. It wouldn't have been possible for me to be where I am right now unless Ron Hart had taken the time and the trouble to teach me his vision of science."

It may still be too early to know whether we will realize Don Yarborough's visionary proclamation that "we are either the last generation to die or the first one to live forever," but it is clear that we are living through the first period in history in which human beings will shape their own evolution. We have tripled our life span since the dawn of modern civilization three thousand years ago, mostly through better nutrition and sanitation and the elimination of childhood diseases. In the past few years, millions of Americans have stopped smoking, and started exercising and dieting their way to increased fitness, health, and longevity.

Today we are entering a new era in which the laboratory explorations detailed here are being translated into the first scientifically based antiaging approaches that are designed neither to prevent nor treat disease, but to raise our cellular functioning to a higher level and add decades to life span. This will happen in several stages. First we will continue the trend toward life-style modifications, but with far greater sophistication. Now we eschew cholesterol and saturated fats, but we are learning about other dietary substances that have adverse effects. Gerontologists, such as Denham Harman, have long pointed out the dangers of polyunsaturated fats that add fuel to the free-radical fire. We are also beginning to appreciate, as Ames warned in his *Science* article, that "natural" or "organic" does not necessarily mean better. Vegetables like alfalfa sprouts can be liberally laced with carcinogens and mutagens, while others, like cabbage, contain substances that inhibit mutation and cancer. As new knowledge becomes available, we will be able to separate friend from foe on our dinner plate with pinpoint accuracy. "The concern with 'proaging' substances should extend beyond food to drugs and chemicals that are in our environment," says Regelson. He points out that Lipetz and Smith-Sonneborn found that nalidixic acid and novobiocin, which interfere with DNA supercoiling, shorten life span and accelerate senescence in paramecia. "Regardless of the theory," says Regelson, "whether you are on pro-oxidants and free radicals or DNA supercoiling and repair, we now have the capacity to search for proaging substances and eliminate them from our environment."

The second stage will be a much greater degree of intervention either through diet or supplementation. This could mean either the diet-restriction regime advocated by Walford, or, if Ames's hunch is right that excess food is shortening life, then perhaps less heroic efforts are needed to achieve the same thing. The other possibility is supplementation with antioxidants along the lines suggested by Cutler. With the Ames assay for oxidative DNA damage, Lipetz's measurement of chromatin DNA repair, or the *in vivo* tests now being developed by Cutler and others, we will be able to assess and compare the effectiveness of various antiaging treatments.

The third stage involves the use of pharmaceuticals—hormones, or other bodily substances, as well as synthetic drugs that would raise repair, stabilize supercoiling, maintain the differentiated state of cells, and/or work on other levels to improve organ-system function. The compounds covered in this book, like DHEA and its derivatives, and the cytokinetins being tested by Lipetz and Smith-Sonneborn, represent a fraction of the interventions in the aging process now being tested. These range from extracts of the thymus gland for enhanced immune-system function, to ubiquinone, a component of all body cells, for better cardiac function, to safer estrogen replacements for postmenopausal women, and memory stimulators for Alzheimer victims.

The fourth stage involves the whole promise of genetic engineering. The first use in gerontology will probably be diagnostic—determining which genes are actually involved in the aging process. Within the decade, scientists expect to see the first treatments for inborn genetic defects. Once the techniques have been worked out, the possibility will exist for not just correcting nature's mistakes, but improving on the blueprint, adding genes for DNA repair, for example, or free-radical scavenging, or a better mix of enzymes for metabolizing carcinogenic compounds.

Finally, we may not only be able to stop the clock, we might even set it back. As Smith-Sonneborn's earlier research, in which she used UV light to induce a higher rate of repair in paramecia, showed, it might be possible to erase some of the accumulated deficits of age.

For the present, Regelson believes that we have enough information now to work out approaches that will add thirty years of useful life to our time on Earth. "This means we will move survival closer to the upper limit of about 119 years. I don't think we will go the Walford route and change our habits that dramatically. I think we will find physiological mechanisms for doing this with pharmacology."

Ames agrees: "I think we are going to understand cancer and aging very quickly, perhaps within the next decade. So much fundamental biology is being sorted out. And lots of good people are starting to work on aging, lots of good people are working on cancer, and new information is coming in at a fantastic rate. So I think that people are going to figure out the cause of colon cancer, of stomach cancer, of breast cancer. Biology is going like a rocket and technology is going like a rocket. It is clear that with new knowledge we are going to be able to intervene in lots of ways."

Five years after the 1979 Gordon Research Conference on Aging, which, for the first time, brought together all the work correlating aging and DNA repair and protective systems, another extraordinary gathering of gerontologists from around the world was held. This time it was a symposium on "The Molecular Basis of Aging," held at the Brookhaven National Laboratory in October 1984. Opening and closing the meeting was Dick Setlow, the man who started it all with his discovery of DNA repair. As befits a conference on the genetic nuts and bolts of aging, talks on DNA supercoiling, repair, and gene expression and differentiation dominated, but there were also nonmolecular topics: diet restriction, DHEA, and the role of enzymes. Where the last Gordon Conference had ended with the participants split into factions, this one concluded with a new sense of integration among the various studies of the inner workings of the cell and of the body's visible expression of these workings, between the DNA and the hormones and the immune system.

The mood was one of reconciliation, not just of the science, but of the scientists. It was a public acknowledgment of the contributions of two gerontologists—Sacher, who was dead, and Cutler, who was present at the conference—and it helped lift a shadow that had hung over the latter's life for so long.

Leonard Hayflick, one of three rapporteurs assigned to summarize the proceedings and suggest future research directions, first paid homage to the "terribly neglected theory, championed by the late George Sacher," of longevity-assurance genes. "That's the opposite side of the coin [from most aging theories]," he pointed out. "Instead of looking for changes that cause age processes to occur, Sacher argues that we should be looking for changes that have permitted greater longevity."

Ron Hart, as the last rapporteur, then took the opportunity to set the record straight. "Not only Sacher, Dick Cutler and several other people have approached aging from the longevity-assurance standpoint," he noted, adding that he was heartened by the fact that "Dick has continued on his comparative-evolutionary approach to aging and I think this must be encouraged and supported."

In his closing remarks, Hart said, "The field of gerontology has suffered from ticky-tacky boxes," where the various theories of aging—cellular, molecular, immune, neuroendocrine—were separated from one another. "As we look back, we see it was extremely naive. However, at this meeting, we seem to have a far greater integration of ideas and concepts and find greater commonality of approaches and underlying ideas than we were ever able to do or achieve through all the integrative theories and concepts that have been postulated in the past."

For the future, he suggested that his colleagues start looking at how the various pieces of research interact, examine diet restriction with the tools of molecular biology, study how hormones affect gene expression. "Now that the quality of science has improved so it is equal to or better than most other fields, now that we have ourselves out of the boxes, there is hope we will be able to do some of the interdisciplinary studies which have so long been needed, and for which the methodology has been available for such a short time."

It is a time for optimism. The theoretical groundwork has been laid, the techniques are available, fruitful collaborations between scientists are under way. Now it is up to us, who live in the nuclear age, to support the research that will give new meaning to a word we so often hear today—survival, not in terms of sustaining life after or in spite of a disaster, but in terms of a healthier, vastly extended life for the human species.

Bibliography

Although this book is based primarily on personal interviews, journal articles and books were used to supplement the information. The following references are offered as a guide to anyone who wishes to follow up on a particular subject in greater detail.

Introduction
Hayflick, L. "On the Facts of Life." *Executive Health*, June 1978.

Judson, H. F. *The Eighth Day of Creation*. New York: Simon & Schuster, 1979.

Moment, G. B. "The Ponce de León Trail Today." In *The Biology of Aging*, edited by J. A. Behnke, C. E. Finch, and G. B. Moment. New York: Plenum Press, 1978.

Chapter One: DNA—The Imperfect Molecule
Avery, O. T.; MacLeod, C. M.; and McCarty, M. "Induction of Transformation by a Deoxyribonucleic Acid Fraction from Pneumococcus Type III." *The Journal of Experimental Medicine* 79 (1944): 137–58.

Beukers, R., and Berends, W. "Isolation and Identification of the Irradiation Product of Thymine." *Biochimica et Biophysica Acta* 41 (1960): 550–51.

Boyce, R. P., and Howard-Flanders, P. "Release of Ultraviolet Light-Induced Thymine Dimers from DNA in E. Coli K-12." *Proceedings of the National Academy of Sciences* 51 (1964): 293–300.

Burnet, F. M. *Intrinsic Mutagenesis: A Genetic Approach to Ageing*. New York: John Wiley & Sons, 1974.

_____. *Endurance of Life: The Implications of Genetics for Human Life*. New York: Cambridge University Press, 1978.

Carrel, A. "On the Permanent Life of Tissues Outside of the Organism." *The Journal of Experimental Medicine* 15 (1912): 516–28.

_____. "Contributions to the Study of the Mechanism of the Growth of Connective Tissue." *The Journal of Experimental Medicine* 18 (1913): 287–98.

_____. *Man the Unknown*. New York: Harper & Row, 1935.

Comfort, A. *Ageing: The Biology of Senescence*. London: Routledge and Kegan Paul Ltd., 1964.

Edwards, W. S. *Alexis Carrel: Visionary Surgeon*. Springfield, Ill.: Charles C. Thomas, 1974.

Eisley, L. *Darwin's Century*. New York: Doubleday & Company, 1958.

Everitt, A. V. "The Hypothalamic-Pituitary Control of Ageing and Age-Related Pathology." *Experimental Gerontology* 8 (1973): 265–77.

Finch, C. E. "The Brain and Aging." In *The Biology of Aging*, edited by Behnke *et al*. New York: Plenum Press, 1978.

Hart, R. W., and Setlow, R. B. "Correlation Between Deoxyribonucleic Acid Excision Repair and Life-Span in a Number of Mammalian Species." *Proceedings of the National Academy of Sciences* 71 (1974): 2169–73.

Hayflick, L. "The Serial Cultivation of Human Diploid Cell Strains." *Experimental Cell Research* 25 (1961): 585–621.

———. "The Limited In Vitro Lifetime of Human Diploid Cell Strains." *Experimental Cell Research* 37 (1965): 614–36.

———. "Biomedical Gerontology: Current Theories of Biological Aging." *The Gerontologist* 14 (1974): 454–58.

Hill, R. F. "A Radiation-Sensitive Mutant of *Eschericia coli.*" *Biochimica et Biophysica Acta* 30 (1958): 636–37.

Hollaender, A., and Emmons, C. W. "Wavelength Dependence of Mutation Production in the Ultraviolet with Special Emphasis on Fungi." In *Cold Spring Harbor Symposium on Quantitative Biology,* vol. 9, 179–86. New York: Long Island Biological Association, 1941.

Jacob, F. *The Logic of Life: A History of Heredity.* New York: Vintage Books, 1976.

Kirkwood, T. B. L., and Cremer, T. "Cytogerontology Since 1881: A Reappraisal of August Weismann and a Review of Modern Progress." *Human Genetics* 60 (1982): 101–21.

Kuhn, T. S. *The Structure of Scientific Revolutions.* 2d ed. Chicago: University of Chicago Press, 1970.

Martin, G. M.; Sprague, C. A.; and Epstein, C. J. "Replicative Lifespan of Cultivated Human Cells: Effects of Donor's Age, Tissue and Genotype." *Laboratory Investigations* 23 (1970): 86–92.

Moment, G. B. "The Ponce de León Trail Today." In *The Biology of Aging,* edited by Behnke *et al.* New York: Plenum Press, 1978.

Orgel, L. "The Maintenance of Accuracy of Protein Synthesis and Its Relevance to Aging." *Proceedings of the National Academy of Sciences* 49 (1963): 517–21.

———. "Aging of Clones of Mammalian Cells." *Nature* 243: 441–45.

Price, G. B.; Modak, S. P.; and Makinodan, T. "Age-Associated Changes in the DNA of Mouse Tumor." *Science* 191 (1971): 917–20.

Rosenfeld, A. *Prolongevity.* New York: Avon Books, 1977.

Schneider, E. L., and Mitsui, Y. "The Relationship Between In Vitro Cellular Aging and In Vivo Human Age." *Proceedings of the National Academy of Sciences* 73 (1976): 3584–88.

Setlow, R. B., and Setlow, J. K. "Evidence that Ultraviolet-Induced Thymine Dimers in DNA Cause Biological Damage." *Proceedings of the National Academy of Sciences* 48 (1962): 1250–57.

———, and Carrier, W. L. "The Disappearance of Thymine Dimers from DNA: An Error-Correcting Mechanism." *Proceedings of the National Academy of Sciences* 51 (1964): 226–31.

Smith, J. M. "Review Lectures on Senescence: 1. The Causes of Ageing." *Proceedings of the Royal Society* 157 (1962): 115–27.

Stent, G. S., and Calendar, R. *Molecular Genetics: An Introductory Narrative.* 2d ed. San Francisco: W. H. Freeman, 1978.

Strehler, B. *Times, Cells and Aging.* New York: Academic Press, 1962.

Szilard, L. "On the Nature of the Aging Process." *Proceedings of the National Academy of Sciences* 45 (1959): 30–45.

Upton, A. C. "Ionizing Radiation and the Aging Process. A Review." *Journal of Gerontology* 12 (1957): 306–13.

_____.; Kastenbaum, M. A.; and Conklin, J. W. "Age-Specific Death Rates of Mice Exposed to Ionizing Radiation and Radiomimetic Agents." In *Symposium on Cellular Basis and Aetiology of Late Somatic Effects of Ionizing Radiations*, edited by R. J. Harris, 285–94. New York: Academic Press, 1963.

Watson, J. D., and Crick, F. H. C. "A Structure for Deoxyribose Nucleic Acid." *Nature* 171 (1953): 737–38.

Watson, J. D. *Molecular Biology of the Gene.* 2d ed. New York: W. A. Benjamin, 1970.

Weismann, A. *Essays upon Heredity and Kindred Biological Problems.* 2d. ed. Oxford: Claredon Press, 1892.

Wilkins, R. J., and Hart, R. W. "Preferential DNA Repair in Human Cells." *Nature* 247 (1974): 35–36.

Witkowski, J. A. "Alexis Carrel and the Mysticism of Tissue Culture." *Medical History* 23 (1979): 279–96.

_____. "Dr. Carrel's Immortal Cells." *Medical History* 24 (1980): 129–42.

Chapter Two: New Evidence

Ames, B. N.; Durston, W. E.; Yamasaki, E.; and Lee, F. D. "Carcinogens Are Mutagens: A Simple Test System Combining Liver Homogenates for Activation and Bacteria for Detection." *Proceedings of the National Academy of Sciences* 70 (1973): 2281–85.

Burnet, F. M. *Intrinsic Mutagenesis: A Genetic Approach to Ageing.* New York: John Wiley & Sons, 1974.

Miller, E. C., and Miller, J. A. "Mechanisms of Chemical Carcinogenesis: Nature of Proximate Carcinogens and Interactions with Macromolecules." *Pharmacological Reviews* 18 (1966): 805–38.

Schwartz, A. "Correlation Between Species Life Span and Capacity to Activate 7.12-dimethybenz(a)anthracene to a Form Mutagenic to a Mammalian Cell." *Experimental Cell Research* 94 (1975): 445–47.

Chapter Three: "Not Why Do We Die, But Why Do We Live So Long?"

Cleaver, J. E. "Defective Repair Replication of DNA in Xeroderma Pigmentosum." *Nature* 218 (1968): 652–56.

_____, and Trosko, J. E. "Absence of Excision of Ultraviolet-Induced Cyclobutane Dimers in Xeroderma Pigmentosum." *Photochemistry and Photobiology* 11 (1970): 547–50.

Hart, R. W.; Sacher, G. A.; and Hoskins, T. L. "DNA Repair in a Short- and a Long-Lived Rodent Species." *Journal of Gerontology* 34 (1979): 808–17.

_____, and Trosko, J. E. "DNA Repair Processes in Mammals." In *Interdisciplinary Topics in Gerontology*, edited by R. G. Cutler, vol. 9. Basel: S. Karger, 1976.

Regan, J. D.; Trosko, J. E.; and Carrier, W. L. "Evidence for Excision of Ultra-

violet-Induced Pyrimidine Dimers from the DNA of Human Cells In Vitro."
Biophysical Journal 8 (1968): 319–25.

Sacher, G. A. "Evolutionary Theory in Gerontology." *Perspectives in Biology and Medicine* 25 (1982): 339–53.

———. "On the Statistical Nature of Mortality with Especial Reference to Chronic Radiation Mortality." *Radiology* 67 (1956): 250–57.

———. "Relation of Lifespan to Brain Weight and Body Weight in Mammals." In *Ciba Foundation Colloquia on Ageing*, edited by G. E. W. Wolstenholme and M. O'Connor, vol. 5, 115–33. London: Churchill, 1959.

———, and Hart, R. W. "Longevity, Aging, and Comparative Cellular and Molecular Biology of the House Mouse, *Mus musculus*, and the White-Footed Mouse, *Peromyscus leukopus*." In *Genetic Effects on Aging*, edited by D. Bergsma and D. E. Harrison, vol. 14. Birth Defects: Original Article Series, The National Foundation–March of Dimes, 71–96. New York: Alan R. Liss, 1978.

Trosko, J. E., and Chang, C. C. "Genes, Pollutants and Human Diseases." *Quarterly Reviews of Biophysics* 11 (1978): 603–27.

———, and Hart, R. W. "DNA Mutation Frequencies in Mammals." In *Interdisciplinary Topics in Gerontology*, edited by R. G. Cutler, vol. 9. Basel: S. Karger, 1976.

Chapter Four: Biochemistry Rather Than Brains

Crowley, C., and Curtis, H. J. "The Development of Somatic Mutations in Mice with Age." *Proceedings of the National Academy of Sciences* 49 (1963): 626–28.

Curtis, H. J. "Biological Mechanisms Underlying the Aging Process." *Science* 141 (1963): 686–98.

Cutler, R. G. "Transcription of Reiterated DNA Sequence Classes Throughout the Lifespan of the Mouse." In *Advances in Gerontological Research*, edited by Bernard Strehler, vol. 4. New York and London: Academic Press, 1972.

———. "Evolution of Human Longevity and the Genetic Complexity Governing Aging Rate." *Proceedings of the National Academy of Sciences* 72 (1975): 4664–68.

———. "Nature of Aging and Life Maintenance Processes." In *Interdisciplinary Topics in Gerontology*, edited by R. G. Cutler, vol. 9. Basel: S. Karger, 1976.

Harman, D. "Aging: A Theory Based on Free Radical and Radiation Chemistry." *Journal of Gerontology* 11 (1956): 298–300.

———. "The Aging Process." *Proceedings of the National Academy of Sciences* 78 (1981): 7124–28.

Medawar, P. B. "Old Age and Natural Death." In *The Uniqueness of the Individual.* 2d ed., rev. New York: Dover Publications, 1981.

Sacher, G. A. "Molecular Versus Systemic Theories on the Genesis of Ageing." *Experimental Gerontology* 3 (1968): 265–71.

———. "Maturation and Longevity in Relation to Cranial Capacity in Hominid Evolution." In *Primate Functional Morphology and Evolution*, edited by R. Tuttle, vol. 1. The Hague: Mouton Publishers, 1975.

Tolmasoff, J. M.; Ono, T.; and Cutler, R. G. "Superoxide Dismutase: Correlation with Lifespan and Specific Metabolic Rate in Primate Species." *Proceedings of the National Academy of Sciences* 77 (1980): 2777–81.

Chapter Five: A Supergene for Aging?

Liu, R. K., and Walford, R. L. "The Effect of Lowered Body Temperature on Lifespan and Immune and Non-immune Processes." *Gerontologia* 18 (1972): 363–88.

McCay, C. M.; Crowell, M. F.; and Maynard, L. A. "The Effect of Retarded Growth Upon the Length of Life Span and Upon the Ultimate Body Size." *The Journal of Nutrition* 10 (1935): 63–79.

Medawar, P. B., and Medawar, J. S. *The Life Science: Current Ideas of Biology.* New York: Harper & Row, 1977.

Meredith, P. J., and Walford, R. L. "Effect of Age on Response to T- and B-Cell Mitogens Congenic at the H-2 Locus." *Immunogenetics* 5 (1977): 109–28.

Paffenholz, V. "Correlation Between DNA Repair of Embryonic Fibroblasts and Different Lifespan of 3 Inbred Mouse Strains." *Mechanisms of Ageing and Development* 7 (1978): 131–50.

Smith, G. S., and Walford, R. L. "Influence of the Main Histocompatibility Complex on Ageing in Mice." *Nature* 270 (1977): 727–29.

Stent, G. S., and Calendar, R. *Molecular Genetics: An Introductory Narrative.* 2d ed. San Francisco: W. H. Freeman, 1978.

Walford, R. L. *The Immunologic Theory of Aging.* Copenhagen: Munksgaard, 1969.

_____. "Antibody Diversity, Histocompatibility Systems, Disease States, and Ageing." *The Lancet* 2 (1970): 1226–29.

_____. Introduction to special issue on "Immunology and Aging." *Gerontologia* 18 (1972): 243–46.

_____. "Immunologic Theory of Aging: Current Status." *Federation Proceedings* 33 (1974): 2020–27.

_____, and Bergmann, K. "Influence of Genes Associated with the Main Histocompatibility Complex on Deoxyribonucleic Acid Excision Repair Capacity and Bleomycin Sensitivity in Mouse Lymphocytes." *Tissue Antigens* 14 (1979): 336–42.

Chapter Six: "Life Extension Is In"

Hart, R. W.; Setlow, R. B.; and Woodhead, A. D. "Evidence that Pyrimidine Dimers in DNA Can Give Rise to Tumors." *Proceedings of the National Academy of Sciences* 74 (1977): 5574–78.

Preer, J. R., Jr. "Nuclear and Cytoplasmic Differentiation in the Protozoa." In *Developmental Cytology,* edited by W. Rudnick. New York: Ronald Press, 1959.

Smith-Sonneborn, J. "Age Correlated Sensitivity to Ultraviolet Radiation in *Paramecium.*" *Radiation Research* 46 (1971): 64–69.

_____. "DNA Repair and Longevity Assurance in *Paramecium tetraurelia.*" *Science* 203 (1979): 1115–17.

Sonneborn, T. M. "The Relation of Autogamy to Senescence and Rejuvenescence in *Paramecia aurelia.*" *Journal of Protozoology* 1 (1954): 38–53.

_____, and Schneller, M. "Age Induced Mutations in *Paramecium.*" In *Biology of Aging,* edited by B. L. Strehler. Baltimore: Waverly Press, 1955.

Woodruff, L. L. *"Paramecium aurelia* in pedigree culture for twenty-five years." *Transactions of the American Microscopy Society* 51 (1932): 196–98.

Chapter Seven: Bringing It All Together

Adelman, R. C., and Britton, G. W. "The Impaired Capability for Biochemical Adaptation During Aging." *Bioscience* 25 (1975): 639–43.

Benditt, E. P., and Benditt, J. M. "Evidence for a Monoclonal Origin of Human Atherosclerotic Plaques." *Proceedings of the National Academy of Sciences* 70 (1973): 1753–56.

Brash, D. E., and Hart, R. W. "Molecular Biology of Aging." In *The Biology of Aging,* edited by Behnke *et al.* New York: Plenum Press: 1978.

Bulbrook, R. D., *et al.* "A Comparison Between the Urinary Steroid Excretion of Normal Women and Women with Advanced Breast Cancer." *The Lancet* 2 (1962): 1235–37.

———. "Abnormal Excretion of Urinary Steroids by Women with Early Breast Cancer." *The Lancet* 2 (1962): 1238–40.

Bulbrook, R. D.; Hayward, J. L.; and Spicer, C. C. "Relation Between Urinary Androgen and Corticoid Excretion and Subsequent Breast Cancer." *The Lancet* 2 (August): 395–98.

Burnet, F. M. *Immunological Surveillance.* London: Cambridge University Press, 1978.

Cristofalo, V. J., and Kabakjian, J. R. "Lysosomal Enzymes and Aging In Vitro: Subcellular Enzyme Distribution and Effect of Hydrocortisone on Cell Lifespan." *Mechanisms of Ageing and Development* 4 (1975): 19–28.

Denckla, W. D. "Role of the Pituitary and Thyroid Glands in the Decline of Minimal 02 Consumption with Age." *The Journal of Clinical Investigations* 53 (1974): 572–81.

———. "Aging, Dying and the Pituitary." In *Biological Mechanisms in Aging,* edited by R. T. Schimke. Bethesda: NIH Publication No. 81–2194, June 1981.

Finch, C. E. "Neural and Endocrine Mechanisms in Aging." In *Biological Mechanisms in Aging,* edited by R. T. Schimke. Bethesda: NIH Publication No. 81–2194, June 1981.

Hart, R. W.; D'Ambrosio, S. M.; and Ng, K. J. "Longevity, Stability and DNA Repair." *Mechanisms of Ageing and Development* 9 (1979): 203–23.

Loeb, L. A.; Silber, J. R.; and Fry, M. "Infidelity of DNA Replication in Aging." In *Biological Mechanisms in Aging,* edited by R. T. Schimke. Bethesda: NIH Publication No. 81–2194, June 1981.

Martin, G. M. "Genetic Syndromes in Man with Potential Relevance to the Pathobiology of Aging." In *Genetic Effects on Aging,* edited by D. Bergsma and D. E. Harrison, vol. 14. Birth Defects: Original Article Series, The National Foundation–March of Dimes, pp. 5–39. New York: Alan R. Liss, 1978.

———. *et al.* "Replicative Lifespan of Cultivated Human Cells: Effects of Donor's Age, Tissue and Genotype." *Laboratory Investigations* 23 (1970): 86–92.

Peto, R. "Epidemiology, Multistage Models, and Short-Term Mutagenicity Tests." In *Origins of Human Cancer, Book C,* edited by H. H. Hiatt, J. D. Watson, and J. A. Winsten. Cold Spring Harbor Conferences on Cell Proliferation. New York: Cold Spring Harbor, 1977.

Schwartz, A. G. "Inhibition of Spontaneous Breast Cancer Formation in Female C3H (Avy/a) Mice by Long-Term Treatment with Dehydroepiandrosterone." *Cancer Research* 39 (1979): 1129–32.

_____. "Protective Effect of Dehydroepiandrosterone Against Aflatoxin B_1- and 7.12-Dimethylbenz(a)anthracene-Induced Cytotoxicity and Transformation in Cultured Cells." *Cancer Research* 35 (1975): 2482–87.

Tolmasoff, J. M.; Ono, T.; and Cutler, R. G. "Superoxide Dismutase: Correlation with Lifespan and Specific Metabolic Rate in Primate Species." *Proceedings of the National Academy of Sciences* 77 (1980): 2777–81.

Yen, T. T., *et al.* "Prevention of Obesity in Avy/a Mice by Dehydroepiandrosterone." *Lipids* 12 (1977): 409–13.

Chapter Eight: Taking It One Step Further

Bauer, W. R.; Crick, F. H. C.; and White, J. H. "Supercoiled DNA." *Scientific American* 243 (1980): 118–33.

Hart, R. W., and Setlow, R. B. "DNA Repair in Late-Passage Human Cells." *Mechanisms of Ageing and Development* 5 (1976): 67–77.

Holliday, R., and Tarrant, G. M. "Altered Enzymes in Aging Human Fibroblasts." *Nature* 238: 26–30.

Lipetz, P. D., *et al.* "Determination of DNA Superhelicity and Extremely Low Levels of DNA Strand Breaks in Low Numbers of Nonradiolabeled Cells by DNA—4'6-Diamidino-2-phenylindole Fluorescence in Nucleoid Gradients." *Analytical Biochemistry* 121 (1982): 339–48.

_____. "DNA Superstructure, Differentiation, and Aging." In *Biological Mechanisms in Aging*, edited by R. T. Schimke. Bethesda: NIH Publication No. 81-2194, June 1981.

Martin, G. M., *et al.* "Do Hyperplastoid Cell Lines 'Differentiate Themselves to Death'?" *Advances in Medicine and Biology* 53 (1975): 67–90.

Pendergrass, W. R.; Martin, G. M.; and Bornstein, P. "Evidence Contrary to the Protein Error Hypothesis for In Vitro Senescence." *Journal of Cellular Physiology* 87: 3–13.

Chapter Nine: Life Extension 1: Supercoils

Lipetz, P. D.; Galsky, A. G.; and Stephens, R. E. "Relationship of DNA Tertiary and Quaternary Structure to Carcinogenic Processes." *Advances in Cancer Research* 36 (1982): 165–210.

Sinden, R. R.; Carlson, J. O.; and Pettijohn, D. E. "Torsional Tension in the DNA Double Helix Measured with Trimethylpsoralen in Living *E. coli* Cells: Analogous Measurements in Insect and Human Cells." *Cell* 21: 773–83.

Smith-Sonneborn, J.; Lipetz, P. D.; and Stephens, R. E. "*Paramecium* Bioassay of Longevity Modulating Agents." In *Intervention in the Aging Process, Part B: Basic Research and Preclinical Screening*, edited by W. Regelson and F. M. Sinex. New York: Alan R. Liss, 1983.

Trosko, J. E., and Chang, C. C. "An Integrative Hypothesis Linking Cancer, Diabetes and Atherosclerosis." *Medical Hypotheses* 6 (1980): 455–468.

Worcel, A.; Strogatz, S.; and Riley D. "Structure of Chromatin and the Linking
Number of DNA." *Proceedings of the National Academy of Sciences* 78 (1981):
1461–65.

Yew, F. H., and Johnson, R. T. "Ultraviolet-Induced DNA Excision Repair in
Human B and T Lymphocytes. III. Repair in Lymphocytes from Chronic
Lymphocytic Leukemia." *Journal of Cell Science* 39 (1979): 329–37.

Chapter Ten: Life Extension 2: Supergenes

Braun, W. E. *HLA and Disease: A Comprehensive Review*. Boca Raton, Fla.: CRC
Press, 1979.

Cutler, R. G. "Longevity Is Determined by Specific Genes: Testing the Hypothesis." In *Testing the Theories of Aging*, edited by R. Adelman and G. Roth. Boca
Raton, Fla.: CRC Press, 1982.

Fahmy, M. J., and Fahmy, O. G. "Intervening DNA Insertions and the Alteration
of Gene Expression by Carcinogens." *Cancer Research* 40 (1980): 3374–82.

————. "Altered Control of Gene Activity in the Soma by Carcinogens." *Mutation Research* 72 (1980): 165–72.

Hall, K. Y.; Bergmann, K.; and Walford, R. L. "DNA Repair, H-2, and Aging in
NZB and CBA Mice." *Tissue Antigens* 16 (1980): 104–10.

Hassan, H. M., and Fridovich, I. "Superoxide, Hydrogen Peroxide, and Oxygen
Tolerance of Oxygen-Sensitive Mutants of *Eschericia Coli*." *Review of Infectious
Diseases* 1 (1979): 357–69.

Munkrees, K. D. "Biochemical Genetics of Aging of *Neurospora crassa* and
Podospora anserina: A Review." In *Age Pigments*, edited by R. S. Sohal. Amster-
dam: Elsevier/North-Holland Biomedical Press, 1981.

Murad, F., *et al.* "Guanylate Cyclase: Activation by Azide, Nitro Compounds, Ni-
tric Oxide, and Hydroxyl Radical and Inhibition by Hemoglobin and Myoglo-
bin." In *Advances in Cyclic Nucleotide Research*, edited by W. J. George and L. J.
Ignarro, vol. 9. New York: Raven Press, 1978.

————. "Properties and Regulation of Guanylate Cyclase and Some Proposed
Functions for Cyclic GMP." In *Advances in Cyclic Nucleotide Research*, edited by
W. J. George and L. J. Ignarro, vol. 2. New York: Raven Press, 1979.

Novak, R. "Gene Affecting Superoxide Dismutase Activity Linked to the Histocompatibility Complex in H-2 Congenic Mice." *Science* 207 (1980): 86–87.

Ono, T., and Cutler, R. G. "Age-Dependent Relaxation of Gene Repression: Increase of Endogenous Murine Leukemia Virus-related and Globin-related RNA
in Brain and Liver of Mice." *Proceedings of the National Academy of Sciences* 75
(1978): 4431–35.

Walford, R. L. "Immunology and Aging." *American Journal of Clinical Pathology*
74 (1980): 247–53.

————. *Maximum Life Span*. New York: W. W. Norton & Company, 1983.

Chapter Eleven: "The Cell Controls Its Own Destiny"

Doolittle, R. F., *et al.* "Simian Sarcoma Virus Onc Gene, V-sis, Is Derived from the Gene (or Genes) Encoding a Platelet-Derived Growth Factor." *Science* 221 (1983): 275–77.

Frank, J. P., and Williams, J. R. "X-ray Induction of Persistent Hypersensitivity to Mutation." *Science* 216 (1982): 307–08.

Harrison, D. E. "Is Limited Cell Proliferation the Clock That Times Aging?" In *The Biology of Aging,* edited by Behnke *et al.* New York: Plenum Press, 1978.

Holliday, R., and Pugh, J. E. "DNA Modification Mechanisms and Gene Activity During Development." *Science* 187 (1975): 226–32.

Schneider, E. L.; Tice, R. R.; and Kram, D. "Bromodeoxyuridine Differential Chromatid Staining Technique: A New Approach to Examining Sister Chromatid Exchange and Cell Replication Kinetics." *Methods of Cell Biology* 20 (1978): 379–409.

Stephens, R. E., and Lipetz, P. D. "Higher Order DNA Repair in Human Peripheral Leukocytes: A Factor in Aging and Cancer?" In *Intervention in the Aging Process, Part B: Basic Research and Preclinical Screening.* New York: Alan R. Liss, 1983.

Wilkins, R. J., and Hart, R. W. "Preferential DNA Repair in Human Cells." *Nature* 247 (1974): 35–36.

Williams, J. R. "Alteration in DNA/Chromatin Structure During Aging." In *Intervention in the Aging Process, Part B: Basic Research and Preclinical Screening.* New York: Alan R. Liss, 1983.

Chapter Twelve: Life Extension—The Long and the Short of It

Ames, B. N., *et al.* "Carcinogens Are Mutagens: A Simple Test System Combining Liver Homogenates for Activation and Bacteria for Detection." *Proceedings of the National Academy of Sciences.* 70 (1973): 2281–85.

Ames, B. N.; Cathcart, R.; Schwiers, E.; and Hochstein, P. "Uric Acid Provides an Antioxidant Defense in Humans Against Oxidant-and Radical-Caused Aging and Cancer: A Hypothesis." *Proceedings of the National Academy of Sciences* 78 (1981): 6858–62.

Ames, B. N. "Dietary Carcinogens and Anticarcinogens: Oxygen Radicals and Degenerative Diseases." *Science* 221 (1983): 1256–66.

Andres, R. "Effect of Obesity on Total Mortality." *International Journal of Obesity* 4 (1980): 381–86.

Belloc, N. "Relationship of Health Practices and Mortality." *Preventive Medicine* 2 (1973): 67–81.

Breslow, L., and Enstrom, J. E. "Persistence of Health Habits and Their Relationships to Mortality." *Preventive Medicine* 9 (1980): 469–83.

Cathcart, R.; Schweirs, E.; Saul, R. L.; and Ames, B. N. "Thymine Glycol and Thymidine Glycol in Human and Rat Urine: A Possible Assay for Oxidative DNA Damage." *Proceedings of the National Academy of Sciences* 81 (1984): 5633–37.

Cutler, R. G. "Longevity Is Determined by Specific Genes: Testing the Hypothesis." In *Testing the Theories of Aging,* edited by R. Adelman. Boca Raton, Fla.: CRC Press, 1982.

Hollstein, M. C.; Brooks, P.; Linn, S.; and Ames, B. N. "Hydroxymethyluracil DNA Glycosylase in Mammalian Cells." *Proceedings of the National Academy of Sciences* 81 (1984): 4003–7.

Kiecolt-Glaser, J. K.; Stephens, R. E.; Lipetz, P. B.; Speicher, C. E.; and Glaser, R. "Distress and DNA Repair in Human Lymphocytes." *Journal of Behavioral Medicine,* in press.

Index

Aaronson, Stuart A., 234
abiotrophic disorders, 130,135, 210, 250
accelerated aging, human syndromes of, 130, 135, 210, 250
Adelman, Richard, 136
adrenal gland, 145
Advances in Gerontological Research, 82
aflatoxin, 132, 138, 139
age-related diseases, 6, 7, 20, 21, 50, 105, 127, 135, 140, 142, 209, 239
   see also individual diseases, e.g., arteriosclerosis; cancer; diabetes
"Aging at the Molecular and Cellular Levels," 84
aging research, *see* age-related diseases; antioxidants; DHEA; DNA repair; DNA supercoiling; "few genes" theory of life span; hormones; immune system; life extension; "somatic mutation" theory; *names of individual researchers*
Alzheimer's disease, 214, 239, 261
American Academy for the Advancement of Science, 51
American Aging Association, 90, 237–38, 242
American Association for the Advancement of Science, 73
American Cancer Society, 140
Ames, Bruce, 50, 241–50, 252, 260, 261–62
   Ames test, 241, 242–43

test to measure oxygenation damage to DNA, 247–49, 250, 254, 261
Amos, D. Bernard, 100
Amos, Harold, 45–46
Andres, Reubin, 249
Animal Medical Center, 257
antibodies, 98–99, 100, 168
antioxidants, 91, 126, 132, 209, 215, 245–47, 251–54, 258
   catalase, 209, 211, 215
   peroxidase, 215
   superoxide dismutase (SOD), 92–93, 129, 132, 147–48, 205–206, 207, 209, 210, 211, 213–14, 215, 245, 257, 262
   testing and correcting for deficiencies in, 247–49, 254, 261
   uric acid, 245–47
Applezweig, Norman, 143
Argonne National Laboratory, 76, 174
   Sacher's work at, 22–23, 54, 55, 60, 71–73, 84, 88
Argonne University Associates Biology Committee, 38–39
Aristotle, 58
arteriosclerosis, 6, 50, 133–34, 135, 142
arthritis, 6, 50, 135
   rheumatoid, 99, 209
Association of German Naturalists, 14
Atanasoff, Dr. John, 87
atherosclerosis, 239
Atomic Energy Commission, 56, 66